"I've heard folic acid can prevent anemia and birth defects—and help reduce the risk of heart disease. What kinds of food should I eat to make sure I'm getting enough?"

"Osteoporosis is said to account for more than a million broken bones every year. . . . Maybe I should be thinking of getting more calcium!"

"I'm trying and trying to lose weight. Am I doing something wrong? Could there be hidden fat in my food that I don't know about?"

Everybody's talking about nutrition these days . . . but it's not always easy to get the facts. Here in one comprehensive, convenient volume, you can find the facts you need on:

CALORIES • FAT • PROTEIN • CARBOHYDRATES • DIETARY FIBER • SODIUM • FOLIC ACID • ANTIOXIDANTS • CALCIUM

The Nutrition Doctor's A-to-Z Food Counter

THE
NUTRITION DOCTOR'S
A-TO-Z
FOOD COUNTER

Dr. Ed Blonz

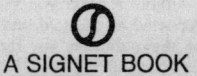

A SIGNET BOOK

SIGNET
Published by the Penguin Group
Penguin Putnam Inc., 375 Hudson Street,
New York, New York 10014, U.S.A.
Penguin Books Ltd, 27 Wrights Lane,
London W8 5TZ, England
Penguin Books Australia Ltd, Ringwood,
Victoria, Australia
Penguin Books Canada Ltd, 10 Alcorn Avenue,
Toronto, Ontario, Canada M4V 3B2
Penguin Books (N.Z.) Ltd, 182–190 Wairau Road,
Auckland 10, New Zealand

Penguin Books Ltd, Registered Offices:
Harmondsworth, Middlesex, England

First published by Signet, an imprint of Dutton NAL,
a member of Penguin Putnam Inc.

First Printing, January, 1999
10 9 8 7 6 5 4 3 2 1

ACKNOWLEDGMENTS

My sincere thanks to my wife, Kay, without whom this project would not have been possible. Thanks also to our son, Josh, for giving us the time and understanding to complete this project. Finally, best wishes to all my friends and readers for their continued support and encouragement.

NOTE

Research about human nutrition is constantly evolving. While the author has made every effort to include the most accurate and up-to-date information in this book, there can be no guarantee that what we know about this complex subject won't change with time. Please keep in mind that this book is not intended for the purpose of self-diagnosis or self-treatment. The reader should consult his or her physician regarding all health concerns before undertaking any major dietary changes. The author and publisher of this book are not physicians and are not licensed to give medical advice. The author and publisher disclaim any liability arising directly or indirectly from the use of this book.

Contents

How to Use This Book

From Abalone to Zwieback

The Nutrition Doctor's A-to-Z Food Counter lists more than 10,000 of the most common foods in alphabetical order. It is a comprehensive guide to generic and brand-name foods in a user-friendly format. It gives you all-in-one convenience by listing the following key nutrients:

Calories
Fat
Protein
Carbohydrate
Fiber
Sodium

But this book also goes one step further by identifying those foods that are a good source of the following health-related nutrients:

Folic Acid
Antioxidants
Calcium

The Nutrition Doctor's A-to-Z Food Counter is specifically designed to let you see which types of foods have the highest levels of these important nutrients. It will also let you compare content among similar foods, and help you make more healthful food choices. The book uses standardized servings sizes similar to those used on food packages. Values are rounded to the nearest whole number, and fats are to the nearest tenth of a gram. Whenever possible, similar foods have been listed in comparable portion sizes. If a product is dispensed as single-serving items, the data will be for one item. Be alert to the fact that differences in nutrient content might be due to the fact that one company's "item" might be significantly larger than another's.

We have alphabetized the listings for easy reference, and used cross references for those foods that are known under more than one name. As you look through the listings, you'll see that there may be variations in nutrient content—even among similar types of foods. This can be due to the fact that different manufacturers rely on different raw materials to make their product, or because different analytical laboratories were used to perform the nutritional analysis.

The basic knowledge you can gain from this book will help you to form a nutrition agenda and shopping strategy. In this context, *The Nutrition Doctor's A-to-Z Food Counter* is invaluable in helping you to decide which products are best for you and your family.

THE F-A-C GUIDE TO GOOD NUTRITION

F = Folic Acid

To receive an F in the FAC column a
food portion must contain at least 40
micrograms of folic acid

Folic acid plays a key role in helping prevent anemia and
certain types of birth defects. New research evidence has
now found that this B vitamin can also play a role in de-
creasing the risk of heart disease. What's encouraging about
folic acid's laudatory talents is that they don't rely on mega-
dose amounts. You can get all the folic acid you need from
a healthy diet. But, unfortunately, surveys indicate that
folic-acid-containing foods are apparently in dangerously
short supply on the average U.S. plate. The best food
sources for folic acid include dark green leafy vegetables;
citrus fruit, such as oranges; tomatoes; strawberries; beans;
liver; peanuts; and folic-acid-fortified cereals.

What's so special about folic acid?

The body is in a constant state of flux with cells being
replaced on a regular basis. The raw material for this cellular "turnover" comes, in part, from the body's own recy-
cling system and partially from newly received materials.
Folic acid, also called folate, is a key ingredient in a type
of construction shuttle service that moves the body's single
carbon "bricks" from one compound to another. Folate
also plays a role in the synthesis of DNA and RNA, the
genetic material involved in cell division and reproduction.

As you would imagine, when the construction of new
cells and tissues goes awry, or is forced to slow down, there
can be serious repercussions.

When folate is in short supply, one of the first places
problems occur is in the blood. In cellular terms, the life
span of the doughnut-shaped red blood cell is relatively

short, each cell being replaced every 120 days. Because of this short life span, they are among the first cells in the body to suffer from a folic acid deficiency. Without folate, red blood cells are not made in sufficient numbers and a type of anemia results.

Giving a folic acid supplement or adding folate-rich foods can bring about a dramatic recovery in those suffering from a folate-deficiency anemia.

The outlook, however, isn't as promising if there's a folate deficiency during pregnancy.

Following conception, the developing fetus begins to lay down the groundwork for many bodily systems. One of the first to develop is the nervous system, and folic acid plays a key role. The catch, though, is that folate must be present during the first few weeks after conception—a time at which most women are unaware they're even pregnant. If there's insufficient folate during this crucial period, mistakes can be made in the formation of the nervous system. Unfortunately, no amount of folate can make up for these structural abnormalities once that period has passed. Spina bifida is a type of birth defect, in which one or more of the vertebra of the spinal column fail to develop properly. It affects approximately 1 out of every 1,000 babies born. It is estimated that as much as 75 percent of all cases of spina bifida are attributable to a folate deficiency during those first few weeks of pregnancy. This makes it especially important for all women to have adequate folic acid in their diets *before* the pregnancy even begins. The problem is that less than half of all pregnancies are planned.

The U.S. Public Health Service recommends that all women of childbearing age who are capable of becoming pregnant should make sure they consume at least 400 micrograms of folic acid per day. The second National Health and Nutrition Education Survey (NHANES II) of food consumption found the average folic acid intake to be 200 micrograms per day—half of the Public Health Service guideline amount.

Scientists have discovered that if the body doesn't have enough folic acid, a chemical called homocysteine begins to accumulate. A number of studies have indicated that as the level of homocysteine rises, so to does the risk of heart disease.

A recent study in the *New England Journal of Medicine* looked at 1,041 elderly men and women. The scientists at the USDA's Human Nutrition Research Center on Aging at Tufts University found that those with the highest levels of homocysteine in their bloodstream were twice as likely to have significant narrowing of the arteries in the neck, amounting to as much as a 25 percent loss of the inner diameter. Such a decrease in blood flow would be a serious harbinger to heart disease and stroke.

To help reduce all these serious yet avoidable health risks, the government has mandated the fortification of enriched cereal grains with 140 micrograms of folate for every 100 grams (3.5 ounces) of grain. This is twice the level needed to replace the folate that is lost during milling. The cereal grains affected include the flours from wheat, rice, corn, rye, barley, triticale, and buckwheat, as well as cornmeal, rice, farina, and macaroni or pasta.

A study in the *American Journal of Public Health* affirmed how grain fortification could prevent hundreds of birth defects every year. Efforts must be made to assure that folate-rich foods make a regular appearance at the table. It is also the reason why we indicate those foods that provide at least 40 micrograms of folate per serving with the letter "F" in our FAC column.

A = Antioxidants

> To receive an A in the FAC column a food
> portion must contain at least 20 percent of
> the 1989 Adult Recommended Daily Allow-
> ance (RDA) for
> ### Vitamin A
> ### β carotene
> ### Vitamin C
> ### OR Vitamin E

Mother Told You to Eat Your Fruits and Vegetables

If there's ever been a family of compounds to crow about,
it's the antioxidant. These compounds, found in fruits, vegetables, and grains, have garnered an excellent reputation
among health scientists—and with good reason.

Studies looking for links between diet and disease consistently find that the incidence of killer diseases, such as heart
disease and certain cancers, goes down as the consumption
of fruits and vegetables increases. Over the years scientists
have been trying to learn more about this effect. Is it something in these foods, or just the fact that the more fruits
and vegetables you eat, the less room you might have for
other, less healthful fare? The answer has to do with the
presence of antioxidants.

What Do They Do?

It all has to do with oxygen, the oxygen we breathe to
stay alive, and the same oxygen that rusts a nail when it
is left exposed to the elements. Obviously, we need oxygen to stay alive. But it turns out that oxygen, in the
wrong place at the wrong time, can do serious damage
to the body. The problem comes when the oxygen reacts

and forms "free radicals," compounds that damage cells and are believed to be involved in the development of heart disease, cancer, aging, and a host of other ailments. The fat in your bloodstream is a key target for this type of reaction.

Think about it. If fat is a target, the more fat you have in your bloodstream, the greater the likelihood that free radicals and oxidized fats will form and damage will result. It's a very solid rationale behind the wisdom of a low-fat diet. But if this is the case, how do we explain the apparent healthfulness of the consumers of the "Mediterranean diet"—people in Greece, Italy, France, and other countries—who routinely have higher intakes of fat than us, yet can boast health statistics that put us to shame? It turns out that the body has a defense system that can help prevent this type of "oxidation" from causing harm. But to be at its best, the body depends on a daily supply of antioxidant nutrients from the diet. If you examine the diets of these cultures you will find that they also have a hefty intake of dietary antioxidants from their daily intake of fresh fruits, vegetables, and grains. Here in this country we eat a high-fat diet, but fail to get the antioxidant nutrients we need.

Look for items with the letter "A" in the FAC column for foods high in antioxidants.

It is recommended that you aim for three to five servings of vegetables and two to four servings of fruits every day. Although this may sound imposing, it's not when you consider that a typical serving is a medium piece of fruit, 1 cup of a leafy vegetable, ½ cup of fruit or cooked vegetables, ¼ cup of dried fruit, or 6 ounces of a fruit or vegetable juice.

Vitamin A and the Carotenes

We get Vitamin A from the foods we eat in two separate forms. The first is the preformed, "active" vitamin A itself, and the second are the carotenes, compounds that animal organisms are able to change into the "active" vitamin A. We find the preformed vitamin A in foods of animal origin, such as dairy products, eggs, and organ meats. You can also find this form of the vitamin A in vitamin-fortified foods, such as breakfast cereals. The carotenes are found in most yellow and green vegetables and fruits.

Vitamin E

Nature uses vitamin E to protect its plant seed oils, the energy source used by the developing seed to sprout, send down its roots, and grow to the point that it can begin producing energy on its own. That's why we find the highest concentrations of vitamin E in foods like sunflower seeds, wheat germ, and almonds. Among vegetables, kale and sweet potatoes are the best sources. Aside from these natural food sources, you can always get a Recommended Daily Allowance (RDA) through vitamin-fortified cereals.

Vitamin C

In addition to its role as an antioxidant, vitamin C, also called ascorbic acid, is needed for protein metabolism and the immune system, as well as for healthy gums, healing of wounds, and making collagen (the "cement" that holds body cells together). You can find vitamin C in fruits and vegetables, especially citrus fruits, peppers, melons, berries, brussels sprouts, green vegetables, tomatoes, and potatoes.

C = Calcium

To receive a C in the FAC column a
food portion must contain at least 200
milligrams of calcium (20 percent of the
Reference Daily Intake as found on the
food label)

The human skeleton is destined to turn into a fragile shell
if we deprive it of the raw materials it needs. The key
weight-bearing bones in the body are the hip, upper thigh,
and spine. If the mineral content of these bones dips too
low, they lose their ability to support the body and can
snap or begin to crumble without warning. This condition
is called osteoporosis (os-tee-oh-pore-OH-sis).

At present osteoporosis is incurable. It's believed to account for more than a million broken bones every year and
is indirectly involved in one in five deaths in people over
70. It's estimated that one-third of the postmenopausal
women in this country suffer from this disease.

The strength and long-term health of the body's precious
framework depend to a large degree on our diet. Calcium,
the most plentiful mineral in the body, tops the list. Its role
in our bones is only one of calcium's responsibilities.

Prevention Is a Long-Term Proposition

Like an active bank account, the bones of our skeleton,
despite their solid feel, are involved in a continuous process of mineral deposits and withdrawals. Childhood, ad-
olescence, and early adulthood—up to about age 35—
are the critical times to "bone up" on dietary calcium.
It is during these periods that the body has the capacity

to save its dietary calcium. The amount of savings, however, depends entirely on the calcium in the diet, and the importance of this cannot be overemphasized.

Once we hit our thirties the body's automatic teller begins to shift gears. Our dietary deposits are no longer able to keep pace with the withdrawals, no matter how much calcium we eat. The third decade of life is the start of a slow but continuous erosion of the skeleton. From that point on, diet helps determine how fast this deterioration occurs.

Best Food Sources

When dietary sources of calcium are discussed, milk and milk products tend to hold center stage. Dairy products represent more than 75 percent of the calcium in the American diet. One 8-ounce glass of skim milk contains about 302 milligrams of calcium; that's 25 percent of the RDA for a teenager or young adult. You will find as you look through the book that milk products are not the only source of calcium.

This is important to know because many people either don't care for or can't tolerate dairy products because of either lactose intolerance or an allergy to milk. For lactose intolerance, there are remedies available. For a milk allergy, however, you will have to get calcium elsewhere. There are plenty of foods besides dairy that contain calcium. It is found in green leafy vegetables, small fish with edible bones, broccoli, dried fruits, legumes, and nuts. Other options include calcium-fortified foods, such as cereal or orange juice.

Calories

Calories are units of energy. Although it is not considered a nutrient, energy is more important than other nutrients because without it our bodies would grind to an immediate halt. Due to energy's essential nature, the body has become quite good at conserving it, and in times of scarcity, this ability can make the difference between those who survive and those who perish.

A calorie is defined as the amount of heat energy necessary to raise the temperature of 1 gram of water 1 degree Celsius. Technically, when we see the word "calorie" on a food label or in any nonscientific writing, it refers to a kilocalorie (kilo = 1,000), which is often abbreviated as kcal. For the purposes of this book you can consider a calorie to be the equivalent of a kcal, and we use "kcal" for the column headings.

Fats, proteins, carbohydrates, and even alcohol are complex compounds that have a caloric value because it took energy to make them. When we metabolize or burn them, the energy is then released and used by the body. One gram of fat contains approximately 9 calories and 1 gram of protein or carbohydrate contains 4 calories. A gram of alcohol contains 7 calories. Fats contain most calories because they give off the greatest amount of energy when metabolized.

Fat

Fat, a member of the lipid family, is the most concentrated form of energy in all living things; it has more than twice the calories of protein or carbohydrates. The human body—like other mammals—is designed to turn virtually all its excess dietary calories into fat and store it as an energy reserve.

Fat provides insulation for the body and padding around sensitive internal organs. Several nutrients are found in fat, including vitamins A, E and K, and the essential fatty acids. When eaten, fats slow the rate at which the stomach empties, causing a feeling of fullness and satisfaction. And let us not forget a most important quality, namely that fat contributes some of the most wonderful tastes and textures in our food.

The individual fatty acids resemble chains ranging in length from 8 to 25 links. Fats come in three basic types: saturated, monounsaturated, and polyunsaturated. The fats and oils in our diet are made up of different proportions of these three types.

Fat sources that are primarily saturated are found in animal products such as butter, lard, eggs, meat, and poultry. Vegetable sources that contain a high proportion of saturated fat include coconut oil, palm oil, palm-kernel oil, and cocoa butter.

Oils that are primarily monounsaturated include olive oil, canola (rapeseed), almond, avocado, and peanut oils.

Polyunsaturated fat is found in the oils of seeds and some nuts, including corn, soy, safflower, sesame, and walnut. Fish oils also contain relatively high concentrations of polyunsaturated fat, making them unique in the animal world. Polyunsaturated fat is the only type of fat known to be required by the body.

Does Our Fat Intake Increase the Risk of Disease?

There's been a great deal of mudslinging in the fat arena, so if you are bewildered by the roles and risks of fats, you're not alone. There is nothing inherently "wrong" with fat, but scientific studies have found a strong association between an overconsumption of fat and the risk of developing our most troublesome health problems, including heart disease and cancer.

One explanation is that fats have a nasty tendency to react and become "oxidized," turning into compounds that can lead to heart disease, cancer, and other degenerative diseases. The higher one's fat consumption, the greater the risk. Moreover, our bodies have a defense system that can prevent this from happening. Our defenses depend on a healthful diet that contains plenty of antioxidant nutrients. These nutrients, found in vegetables, fruits, and grains, include vitamins A, E, and C, and the carotenoids, as well as a wide variety of naturally occurring plant compounds (phytochemicals) found in whole foods. Scientists are only beginning to understand what it is about healthful foods that make them so good for us.

Consider also that in other countries, such as those in the Mediterranean, people consume higher levels of fat and yet they have health statistics that put Americans to shame. The answer is that their diet focuses on fresh whole foods.

It is also important to stay away from processed food fats that are made via partial hydrogenation, the process by which a vegetable oil is changed from a liquid oil to a semisolid fat. Partial hydrogenation does more than harden the oil, it creates *trans* fatty acids, a type of aberrant fat that is linked to major diseases such as heart disease and cancer. You will find partially hydrogenated oils in shortening, nondairy creamers; stick margarines; snack foods, such as doughnuts, chips, and pastries; and deep-fried foods, such as french fries. If there is one fat to avoid entirely, this is it. Read the ingredient statement on the food label to find out whether it is present.

The more you understand about the key players in the

fat saga, the greater your appreciation for the need to emphasize fresh fruits, vegetables, grains, and nuts. With this style of eating you give your body the antioxidant nutrients it needs to protect itself. That is one of the reasons why, in addition to listing how much fat a food contains, we also tell you which foods are a good source of the antioxidant nutrients. You will find these foods by looking for the "A" in the column at the right-hand side of the page.

Protein

The word protein comes from the Greek *proteos*, which means "to come first." It's a fitting name because protein is a primary ingredient in every cell of the body. Protein is needed to make hair, skin, nails, muscles, organs, blood cells, nerve, bone and brain tissue, enzymes, hormones, antibodies, chemical messengers, and the DNA and RNA used to form the genetic code of life. That's quite a lineup!

All proteins are made from building blocks called amino acids. While there are many different types of protein, there are only about 22 kinds of amino acids. Of these 22, our body can manufacture all but nine. The reason we need protein in our diet is to supply these nine essential amino acids (EAAs). Because most dietary proteins are too large to be absorbed, the body uses its digestive enzymes to separate the food proteins into their individual amino-acid building blocks; only then can they be absorbed and used by the body as raw materials to make the variety of proteins necessary for good health.

Too Little Protein Can Cause Problems

In the developing countries of Africa, Asia, and South America, protein foods are scarce, and deficiencies, when present, can be life-threatening. For generally well-nourished people, a protein intake below required levels will not pose problems if it's only for a day or two now and then. But if the body consistently fails to get enough protein, it will begin showing signs of deficiency.

Depending on the length and degree, symptoms of an ongoing protein deficiency could include: increased susceptibility to disease, fatigue, anemia, hair and skin problems, mental confusion, pallor, digestive disturbances, muscle wasting, weight loss, and eventually death.

Too Much of a Good Thing

As essential as protein is, an excess can cause problems—in the United States, overconsumption is more the norm than the exception. The average individual does not benefit from extra protein, mainly because there is no way to store it for later use. Because the body has an ability to use protein for energy (1 gram of protein yields 4 calories), whenever we overindulge on protein, the body takes the excess, turns it into fat, and stashes it away as stored energy.

What If You Don't Eat Meat?

Most foods have some amino acids. Animal proteins, such as meat, fish, eggs, and dairy products, are complete proteins because they contain all the EAAs. With the exception of soybeans, vegetable proteins such as those from grains and legumes are incomplete proteins because they lack one or more EAAs. You can easily meet your daily protein requirement by eating only vegetable proteins, however, by combining different foods so that sufficient amounts of all the EAAs are consumed.

There are three basic types of vegetable protein: whole grains, such as rice, corn, oats, and barley; legumes, such as beans and lentils; and nuts and seeds, such as almonds and peanuts, and sunflower and sesame seeds. By planning your meals to include foods from two or more of these groups, you end up creating a complete protein. For example, by eating both rice (grains) and beans (legumes), you supply the body with the daily EAAs it needs.

Putting together this type of "complementary protein" is the essence of vegetarianism. At one time, it was thought that the body needed all the EAAs to be consumed at the same meal. Recently, however, scientists have determined that the body can successfully make protein so long as the full complement of EAAs is present over the course of a day.

How Much Do You Need?

A quick way to estimate your daily protein requirement is to count 11 grams of protein for every 30 pounds of body weight. By this method, a 150-pound adult needs about 55 grams of protein per day. (Note: If you're overweight, use your ideal body weight for this calculation.) Pregnant women should add an extra 10 grams of protein per day, and nursing mothers an extra 12 to 15 grams during the first 6 months. Requirements for children are higher.

Carbohydrates

The word carbohydrate comes from the Latin *carbo* for carbon, and *hydras*, which refers to the combining with water. As a group, carbohydrates represent the body's most important source of energy. There are three basic types: simple carbohydrates, complex carbohydrates, and fiber.

Simple and Sweet

The most important carbohydrate is glucose (also called blood sugar). Glucose is the body's basic fuel: it's the preferred fuel of the brain and nervous system, and the only fuel that the red blood cells can use. Indeed, there are entire body systems dedicated specifically to maintaining the level of glucose in the blood.

Glucose is referred to as a single sugar because it exists as individual, unattached units. Other common single sugars in our diet include fructose, also called fruit sugar, and galactose.

Simple carbohydrates can also be double sugars, which are two single sugars connected to one another. The most common of these is sucrose, or table sugar (glucose and fructose); lactose, or milk sugar (glucose and galactose); and maltose (glucose and glucose), which is found in grains and malt beverages such as beer. What simple carbohydrates share is sweetness; they stimulate the sweet taste receptors on the tongue.

It's All in the Build

Although glucose is a "single" sugar, it serves as the building block for the complex carbohydrates, which are found in grains, legumes, and potatoes. These complex carbohydrates, or starches, consist of hundreds to thousands of glucose units connected to each other in straight-line or branched formations. They are too large to be absorbed through the wall of the digestive tract, so the body releases a set of enzymes designed to break the starch apart, piece by glucose piece.

Cellulose is a complex carbohydrate that is found in hay and wood pulp as well as many vegetables. It is also made from glucose. The big difference, though, between a meal of mashed potatoes and one of mashed wood is that the body lacks the enzymes needed to separate the complex of glucose units of cellulose. As a result, the starch gets digested and absorbed, while the cellulose passes through the system unabsorbed. Because the body cannot digest cellulose, this complex carbohydrate is classified as a dietary fiber.

The Fuel with Something Extra

Normally, muscles require oxygen from the bloodstream when they work. This is why our breathing rate picks up during physical activity. Carbohydrates, though, are exceptional in that they're an anaerobic fuel (an = without; aerobic = requiring oxygen). There's a small amount of stored carbohydrate, called glycogen, in the muscles and liver, and the body relies on this fuel to meet special demands. It's this fuel and the anaerobic ability of carbohydrates that enables us to dash across a room and grab a falling child or sprint down the street to catch a bus. This carbohydrate provides a vital source of energy that keeps the muscles working until the lungs gear up to provide the needed oxygen.

Focus on the Complex

When thinking about carbohydrates in your diet, focus on the complex rather than the simple sugars. Why, if all carbohydrates end up as glucose? The answer is in the nutrient company the different carbohydrates keep. Except for fruits, foods high in simple sugars tend to be high-calorie and often high-fat processed foods, where intense flavor or a sweet taste is the main offering. In contrast, complex carbohydrates are generally found in grains, vegetables, and legumes—whole foods with a wide array of valuable nutrients and fiber.

Fiber

Today, just about every nutrition book and newsletter trumpets the praises of fiber without explaining exactly what it is and what it does. So before you dive into your next bowl of All-Bran, here's a brief look behind the labels.

To start with, dietary fiber, or roughage, is a type of carbohydrate that's found only in plant products such as vegetables, nuts, fruits, and grains. A considerable body of research evidence has accumulated that links an increased fiber intake (25 to 30 grams a day) with positive effects on heart disease, cancer, diabetes, constipation, diarrhea, diverticulitis, hemorrhoids, and ulcerative colitis. With a list like that, it's no wonder we keep hearing how important fiber is for good health. Fiber is good for you!

Fiber's imposing set of talents is made even more impressive when you consider that it doesn't contribute any calories, essential vitamins, or minerals to the body. In fact, it's not digested by the body at all! How can a substance we can't even digest be so healthful? The very fact that you cannot digest it is what turns out to be its greatest asset.

Why Fiber Can't Be Digested

The foods we eat are made up of a complex combination of nutrients and nonnutrient ingredients. In order for your body to absorb and use what's in food, it first has to take the food apart piece by piece. This dis-assembly line is your digestive system, a 26-foot-long muscular tube.

The "workers" along the digestive tract are enzymes, which are chemicals that can break apart the proteins, carbohydrates, or fats in food. Each of the dozen or so enzymes needed to digest a typical meal can perform only one action on one nutrient. For example, one enzyme specializes in splitting big proteins into smaller pieces, but a different one is needed to complete the job.

Fiber is unique because the body lacks the right enzymes to take it apart. This means that instead of being absorbed like the other carbohydrates we eat, fiber becomes part of the bulk that travels through the small intestine into and through the large intestines, and eventually out of the body.

The word "fiber" doesn't refer to one substance; rather, it represents a variety of indigestible materials that are found in plant foods. As it travels through the body, what each type of fiber does depends on how it's built. An important distinction is whether the fiber dissolves in water, so there are two main categories of dietary fiber, insoluble and soluble, and their health benefits differ.

INSOLUBLE FIBER

The most familiar of the insoluble fibers is wheat bran, but this type is also found in vegetables, fruits, and whole grains such as corn, rye, barley, and brown rice. Insoluble fiber increases the bulk and weight of the stool as well as the rate at which food travels through the digestive system. This makes for potential benefits against cancer. Population studies routinely find that the incidence of colon cancer goes down as the intake of insoluble fiber goes up. That's because fiber can effectively dilute or even grab on to potential cancer-causing substances and quickly usher them out of the body. That's some bodyguard!

Insoluble fiber also gets mixed together with the bile salts, the digestive juice produced by the liver that helps with the absorption of dietary fats. Because the liver makes its bile salts from cholesterol, this binding action by insoluble fiber causes more cholesterol to leave the body.

SOLUBLE FIBER

Perhaps the most famous soluble fiber is oat bran, but this type of fiber is also found in rice bran, legumes (beans, lentils, and peas), fruits, and vegetables. Although these fibers dissolve in water, the body cannot absorb them because of their large size. Soluble fiber can't match the ability of insoluble fiber to add bulk. It can, however, improve conditions connected with diabetes because it tends to slow the rate at which the body absorbs sugar. In addition, through a complex series of reactions, soluble fiber has a demonstrated ability to help lower blood cholesterol levels. Fruits and vegetables often contain both soluble and insoluble fibers. This is further testimony to the wisdom behind including them in the diet.

Figuring Your Fiber Strategy

At present, the typical American diet contains about 12 to 15 grams of dietary fiber per day. Most authorities recommend twice this amount, up to at least 25 to 30 grams per day. An adequate fiber intake is an essential part of a healthy diet.

There are many ways to give your body the fiber boost it needs. Key to this is making more fiber-conscious food selections, which comes from knowing where the fiber is—and where it isn't. With the information contained in these pages, you're on your way!

Checking to see how your current diet stacks up is a good first step. By scanning through this book you'll be able to get a good idea where your current diet stands on the fiber scale. Then, take a look at the food categories you normally include in your daily diet and which choices might represent better alternatives.

Sodium

The Latest Shake

A salt shaker is usually nearby whenever food is served, and next to sugar, we add more salt to our food than any other condiment. Salt, which usually refers to table salt, is a chemical compound called sodium chloride. Both sodium and chloride are essential for life. Our health, however, can be maintained with as little as one-tenth of a teaspoon of salt per day. By contrast, an American's average daily intake is 10 to 35 times that amount.

Where does all that salt in our diet come from? It turns out that about 10 percent is naturally present in food, 15 percent is added during cooking and at the table, while a whopping 75 percent comes from processed foods.

We must also factor in the scientific evidence that too much dietary sodium is associated with the risk of high blood pressure. Although the connection between salt and high blood pressure may not be an issue for everyone, there are good reasons to moderate our intake of salt and the sodium it contains. **That is the reason why we have a separate column devoted to sodium.**

Why Is There so much Sodium in Processed Food?

Food manufacturers find salt attractive for several reasons. Besides it role as a flavor enhancer, salt can retard the growth of a variety of microorganisms. In fact, in the days before refrigeration, salting was the only practical way to keep meats and fish from spoiling.

Salt also plays a role in food texture. Processed meats such as bologna, frankfurters, and luncheon meats contain high levels of salt because it helps form and maintain the gel-like consistency. Salt is also abundant in tomato-based products, such as spaghetti and pizza sauce or tomato juice, and it is used widely in cheese and prepared soups.

The Link with High Blood Pressure

Hypertension, or high blood pressure, currently affects about 60 million people in the United States. It is called the silent killer because there are no warning signs until problems such as heart disease, stroke, or kidney disease have already developed. The only real way to detect hypertension is to have your blood pressure checked.

The connection between salt and hypertension was suggested after several population studies compared salt intake with blood pressure. Scientists found that hypertension was rare in societies with a low-salt diet, while in societies with a high-salt diet, hypertension was more common. This finding, along with those from several animal studies, led to a public health policy to lower salt in our diet.

There is some logic to this association. The body rids itself of excess sodium via the urine, but there is an upper limit to how much salt a given amount of urine can contain. The body responds to a high salt intake by increasing our thirst, the added water being needed to dilute the sodium to get it out of the body. (That, by the way, is why drinking ocean salt water actually makes us *more* thirsty.) It may be that the increased blood volume brought about by a high-salt intake contributes to the higher blood pressure.

To Salt or Not?

Unfortunately, science has not yet come up with a way to predict who gets hypertension. The other complicating factor is that not everyone who has hypertension is what's called a "salt-sensitive hypertensive," meaning that their blood pressure goes up or down with their intake of dietary sodium. At present it's known that there is a strong genetic component and that African-Americans are more likely to develop high blood pressure than European-Americans. Therefore, the key is to routinely check your blood pressure, particularly if you are black or obese, have a high alcohol consumption, or tend to be inactive.

If you are at high risk, or are uncertain about your blood pressure, keep your intake of sodium to a minimum. Avoid reaching for the salt before you taste your food. Saltiness is one of our basic tastes, and salt can help bring out the flavor in food. The key, however, is to enjoy the natural flavor of food, not that which sits in the salt shaker.

The recommended upper limit of sodium for adults and children more than 4 years of age is 2,400 milligrams per day.

Reading Labels

Decoding What the Package Says

A Cluttered Past

The marketing of food through commercials and printed
advertisements and on package labels has led to a confusing
melange of hype. It's a phenomenon that parallels advance-
ments in nutrition science. As more people became inter-
ested in the connection between diet and health, food
companies began using labels and advertisements to
make and market "healthful" products. A key event oc-
curred in 1984 when Kellogg advertised that their All-
Bran cereal was useful in the prevention of cancer; pre-
viously, such claims hadn't been permitted by the Food
and Drug Administration (FDA). The difference in this
case was that the Kellogg ads had received the endorse-
ment of the National Cancer Institute, another government organization.

The food industry waited to see whether the FDA would
order Kellogg to change their ads, but as time passed it
became obvious that nothing was going to happen. Other
companies followed Kellogg's lead and a flood of health
claims and messages worked their way into the market-
place, each trying to outdo the other in proclaiming the
healthfulness of their product.

The result was such a hodgepodge of messages and in-
flated claims that in March 1990, the Secretary of Health
and Human Services, Dr. Louis Sullivan, decried the food
label as a "Tower of Babel" in desperate need of reform.
The Nutrition Labeling and Education Act (NLEA) was
passed that year, and a set of label regulations were published in January 1993. These regulations were designed to
bring some order and consistency to the way foods are
labeled.

On Every Package

At present, every package must list the name of the product; the name and address of the company who manufactured, packed, or distributes the product; and the amount of the product contained in the package. Most packages will also have an ingredient list where the ingredients are listed with the most prevalent item (by weight) followed by the remaining items in order of descending weight, but the actual weights of the items are not displayed.

There is also a "nutrition facts" panel, designed to help you place one serving of that food in the context of your total daily diet. It does this by comparing the amount of nutrients in one serving of food with the total amount of fat, carbohydrate, fiber, protein, vitamins, and minerals that should be present in an average daily diet. It's based on the dietary standard called the Daily Value (DV), which is an updated and expanded version of the U.S. Recommended Daily Allowances, or "U.S. RDA," the allowance for vitamins, minerals, and protein that has been used on packaged foods since 1973.

Daily Values for fat, saturated fat, carbohydrate, fiber, and protein are based on the number of calories you eat during the day, while DVs for cholesterol, sodium, and potassium are fixed amounts.

Daily Values

Fat: 30 percent of daily calories
Saturated Fat: 10 percent of daily calories
Carbohydrate: 60 percent of daily calories
Fiber: 11.5 g per 1,000 calories
Protein: 10 percent of daily calories
Cholesterol: 300 mg per day
Sodium: 2,400 mg per day

Table of Daily Values

The bottom half of the new label lists the amounts of fat, saturated fat, cholesterol, sodium, total carbohydrate, and fiber that should be present in an average 2,000-calorie and 2,500-calorie diet. At the very bottom there's a notation that fat contains 9 calories per gram and protein or carbohydrate contains 4 calories per gram.

When reading this information, keep in mind that a 2,000-calorie diet may be excessive for smaller women and children, and a 2,500-calorie diet would provide insufficient calories for larger individuals and those who are physically active. The purpose of these numbers is to let you see how one serving of the food would compare with a typical day's diet.

Nutrition Facts

Serving Size 1/2 cup (114g)
Servings Per Container 4

Amount Per Serving

Calories 260   Calories From Fat 120

% Daily Value*

Total Fat 13g	**20%**
Saturated Fat 5g	**25%**
Cholesterol 30mg	**10%**
Sodium 660mg	**28%**
Total Carbohydrates 31g	**11%**
Dietary Fiber 0g	**0%**
Sugars 5g	
Protein 5g	

Vitamin A	4%	Vitamin C	2%
Calcium	15%	Iron	4%

* Percent Daily Values are based on a 2,000 calorie diet. Your daily values may be higher or lower depending on your calorie needs:

Nutrient	Calories	2,000	2,500
Total Fat	Less than	65g	80g
Sat Fat	Less than	20g	25g
Cholesterol	Less than	300mg	300mg
Sodium	Less than	2,400mg	2,400mg
Total Carbohydrate		300g	375g
Fiber		25g	30g

Calories per gram:
Fat 9 • Carbohydrates 4 • Protein 4

Helping You Shop

The Nutrition Doctor's A-to-Z Food Counter can help you decide on products before you get to the store, but once there you should examine the name, ingredient list, nutrition panel, and preparation instructions on the package. If your decision is between two similar products, examine their ingredients and nutritional panels side by side to see which one offers more of what you seek. Does one have less fat? Is one made with whole grains? Is sugar the number one ingredient or is it further down on the list? Is one fortified with vitamins and minerals that you seek? Is one of the choices a source of folic acid, antioxidants, or calcium as indicated by an F, A, or C in *The Nutrition Doctor's A-to-Z Food Counter*?

And finally, before you toss the desired brand into your cart, check the package for any defects such as water stains, leaks, or bulges that may indicate mishandling or tampering. You should also check for an expiration date to assure you're getting a product that is still safe to eat.

Glossary of Terms Used on Food Labels

FAT

- Fat-Free: Less than ½ g (gram) of fat per serving (or per 50 g of food)
- Low Fat: 3 g of fat or less, per serving (or per 50 g of food)
- Low in Saturated Fat: 1 g of saturated fat or less, per serving (no more than 15 percent of the calories are saturated fat)
- ___Percent Fat Free: Contains the stated percent of nonfat ingredients. This term is allowed only in low-fat, or fat-free foods.
- Low Cholesterol: Less than 20 mg (milligrams) per serving (or per 50 g of food)
- Cholesterol Free: Less than 2 mg of cholesterol *and* no more than 2 mg of saturated fat per serving
- Lean: Less than 10 g fat, less than 4 g saturated fat,

and less than 95 mg cholesterol per 100 g (3½ ounces). (Used on meat, fish, poultry, and game.)
- Extra Lean: Less than 5 g fat, less than 2 g saturated fat, and less than 95 mg cholesterol per 100 g. (Used on meat, fish, poultry, and game.)

CALORIES
- Reduced Calories: A product altered to contain 25 percent fewer calories than the food it's being compared to. (Cannot be used if the other food already meets the requirement for a "low calorie" claim.)
- Calorie Free: Fewer than 5 calories per serving
- Low Calorie: 40 calories or less per serving (and per 50 g of food)
- Light: Contains ⅓ fewer calories or ½ the fat of the usual food. (If the usual food gets more than half its calories from fat, the reduction must be ½ the fat.)

SODIUM
- Sodium Free: Less than 5 mg per serving
- Low Sodium: Less than 140 mg per serving and per 50 g of food
- Very Low Sodium: Less than 35 mg per serving and per 50 g of food
- Reduced Sodium: Contains no more than ¼ the sodium of the comparable food
- Light: Light can be used if the sodium content of a low-calorie, low-fat food has been reduced by half

SUGAR
- Sugar Free: Less than ½ g per serving

GENERAL TERMS
- Free: An amount small enough to have no likely effect on the body
- [Nutrient] Free: Food contains an insignificant amount of the nutrient
- Low: Low enough so that you can have it many times during the day without exceeding dietary guidelines
- Less or Reduced: Contains at least 25 percent less of the named substance than the comparable food

- More: Contains at least 10 percent more of the named nutrient than the comparable food
- High In: One serving must contain at least 20 percent of the daily requirement
- A Source of: One serving must provide 10 to 19 percent of the daily requirement
- Healthy: Must be low in fat and low in saturated fat
- Fresh: Must be raw, not frozen, processed, or preserved in any way (irradiation at low levels is allowed). Other uses, such as "fresh milk" or "freshly baked bread" are still permitted.
- Fresh Frozen: Quickly frozen while still fresh (blanching before freezing is permitted)
- Light: Can be used to describe properties such as taste, texture, and color, but the label must explain the intent, such as "light brown sugar"
- Implied Value: A product cannot claim to be made with an ingredient unless it has enough to be considered a good source of that ingredient. For example, "made with oat bran" can only appear on products that would be considered a good source of fiber.

SYNONYMS
- Free: without, no, zero
- Less: fewer
- Light: lite
- Low: little, few, low source of
- Fresh Frozen: freshly frozen, frozen fresh

About the Data

All the data in these tables are based on the latest available information from a number of sources, including product labels, information gathered from product manufacturers, the U.S. Department of Agriculture (*Agricultural Handbook* No. 11), the Canadian Nutrition Foundation, and the Produce Marketing Association. The database was customized by Nutrition Resource, and the information was retrieved through the use of *Nutritionist IV Diet Analysis software (Version 4.1, First DataBank Division, the Hearst Corporation).*

Abbreviations

OZ = Ounce
SERV = Serving
TBSP = Tablespoon
TSP = Teaspoon
gms = Grams
FF = Fat free
LF = Low fat
NF = Non-fat
RF = Reduced fat
LS = Low sodium
W/ = With
LT = Light
NSA = No sugar added
WW = Whole wheat
COND = Condensed
*PFC = Prepared from condensed
PKG = Package
NV = No value available
Kcal = Calorie
CARB = Carbohydrate
FIBER = Dietary fiber (insoluble plus soluble)
SOD = Sodium
FAC = F = Folic acid, A = Antioxidant, C = Calcium
<1 = Less than 1

(*Used in soups only)

Equivalents

Volume

1 teaspoon = ⅓ tablespoon
1 tablespoon = 3 teaspoons
2 tablespoons = 1 fluid ounce
4 tablespoons = ¼ cup
16 tablespoons = 1 cup
8 fluid ounces = 1 cup
2 cups = 1 pint
2 pints = 1 quart
4 quarts = 1 gallon
1 liter = 1.05 quarts

Mass

1 ounce = 28.35 grams
1 pound = 16 ounces
1 pound = 0.454 kilograms
1 gram = 1,000 milligrams
1 milligram = 1,000 micrograms (µg)
100 grams = 3.5 ounces
1 kilogram = 2.2 pounds

A

	Serv.	K-Cal.	Fat	Prot.	Carb.	Fib.	Sod.	FAC
Abalone								
Raw	3 Oz	89	0.7	15	5	0	256	
Fried	3 Oz	161	5.8	17	9	0	502	
Steamed or Poached	3 Oz	176	1.3	29	10	0	429	
Acorn								
Raw, Shelled	1 Oz	105	6.8	2	12	NV	0	
Dried	1 Oz	145	8.9	2	15	1	0	F
Acorn Flour	1 Oz	142	8.6	2	16	1	0	F

Acorn Squash (See Squash, Winter)

Adzuki Bean (See Bean, Adzuki)

Agar (See Seaweed, Dried)

Ahi Tuna (See Tuna, Yellowfin)

	Serv.	K-Cal.	Fat	Prot.	Carb.	Fib.	Sod.	FAC
Alcoholic Beverages								
Beer								
Budweiser	12 Oz	144	0	1	11	0	12	
Budweiser LT	12 Oz	110	0	1	7	0	12	
Coors	12 Oz	137	0	1	12	0	0	
Coors, LT	12 Oz	103	0	1	5	0	0	
Michelob	12 Oz	156	0	2	14	0	12	
Miller High Life	12 Oz	147	0	1	13	0	7	
Rolling Rock	12 Oz	145	0	0	10	0	0	
Beer, Nonalcoholic								
Cutter	12 Oz	76	0	1	20	0	1	
Sharp's	12 Oz	86	0	1	10	0	5	
Liqueur								
Bourbon	1 Oz	65	0	0	0	0	0	
Brandy	1 Oz	65	0	0	0	0	0	
Coffee/Kahlua	1 Oz	107	0.1	0	11	0	3	
Coffee/Kahlua W/Cream	1 Oz	102	4.9	1	7	0	29	

	Serv.	K-Cal.	Fat	Prot.	Carb.	Fib.	Sod.	FAC
Crème De Menthe	1 Oz	125	0.1	0	14	0	2	
Gin	1 Oz	69	0	0	0	0	0	
Rum	1 Oz	56	0	0	3	0	6	
Rye Whiskey	1 Oz	70	0	0	0	0	0	
Scotch	1 Oz	70	0	0	0	0	0	
Tequila	1 Oz	70	0	0	0	0	0	
Vodka	1 Oz	69	0	0	0	0	0	
Whiskey	1 Oz	69	0	0	0	0	0	
Mixed Drinks								
Alexander	1 Oz	71	0.7	0	3	0	3	
Black Russian	1 Oz	81	0	0	5	0	1	
Bloody Mary	1 Oz	23	0	0	1	0	67	
Daiquiri	1 Oz	56	0	0	2	0	2	
Frozen Daiquiri	1 Oz	54	0	0	2	0	1	
Gibson	1 Oz	67	0	0	0	0	1	
Gimlet	1 Oz	56	0	0	0	0	1	
Gin and Tonic	1 Oz	23	0	0	2	0	1	
Gold Cadillac	1 Oz	91	0.9	0	11	0	4	
Grasshopper	1 Oz	82	1.8	0	8	0	7	
Highball	1 Oz	26	0	0	0	0	4	
Irish Coffee	1 Oz	26	1.3	0	1	0	2	
Long Island Iced Tea	1 Oz	29	0	0	2	0	1	
Mai Tai	1 Oz	73	0	0	7	0	3	
Manhattan	1 Oz	64	0	0	1	0	1	
Margarita	1 Oz	68	0	0	4	0	111	
Martini	1 Oz	63	0	0	0	0	1	
Piña Colada	1 Oz	77	2.5	0	9	0	23	
Rum Cooler	1 Oz	17	0	0	3	0	1	
Rum, Hot Buttered	1 Oz	37	1.4	0	1	0	1	
Sangria	1 Oz	20	0	0	3	0	3	
Scotch W/Soda	1 Oz	27	0	0	0	0	4	
Screwdriver	1 Oz	25	0	0	3	0	0	
Singapore Sling	1 Oz	30	0	0	2	0	4	
Sloe Gin Fizz	1 Oz	16	0	0	0	0	5	
Stinger	1 Oz	92	0.1	0	7	0	1	
Tequila Sunrise	1 Oz	34	0	0	3	0	1	
Tom Collins	1 Oz	16	0	0	0	0	5	
Whiskey Sour	1 Oz	48	0	0	5	0	14	
White Russian	1 Oz	77	0.4	0	5	0	2	
Zombie	1 Oz	58	0	0	2	0	1	
Wine								
Cabernet Sauvignon	4 Oz	88	0	0	1	0	4	
Chablis	4 Oz	84	0	0	2	0	0	
Chardonnay	4 Oz	88	0	0	0	0	0	
Chenin Blanc	4 Oz	88	0	0	2	0	0	
Chianti	4 Oz	92	0	0	2	0	0	
Gewürztraminer	4 Oz	88	0	0	2	0	0	
Marsala	4 Oz	77	0	0	4	0	4	
Port	4 Oz	170	0	0	10	0	0	

	Serv.	K-Cal.	Fat	Prot.	Carb.	Flb.	Sod.	FAC
(Alcoholic Beverages cont.)								
Rosé	4 Oz	88	0	0	3	0	0	
Sauvignon Blanc	4 Oz	80	0	0	1	0	0	
Sherry	4 Oz	128	0	0	4	0	0	
Vermouth, Dry	4 Oz	112	0	0	2	0	0	
Vermouth, Sweet	4 Oz	180	0	0	19	0	0	
Zinfandel	4 Oz	91	0	0	1	0	4	

Alfalfa Seeds

	Serv.	K-Cal.	Fat	Prot.	Carb.	Flb.	Sod.	FAC
Sprouted	1 Cup	10	0.2	1	1	1	2	

Alfredo Sauce (See Pasta Sauce, Alfredo)

Allspice

	Serv.	K-Cal.	Fat	Prot.	Carb.	Flb.	Sod.	FAC
Ground (McCormick)	1 Tsp	6	0	0	1	1	1	

Almond

(1 Oz equals approximately ¼ cup or 25 nuts)

	Serv.	K-Cal.	Fat	Prot.	Carb.	Flb.	Sod.	FAC
Raw								
Chopped, Unblanched	1 Oz	194	17	7	7	4	0	A
(Blue Diamond) Natural	1 Oz	150	13	7	5	3	0	A
(Planters) Sliced	1 Oz	170	15	6	6	NV	0	A
Blanched								
Sliced	1 Cup	615	55	21	20	NV	11	FAC
(Blue Diamond) Whole	1 Oz	150	13	7	5	3	0	A
Dry-Roasted								
Unblanched, Salted	1 Oz	202	17.8	6	8	3	269	A
(Blue Diamond) No Salt	1 Oz	150	13	7	6	3	0	A
(Planters)	1 Oz	170	15	6	6	NV	200	A
Flavored								
Honey-Roasted	1 Oz	214	18	7	10	5	47	A
(Blue Diamond):								
Barbecue	1 Oz	160	16	7	5	3	220	A
Smokehouse	1 Oz	150	14	7	4	3	170	A
Sour Cream/Onion	1 Oz	150	14	7	4	3	140	A
Oil-Roasted								
Whole	1 Cup	970	91	32	25	18	16	FAC
Blanched, Salted	1 Oz	217	20.1	7	6	3	275	A
Unblanched, Salted	1 Oz	243	22.6	8	6	3	306	A

Almond Butter

	Serv.	K-Cal.	Fat	Prot.	Carb.	Flb.	Sod.	FAC
Plain	1 Tbsp	101	9.5	2	3	1	2	A
Plain, Salted	1 Tbsp	99	9.2	2	3	1	70	A
Honey and Cinnamon,								
Salted	1 Tbsp	94	8.1	2	4	1	27	A
Roasted (Maranatha)	1 Tbsp	110	9	4	3	3	0	A

Almond Meal

	Serv.	K-Cal.	Fat	Prot.	Carb.	Flb.	Sod.	FAC
Partially Defatted, Salted	3 Oz	347	15.5	34	25	NV	632	FAC

	Serv.	K-Cal.	Fat	Prot.	Carb.	Fib.	Sod.	FAC
Almond Oil								
(Spectrum)................	1 Tbsp	120	14	0	0	0	0	A
Almond Paste								
(Solo)	2 Tbsp	180	11	4	19	1	0	A
Amaranth								
Raw	1 Cup	7	0.1	1	1	NV	6	A
Boiled, Drained..............	1 Cup	27	0	3	5	NV	28	FAC
Amaranth Grain								
....	1 Cup	729	12.7	28	129	29	41	FAC
Amaranth Flour								
(Arrowhead Mills)	1 Cup	440	6	16	76	8	0	FA
Anasazi Bean (See Bean, Anasazi)								
Anchovy								
Raw, Meat only	1 Oz	37	1.4	2	0	0	30	
Dried, Whole	1 Oz	73	0.9	16	0	0	103	C
Filet, W/Oil, Drained,								
Canned	1 Oz	60	2.8	8	0	0	104	
Paste	1 Tsp	35	2.5	3	0	10	240	
Animal Cracker (See Cookie, Animal Cracker)								
Anise Seed								
Dried (McCormick)	1 Tsp	17	.8	1	2	1	1	
Apple								
Fresh								
W/Skin, 2¾" Diameter...	1 Item	81	0.5	0	21	4	0	
W/Skin, 2¾" Diameter...	8 Oz	134	0.8	0	35	6	0	A
W/Skin, Sliced	1 Cup	64	0.4	0	17	3	0	
W/O Skin, 2¾" Diameter	1 Item	73	0.4	0	19	2	0	
Canned								
Rings (S & W)................	1 Oz	25	0	7	7	1	20	
Sliced (Seneca)..............	1 Cup	90	0	0	22	4	70	
Spiced Crab (S & W).....	1 Oz	35	0	0	8	1	15	
Sweetened (Comstock)..	⅓ Cup	80	0	0	20	1	0	
Crab								
Raw, With Skin	1 Cup	84	0.3	0	22	NV	1	
Frozen								
Baked (Seneca)	1 Item	70	0	0	18	4	0	
Escalloped (Stouffer's) ...	1 Cup	273	4.5	0	56	5	106	A

	Serv.	K-Cal.	Fat	Prot.	Carb.	Flb.	Sod.	FAC
Apple, Dried								
Cooked	1 Cup	143	0.2	1	38	5	50	
Cooked, Sweetened	1 Cup	232	0.2	1	58	5	53	
Uncooked	1 Cup	209	0.3	1	57	7	75	
Uncooked, Sulfured	1 Cup	209	0	1	57	8	75	
Apple Butter								
Cider (Smucker's)	1 Tbsp	45	0	0	11	0	10	
(Eden)	1 Tbsp	20	0	0	5	0	0	
Organic (R.W. Knudsen)	1 Tbsp	13	0	0	3	NV	0	
Apple Chips								
(Seneca)	1 Oz	140	7	0	20	2	15	A
Apple Cider								
Fermented	1 Cup	100	0	0	3	0	0	
Sparkling (Martinelli)	1 Cup	130	0	0	33	NV	7	
W/Spice (R.W. Knudsen)	1 Cup	120	0	0	30	NV	25	
(Tree Top)	1 Cup	120	0	0	29	NV	13	
Apple Juice								
(R.W. Knudsen):								
Clear	1 Cup	110	0	0	28	NV	5	
Natural	1 Cup	120	0	0	30	NV	25	
Original	1 Cup	120	0	0	30	NV	25	
(Kraft) 100% Pure	1 Cup	112	0	0	28	0	7	
(Minute Maid)	1 Cup	112	0	0	28	NV	28	
(Odwalla)	1 Cup	140	0	0	34	0	25	
(Snapple) Apple Crisp	1 Cup	112	0	0	29	0	24	
(Ultra Slim-Fast) Golden	1 Cup	147	1	5	27	3	160	FAC
Apple Juice, Blended								
(R.W. Knudsen):								
W/Apricot	1 Cup	120	0	0	30	NV	35	
W/Banana	1 Cup	120	0	0	30	NV	25	
W/Boysenberry	1 Cup	120	0	0	30	NV	25	
W/Cranberry	1 Cup	120	0	0	30	NV	25	
W/Peach	1 Cup	120	0	0	30	NV	25	
W/Raspberry	1 Cup	120	0	0	30	NV	25	
W/Strawberry	1 Cup	120	0	0	30	NV	25	
(Snapple) W/Cherry	1 Cup	112	0	0	28	NV	64	
(Ultra Slim-Fast)								
W/Cranberry/								
Raspberry	1 Cup	147	1	5	31	3	161	FAC
Apple Juice, Frozen								
Concentrate								
(Seneca)	2 Oz	120	0	0	29	0	10	A
(Tree Top)	2 Oz	120	0	0	29	0	15	A

	Serv.	K-Cal.	Fat	Prot.	Carb.	Fib.	Sod.	FAC
Diluted								
(Seneca)	1 Cup	120	0	0	29	0	10	A
(Tree Top)	1 Cup	120	0	0	29	0	15	A

Apple Pastry (See Pastry, Danish)

Apple Pie (See Pie, Apple)

Apple Strudel (See Pastry, Danish)

Applesauce

	Serv.	K-Cal.	Fat	Prot.	Carb.	Fib.	Sod.	FAC
(Eden)	1 Cup	100	0	0	30	4	30	
(Motts):	1 Cup	200	0	0	52	2	0	
Chunky	1 Cup	180	0	0	46	4	0	
W/Cranberry	1 Cup	220	0	0	54	2	0	
(Seneca):								
Enriched	1 Cup	200	0	0	48	4	0	A
Natural	1 Cup	120	0	0	28	4	0	
(S & W):								
Gravenstein	1 Cup	180	0	0	42	2	10	
Gravenstein, Unsweetened	1 Cup	100	0	0	26	4	10	
(Tree Top):								
Original	1 Cup	200	0	0	50	2	0	A
Unsweetened	1 Cup	140	0	0	36	2	0	A

Apricot

	Serv.	K-Cal.	Fat	Prot.	Carb.	Fib.	Sod.	FAC
Fresh								
Raw	1 Lb	202	1.7	6	47	6	2	FA
Raw, Halves Pitted	1 Cup	74	0.6	2	17	4	2	A
Raw, Pitted	1 Item	17	0.1	0	4	1	0	
Canned W/								
Extra Light Syrup	1 Cup	121	0.3	1	31	4	5	A
Heavy Syrup	1 Cup	214	0.2	1	55	4	28	A
Juice	1 Cup	119	0.1	2	31	4	10	A
Light Syrup	1 Cup	159	0.1	1	42	4	10	A
Water	1 Cup	50	0.1	2	12	3	25	A
Dried								
Cooked, Sulfured	1 Cup	314	0.6	5	81	NV	12	A
Cooked, Sweetened	1 Cup	305	0.4	3	79	11	8	A
Uncooked	1 Cup	381	0.7	6	99	NV	16	A
Uncooked, Sulfured	1 Cup	309	0.6	5	80	12	13	A
Frozen								
Sweetened	1 Cup	237	0.2	2	61	5	10	AC

Apricot Juice—Nectar

	Serv.	K-Cal.	Fat	Prot.	Carb.	Fib.	Sod.	FAC
(Kern)								
W/Mango	1 Cup	152	0	1	37	0	1	A
W/Pineapple	1 Cup	152	0	1	37	0	1	A

	Serv.	K-Cal.	Fat	Prot.	Carb.	Fib.	Sod.	FAC
(*Apricot Juice cont.*)								
(Libby's)	1 Cup	152	0	1	37	0	1	A
(R.W. Knudsen) W/ Apple	1 Cup	120	0	0	30	NV	35	A
Apricot Kernel Oil								
(Spectrum)	1 Tbsp	120	14	0	0	0	0	
Arrowroot Flour								
	1 Cup	457	0.1	0	113	4	3	
Arrowroot Powder								
(Tone)	1 Tsp	10	0	0	2	0	1	
Artichoke, Globe								
Raw	12 Oz	128	0.3	13	26	18	367	FA
Raw, Large	5 Oz	76	0.2	5	17	9	152	FA
Boiled, Medium	4 Oz	60	0.2	4	13	NV	114	FA
Boiled, Small	2.8 Oz	36	0.4	2	7	4	42	FA

Artichoke, Jerusalem (See Jerusalem Artichoke)

	Serv.	K-Cal.	Fat	Prot.	Carb.	Fib.	Sod.	FAC
Artichoke Hearts								
Fresh, Boiled	1 Cup	84	0.3	6	19	9	160	FA
Canned (S & W)	1 Piece	10	0	1	2	0	67	
Frozen (Bird's Eye)	3 Oz	30	0	2	7	0	140	F
Marinated (Progresso)	1 Cup	480	42	3	18	3	871	FA
Marinated (S & W)	1 Oz	20	2	0	2	1	80	
Arugula—Rocket—Rugola								
Raw	1 Cup	5	0.1	1	1	0	5	
Raw	5 Oz	35	0.9	4	5	1	38	FAC
Raw, Leaf	1 Item	1	0.0	0	0	0	1	
Asparagus								
Fresh								
Raw	1 Cup	31	0.3	3	6	3	3	FA
Raw	1 Oz	7	0.2	1	1	3	4	
Raw, Spear	1 Item	3	0	0	0	0	1	
Boiled, Cuts/Tips	1 Cup	45	1	5	8	3	7	FA
Boiled, Spears	1 Cup	43	0.6	5	8	3	20	FA
Canned								
Blended (Del Monte)	1 Cup	40	0	4	6	2	840	FA
Blended (S & W)	1 Piece	3	0	0	1	0	43	
Spears (Del Monte)	1 Cup	40	0	4	6	2	840	FA
Spears (Green Giant)	1 Cup	40	0	4	6	2	34	FA
Frozen								
Cuts (Flav R Pac)	1 Cup	27	0	4	4	3	7	FA
Cuts (Green Giant)	1 Cup	38	0	3	6	2	127	FA

	Serv.	K-Cal.	Fat	Prot.	Carb.	Fib.	Sod.	FAC
Spears (Flav R Pac)	1 Item	3	0	0	0	0	1	
Spears (Seneca)	1 Cup	40	0	4	6	4	440	FA

Asparagus Bean (See Green Bean, Fresh; Yard-Long Bean)

Avocado

	Serv.	K-Cal.	Fat	Prot.	Carb.	Fib.	Sod.	FAC
All Varieties	1 Cup	370	35.2	5	17	12	23	FA
All Varieties	2 Oz	120	12	1	3	2	5	FA
California	1 Item	306	30	4	12	8	21	FA
Florida.............................	1 Item	340	27	5	27	16	15	FA
(Hass)	1 Item	283	32.3	4	1	26	15	FA

Avocado Oil

	Serv.	K-Cal.	Fat	Prot.	Carb.	Fib.	Sod.	FAC
(Hain's)	1 Tbsp	120	14	0	0	0	0	A
(Spectrum)......................	1 Tbsp	120	14	0	0	0	0	A

Awa (See Milkfish)

B

	Serv.	K-Cal.	Fat	Prot.	Carb.	Fib.	Sod.	FAC
Baby Food, Cereal								
Barley								
(Beech-Nut)								
Stage 1, Dry	4 Tbsp	60	0	1	12	1	10	**C**
(Gerber) Dry	4 Tbsp	60	0.5	2	11	1	0	**A**
Mixed Grain								
DRY								
(Beech-Nut) *Stage 2* ..	4 Tbsp	60	1	1	12	1	10	**AC**
(Earth's Best).............	4 Tbsp	55	0.4	2	11	1	0	
(Gerber)	4 Tbsp	60	0.5	2	11	1	0	**A**
(Gerber) W/Banana	4 Tbsp	60	0.5	2	11	1	0	**A**
JARRED								
(Beech-Nut) W/Apple								
Banana, *Stage 2*	4 Oz	90	1	2	19	NV	0	**A**
(Gerber) W/Apple-								
sauce/Banana,								
2nd Foods...............	4 Oz	94	0.7	1	20	1	2	**A**
Oatmeal								
DRY								
(Beech-Nut) W/Ba-								
nana, *Stage 2*...........	4 Tbsp	60	1	1	12	1	0	**AC**
(Gerber)	4 Tbsp	60	1	2	10	1	0	**AC**
JARRED								
(Earth's Best)								
Apple Cinnamon	4 Oz	68	0.7	2	16	2	4	**A**
(Gerber) Apple								
Banana, *2nd Foods*	4 Oz	95	0.9	2	20	2	2	**A**
Rice								
DRY								
(Beech-Nut) *Stage 1* ..	4 Tbsp	60	0	1	12	0	0	**AC**
W/Banana *Stage 2*.....	4 Tbsp	60	0	0	13	0	0	**AC**
JARRED								
(Beech-Nut) W/Apple								
Banana, *Stage 2*.....	4 Oz	90	0	1	20	NV	10	**A**
(Gerber) W/Apple-								
sauce, *2nd Foods*...	4 Oz	100	0	1	23	1	10	**A**

	Serv.	K-Cal.	Fat	Prot.	Carb.	Fib.	Sod.	FAC
W/Mixed Fruit, *3rd* Foods	4 Oz	90	0.2	1	21	0	10	A

Baby Food, Dessert
Apple
(Beech-Nut):

	Serv.	K-Cal.	Fat	Prot.	Carb.	Fib.	Sod.	FAC
Cobbler, *Stage 3*........	4 Oz	94	1	0	19	1	10	A
Dutch, *Stage 2*	4 Oz	100	0	0	22	0	10	A
(Earth's Best) W/Yogurt, Strained	4 Oz	89	0.9	3	16	2	19	A
(Gerber):								
Banana Apple, *2nd* Foods	4 Oz	78	0.1	0	19	1	7	A
Dutch, *2nd Foods*.......	4 Oz	94	0	0	23	2	6	A
W/Banana, *3rd* Foods	4 Oz	87	0	0	20	2	0	A

Banana
(Beech-Nut):

	Serv.	K-Cal.	Fat	Prot.	Carb.	Fib.	Sod.	FAC
Banana W/Pears/ Apples, *Stage 2*	4 Oz	90	0	0	21	1	10	A
W/Pineapple, *Stage 2*	4 Oz	100	0	0	23	0	15	A
(Gerber):								
Banana W/Tapioca, *2nd Foods*..................	4 Oz	88	0.2	0	21	1	4	A
W/Apple, *2nd Foods*...	4 Oz	76	0.1	0	18	1	8	A
W/Vanilla......................	4 Oz	100	1	0	21	0	15	A

Cookie

	Serv.	K-Cal.	Fat	Prot.	Carb.	Fib.	Sod.	FAC
Pretzels, Enriched	1 Item	24	0.1	1	5	0	16	
Teething Biscuits............	1 Item	43	0.5	1	8	0	40	
Zwieback Cookies	1 Item	30	0.7	1	5	0	1	
(Gerber):								
Arrowroot, *Graduates*.	2 Item	25	1	0	4	0	15	
Banana, *Graduates*	1 Item	35	1	<1	6	0	0	
Biter Biscuit, *Graduates*................	1 Item	45	0.5	1	9	0	30	
Pretzel, *Graduates*......	2 Item	25	0	<1	5	0	25	

Custard
(Beech-Nut):

	Serv.	K-Cal.	Fat	Prot.	Carb.	Fib.	Sod.	FAC
Banana, Tropical	4 Oz	110	0	0	24	0	20	A
Vanilla, *Stage 2*	4 Oz	110	0	0	24	0	20	A
(Gerber):								
Cherry Vanilla, *2nd* Foods	4 Oz	78	0.2	0	19	0	7	
Vanilla, *2nd Foods*	4 Oz	108	2	3	20	0	36	

Fruit
(Beech-Nut):

	Serv.	K-Cal.	Fat	Prot.	Carb.	Fib.	Sod.	FAC
Stage 2	4 Oz	80	0	0	19	1	0	A

	Serv.	K-Cal.	Fat	Prot.	Carb.	Fib.	Sod.	FAC
(Baby Food, Dessert cont.)								
(Gerber):								
Blueberry Buckle, *3rd*								
Foods	4 Oz	82	0	0	20	0	29	A
Cherry Cobbler, *3rd*								
Foods	4 Oz	88	0.1	0	21	0	54	A
Hawaiian Delight, *2nd*								
Foods	4 Oz	113	0	1	25	0	23	A
Medley, *2nd Foods*.....	4 Oz	92	0.1	0	21	0	8	A
Peach Cobbler, *2nd*								
Foods	4 Oz	87	0.2	1	21	1	6	A
Peach Cobbler, *3rd*								
Foods	4 Oz	87	0.1	1	21	1	29	A
Strawberry Bar............	1 Item	35	1	0	7	0	10	A
Yogurt								
(Gerber):								
Apple, *2nd Foods*.......	4 Oz	91	1	3	18	1	43	A
Banana, *2nd*								
Foods	4 Oz	85	0.5	1	19	0	18	A
Mixed Fruit, *2nd*								
Foods	4 Oz	89	0.3	1	20	1	18	A
Peach, *2nd Foods*......	4 Oz	87	0.5	1	20	NV	16	A
Pear/Peach, ...	4 Oz	90	1	3	18	NV	42	A

Baby Food, Dinner
Beef
(Beech-Nut):								
Broth, *Stage 1*	4 Oz	144	9.6	13	0	0	64	
Supreme, *Stage 2*......	4 Oz	130	9	2	8	1	45	A
W/Macaroni, *Stage 3*..	4 Oz	87	2	3	15	1	30	A
W/Noodles, *Stage 2* ...	4 Oz	100	6	1	8	2	50	A
(Earth's Best):								
W/Vegetable Pilaf.......	4 Oz	86	2	3	12	1	10	A
(Gerber):								
Vegetable Beef, *2nd*								
Foods	4 Oz	78	3	3	10	3	16	A
W/Beef Gravy, *2nd*								
Foods	4 Oz	122	5	13	6	1	50	
W/Egg Noodle, *2nd*								
Foods	4 Oz	73	2.2	3	10	1	12	A

Chicken
(Beech-Nut):								
W/Broth......................	4 Oz	96	3	13	0	0	88	
W/Rice, *Stage 2*	4 Oz	80	3	1	9	1	50	A
W/Noodles, *Stage 3* ...	4 Oz	74	3	2	9	1	17	A
(Earth's Best):								
W/Sweet Potato,								
Strained	4 Oz	79	0.7	3	12	2	23	A

	Serv.	K-Cal.	Fat	Prot.	Carb.	Fib.	Sod.	FAC
(Gerber):								
Finger Sticks,								
Graduates............	4 Oz	151	8.6	17	2	2	476	
Stew W/Noodles,								
Graduates............	4 Oz	73	3	4	7	1	240	A
Vegetable Chicken,								
2nd Foods	4 Oz	71	2	3	10	3	23	A
W/Chicken Gravy,								
2nd Foods...........	4 Oz	129	7	12	4	0	52	
W/Noodles,								
2nd Foods...........	4 Oz	81	2.2	4	11	2	19	A
W/Noodles, *3rd Foods*	4 Oz	62	1	3	10	1	110	A
W/Rice, *Tropical*	4 Oz	54	1.5	3	8	NV	16	A
Ham								
(Gerber)								
W/Apples, *2nd Foods*	4 Oz	70	1.8	3	10	2	10	
W/Vegetable, *2nd*								
Foods	4 Oz	66	1.8	2	10	1	11	A
Lamb								
Strained	4 Oz	116	5.3	16	0	0	68	A
W/Vegetable, Strained ...	4 Oz	65	1.9	3	10	1	20	A
(Beech-Nut) W/Broth,								
Stage 1	4 Oz	96	4.8	10	0	0	80	
Liver								
Strained	4 Oz	114	4.3	16	2	0	84	FA
Turkey								
(Beech-Nut):								
Supreme, *Stage 2*	4 Oz	90	4	3	9	1	45	A
W/Broth, *Stage 1*........	4 Oz	144	9.6	13	0	0	64	
(Earth's Best):								
W/Vegetable	4 Oz	61	1.2	3	10	2	20	A
(Gerber):								
W/Rice, *2nd Foods*.....	4 Oz	58	1.1	3	9	1	20	A
W/Vegetable, *2nd*								
Foods	4 Oz	55	0.9	2	9	1	12	A
Veal								
(Beech-Nut) W/Broth,								
Stage 1	4 Oz	96	3.2	14	0	0	80	
(Gerber):								
2nd Foods.................	4 Oz	115	5.8	16	0	0	56	A
3rd Foods	4 Oz	122	5.6	18	0	NV	63	A
Baby Food, Fruit								
Apple								
(Beech-Nut) W/Pear/								
Banana, *Stage 2*	4 Oz	70	0	0	16	1	10	A
(Earth's Best):								
Strained.....................	4 Oz	58	0.1	0	14	2	2	A
W/Apricot, Strained.....	4 Oz	53	0.1	1	13	2	3	A

	Serv.	K-Cal.	Fat	Prot.	Carb.	Fib.	Sod.	FAC
(Baby Food, Dessert cont.)								
W/Banana, Strained ...	4 Oz	58	0.1	1	14	2	1	**A**
W/Plum, Strained........	4 Oz	59	0.1	1	14	2	2	**A**
(Gerber) W/Blueberry,								
2nd Foods	4 Oz	57	0	0	14	2	1	**A**
Applesauce								
(Beech-Nut), *Stage 1*.....	4 Oz	70	0	0	15	1	10	**A**
(Gerber) W/Apricot, *2nd*								
Foods	4 Oz	61	0.2	0	14	2	1	**A**
Apricot								
(Beech-Nut) W/Pear/								
Apple, *Stage 2*	4 Oz	70	0	0	16	2	10	**A**
(Gerber) W/Tapioca, *2nd*								
Foods	4 Oz	77	0	0	19	1	5	**A**
Banana								
(Beech-Nut) *Stage 1*	4 Oz	90	0	0	20	1	0	**A**
W/Pear/Apple,								
Stage 2	4 Oz	90	0	0	21	1	10	**A**
(Gerber) W/Tapioca, *2nd*								
Foods	4 Oz	88	0	0	21	1	5	**A**
Peach								
(Beech-Nut) *Stage 1*	4 Oz	60	0	0	14	·2	10	**A**
(Gerber)...........................	4 Oz	70	0	0	16	1	10	**A**
Pear								
(Beech-Nut) *Stage 1*	4 Oz	70	0	0	16	2	0	**A**
W/Pineapple,								
Stage 2	4 Oz	70	0	0	16	2	0	**A**
(Earth's Best) W/								
Raspberry	4 Oz	61	0.1	1	14	3	1	**A**
Plum								
(Beech-Nut) W/Apple/								
Rice, *Stage 2*	4 Oz	90	0	0	18	1	10	**A**
(Gerber) W/Tapioca, *2nd*								
Foods	4 Oz	85	0	0	20	1	4	**A**
Prune								
(Gerber) W/Tapioca, *2nd*								
Foods	4 Oz	87	0	1	20	2	6	

Baby Food, Juice
Apple

	Serv.	K-Cal.	Fat	Prot.	Carb.	Fib.	Sod.	FAC
(Beech-Nut):								
W/Cherry, *Stage 2*......	1 Oz	15	0	0	4	0	3	**A**
W/Cranberry, *Stage 2*	1 Oz	15	0	0	4	0	3	**A**
W/Grape, *Stage 2*	1 Oz	15	0	0	4	0	4	**A**
(Earth's Best)	1 Oz	14	0	0	3	0	1	
W/Grape	1 Oz	14	0	0	3	0	1	
(Gerber):								
W/Carrot, *3rd Foods*...	1 Oz	13	0	0	3	0	3	**A**

	Serv.	K-Cal.	Fat	Prot.	Carb.	Fib.	Sod.	FAC
W/Cherry, *2nd Foods*.	1 Oz	15	0	0	4	0	2	A
W/Cranberry, *2nd Foods*	1 Oz	15	0.1	0	4	0	2	A
W/Grape, *2nd Foods*..	1 Oz	15	0	0	4	0	2	A
W/Peach, *2nd Foods*..	1 Oz	15	0	0	4	0	1	A
W/Plum, *2nd Foods*....	1 Oz	15	0	0	4	0	2	A
W/Prune, *2nd Foods*..	1 Oz	17	0	0	4	0	1	A
Grape								
(Beech-Nut) *Stage 2*	1 Oz	25	0	0	6	0	3	A
White, *Stage 1*............	1 Oz	20	0	0	5	0	0	A
(Gerber) White, *1st Foods*............	1 Oz	20	0	0	5	0	2	A
Mixed Fruit								
(Beech-Nut) *Stage 2*......	1 Oz	18	0	0	4	0	3	A
Tropical Blend, *Stage 2*....................	1 Oz	23	0	0	5	0	1	A
(Gerber) *2nd Foods*.......	1 Oz	15	0	0	4	0	1	A
Punch, *Graduates*.......	1 Oz	17	0	0	4	0	3	A
Orange								
(Beech-Nut) *Stage 3*......	1 Oz	15	0	0	4	0	0	A
(Gerber) *2nd Foods*.......	1 Oz	15	0.1	0	3	0	1	A
W/Carrot, *3rd Foods*...	1 Oz	13	0	0	3	0	3	A
Pear								
(Beech-Nut) *Stage 1*......	1 Oz	15	0	0	4	0	2	A
(Earth's Best)	1 Oz	13	0	0	3	0	0	A
(Gerber) *1st Foods*	1 Oz	15	0	0	4	0	1	A

Baby Food, Vegetable

	Serv.	K-Cal.	Fat	Prot.	Carb.	Fib.	Sod.	FAC
Beet								
(Gerber) *2nd Foods*.......	4 Oz	45	0.1	1	10	2	43	A
Carrot								
(Beech-Nut)								
Stage 1	4 Oz	50	0	0	9	3	60	A
W/Peas, *Stage 2*........	4 Oz	50	0	2	9	2	25	A
Corn								
(Beech-Nut) Creamed, *Stage 2*	4 Oz	90	0	1	18	2	20	A
(Gerber) Creamed, *2nd Foods*..........................	4 Oz	35	0.6	2	14	1	10	A
Green Bean								
(Beech-Nut) *Stage 1*......	4 Oz	35	0	1	7	2	10	A
(Gerber) Creamed, *3rd Foods*..........................	4 Oz	51	0.2	2	10	NV	10	A
Pea								
(Beech-Nut) *Stage 1*......	4 Oz	60	0	4	10	3	0	A
Spinach								
(Gerber) Creamed, *2nd Foods*..........................	4 Oz	54	0.7	4	8	2	32	A

	Serv.	K-Cal.	Fat	Prot.	Carb.	Fib.	Sod.	FAC
(Baby Food, Vegetable cont.)								
Squash								
(Beech-Nut) Butternut,								
Stage 1	4 Oz	50	0	0	10	1	10	A
Vegetable, Mixed								
(Beech-Nut):								
Stage 2	4 Oz	45	0	1	8	3	20	A
Garden, *Stage 2*	4 Oz	50	0	1	9	3	15	A
(Earth's Best):								
Golden Harvest	4 Oz	122	0.4	2	28	2	7	A
Souffle	4 Oz	71	1.7	3	11	2	11	A
(Gerber):								
2nd Foods	4 Oz	56	0.4	1	10	2	18	A
Garden, *2nd Foods*	4 Oz	44	0.5	2	7	3	18	A
W/Cheese, *3rd*								
Foods	4 Oz	50	1.1	2	8	1	51	A
Vegetable W/Meat								
(Gerber):								
W/Bacon, *2nd Foods*	4 Oz	88	3.7	2	11	2	56	A
W/Beef, *2nd Foods*	4 Oz	78	2.7	3	10	3	16	A
W/Chicken, *2nd Foods*	4 Oz	71	2.0	3	10	3	23	A
Bacon								
(All values for cooked bacon)								
Alternative Meat								
Beef (John Morrel)	1 Slice	50	3.5	4	1	0	320	
Beef (Sizzlean)	1 Slice	35	2.5	3	0	0	240	
Pork, Cured (Sizzlean)	1 Slice	55	4.5	3	1	0	245	
Pork, 80% FF (Louis Rich)	1 Slice	17	1	1	0	0	90	
Turkey (Louis Rich)	1 Slice	30	2.5	2	0	0	190	
Canadian								
(Hormel)	1 Slice	35	1.5	6	0	0	305	
(Light & Lean)	1 Slice	17	0.5	3	0	0	NV	
(Oscar Mayer)	1 Slice	25	0.8	4	0	0	310	
Ham								
(Black Label):								
	1 Slice	40	3.5	3	0	0	165	
LS	1 Slice	40	3.5	3	0	0	105	
(Hormel): Microwave	1 Slice	35	2.5	3	0	0	115	
(Old Smokehouse)	1 Slice	40	3.5	3	0	0	140	
(Oscar Mayer):								
	1 Slice	30	2.5	2	0	0	125	
1/8" Thick	1 Slice	60	5	4	0	0	250	
Reduced Sodium	1 Slice	30	2	2	0	0	85	
(Range Brand)	1 Slice	50	4.5	4	0	0	230	
(Red Label)	1 Slice	40	3.5	3	0	0	115	
Bacon Alternative, Vegetarian								
Patties (Morningstar)	1 Item	68	2.8	8	2	2	264	

	Serv.	K-Cal.	Fat	Prot.	Carb.	Fib.	Sod.	FAC
Strips (Morningstar)........	2 Item	60	4.5	2	2	0	220	
Stripples (Worthington) ..	1 Item	28	2.2	1	1	0	110	
Veggie Bacon (Yves)	2 Oz	76	0	16	3	1	549	

Bacon Bits

	Serv.	K-Cal.	Fat	Prot.	Carb.	Fib.	Sod.	FAC
(Bacos)	1 Tbsp	30	1	3	2	0	130	
(Hormel)...........................	1 Tbsp	30	1.5	3	0	0	250	
(Oscar Mayer)	1 Tbsp	25	1.5	3	0	0	220	

Bagel
Cinnamon Raisin

	Serv.	K-Cal.	Fat	Prot.	Carb.	Fib.	Sod.	FAC
(Thomas).....................	1 Item	160	1	6	36	1	290	
Egg (Lender's).................	1 Item	160	1.5	6	30	1	320	
Egg (Thomas)	1 Item	170	1.5	7	35	2	280	
Multigrain (Thomas)	1 Item	170	1.5	6	35	1	310	
Oat Bran, 4"	1 Item	181	0.9	8	38	3	360	
Onion (Lender's)	1 Item	160	0.5	6	31	1	310	
Onion (Natural Ovens)...	1 Item	230	2	12	57	2	300	F
Onion (Thomas)	1 Item	170	1.5	6	35	2	300	
Plain (Lender's)	1 Item	150	0.5	6	30	1	320	
Plain (Natural Ovens)	1 Item	230	2	12	60	2	300	F
Plain (Thomas)...............	1 Item	160	1	6	35	2	320	
Plain, Toasted	1 Item	195	1.1	7	38	2	379	
Poppy Seed, 4"...............	1 Item	195	1.1	7	38	2	379	
Sesame Seed, 4"...........	1 Item	195	1.1	7	38	2	379	
Whole Grain (Natural Ovens)	1 Item	170	2	9	48	8	210	FC

Baked Beans, Canned (See Beans, Baked, Canned)

Baking Mix
(Ener-G):

	Serv.	K-Cal.	Fat	Prot.	Carb.	Fib.	Sod.	FAC
Basic, Dairy-Free........	1 Cup	396	0.3	10	88	2	1,148	
Corn, Gluten-Free.......	1 Cup	446	1.9	9	99	2	324	C
Oat	1 Cup	376	7.7	10	7	12	276	C
Potato, Gluten-Free	1 Cup	878	0	0	226	0	420	C
Rice, Low Sodium	1 Cup	507	2.0	9	111	3	6	
Rice, Regular..............	1 Cup	528	1.8	9	97	3	283	C
White Rice	1 Cup	659	15.4	5	124	2	833	
(Krusteaz) Basic	1 Cup	540	18	12	81	NV	1380	C

Baking Powder

	Serv.	K-Cal.	Fat	Prot.	Carb.	Fib.	Sod.	FAC
Double-Acting...............	1 Tsp	2	0	0	1	0	488	C
LS	1 Tsp	5	0	0	2	0	5	C
(Calumet)......................	1 Tsp	0	0	0	0	0	400	C

	Serv.	K-Cal.	Fat	Prot.	Carb.	Fib.	Sod.	FAC
Baking Soda								
(Arm & Hammer)............	1 Tsp	0	0	0	0	0	952	
Balsam Pear (See Bitter Melon)								
Bamboo Shoots								
Raw	1 Cup	41	0.5	4	8	3	6	
Raw	1 Oz	8	0	1	2	1	1	
Boiled..............................	1 Cup	14	0.3	2	2	1	5	
Canned, Drained	1 Cup	25	0.5	2	4	2	9	
Canned (La Choy)	1 Tbsp	1	0	0	0	0	0	
Banana								
Raw	1 Cup	216	1.1	2	55	4	2	FA
Raw (4 Oz).....................	1 Item	105	0.6	1	27	3	1	A
Raw, Red (3 Oz)............	1 Item	90	0.2	1	23	1	1	A
Batter-Dipped	1 Item	312	20.9	3	31	2	159	
Banana Chips	2 Oz	294	20	1	33	4	3	A
Banana Flakes	1 Tbsp	22	0.1	0	5	0	0	
Smoked	1 Oz	96	0.1	1	22	0	238	
Banana Nectar								
(Libby's)	1 Cup	132	0	0	32	0	24	A
W/Pineapple (Kern's)	1 Cup	152	0	0	32	0	3	A
Barbecue Sauce								
(Bullseye):								
Original..........................	1 Tbsp	30	0	0	7	0	115	
(Cripple Creek):								
Pork...............................	1 Tbsp	20	1	3	2	0	57	
(Hunt's):								
Dijon	1 Tbsp	19	0.2	0	4	0	200	
Hickory	1 Tbsp	19	0	0	5	1	205	
Hickory/Brown Sugar..	1 Tbsp	37	0.1	0	9	0	191	
Honey Mustard	1 Tbsp	24	0.1	0	6	0	225	
Hot & Spicy	1 Tbsp	24	0.1	0	6	0	225	
LT..................................	1 Tbsp	12	0.1	0	3	0	85	
Mesquite	1 Tbsp	20	0.2	0	5	0	180	
Original, Bold..............	1 Tbsp	23	0.1	0	5	0	158	
Teriyaki	1 Tbsp	23	0.0	0	6	0	176	
(KC Master):								
Original..........................	1 Tbsp	30	0	0	7	0	105	
(Kraft):								
Garlic.............................	1 Tbsp	20	0	0	5	0	210	
Hickory Smoke	1 Tbsp	20	0	0	5	0	220	
Hickory, *Thick N Spicy*	1 Tbsp	25	0	0	6	0	220	
Honey, *Thick N Spicy*	1 Tbsp	30	0	0	7	0	175	
Italian Seasonings	1 Tbsp	23	0.3	0	5	0	140	
Mesquite Smoke..........	1 Tbsp	20	0	0	5	0	205	

	Serv.	K-Cal.	Fat	Prot.	Carb.	Fib.	Sod.	FAC
Onion Bits	1 Tbsp	25	0	0	6	0	170	
Original	1 Tbsp	20	0	0	5	0	230	
Original, *Thick N Spicy*	1 Tbsp	25	0	0	6	0	220	
(Lea & Perrins):								
Original	1 Tbsp	25	0	1	7	0	62	
(Leon's):								
Original	1 Tbsp	23	0	0	5	0	150	
(Open Pit):								
Hickory Flavor	1 Tbsp	25	0	0	6	0	190	
Original	1 Tbsp	25	0	0	6	0	245	
Barley								
(Values for uncooked unless indicated)								
Dry	1 Cup	651	4.2	23	135	32	22	F
Pearled, LT	1 Cup	704	2.3	20	155	31	18	F
Pearled, LT, Cooked	1 Cup	193	0.7	4	44	6	5	
Flakes, Rolled (Arrow head Mills)	1 Cup	330	3	12	84	15	0	
Pearled (Arrowhead Mills)	1 Cup	680	2	20	148	24	0	F
Scotch, Med. Pearled, Reg. (Quaker)	1 Cup	680	4	20	148	20	0	F
Scotch-Pearled, Quick Cook (Quaker)	1 Cup	511	3	15	111	15	0	
Barley Flour								
(Arrowhead Mills)	1 Cup	300	2	12	76	12	0	F
(Ener-G) Waxy, Organic	1 Oz	89	0.3	3	22	4	3	
Barracuda								
Raw	3 Oz	81	1	16	0	0	NV	
Broiled	3 Oz	135	5	20	0	0	300	
Fried, Breaded	3 Oz	168	7.5	20	4	0	255	
Basil								
Fresh, Chopped	1 Tbsp	1	0	0	0	0	0	
Fresh, Chopped	2 Cup	23	.5	2	4	3	4	FA
Dried (McCormick)	1 Tsp	3	0	0	1	0	0	
Bass								
Freshwater, Raw	3 Oz	97	3.1	16	0	0	60	
Sea, Raw	3 Oz	82	1.7	16	0	0	35	
Striped, Raw	3 Oz	83	2.0	15	0	0	59	
Freshwater, Broiled	3 Oz	118	3.8	20	0	0	71	
Sea, Broiled	3 Oz	105	2.2	27	0	0	60	
Striped, Broiled	3 Oz	105	2.5	19	0	0	75	
Bay Leaf								
Crumbled	1 Tsp	2	0.1	0	0	0	0	

	Serv.	K-Cal.	Fat	Prot.	Carb.	Flb.	Sod.	FAC

Bean (Also See Green Bean, Wax Bean)
Adzuki

	Serv.	K-Cal.	Fat	Prot.	Carb.	Flb.	Sod.	FAC
Boiled	1 Cup	294	0.2	17	57	NV	19	F
Dried	1 Cup	648	1.0	39	124	25	10	F
Dried (Arrowhead Mills)	2 Oz	190	1	13	35	14	3	F
Organic, Canned (Eden)	1 Cup	220	0	14	38	10	20	F

Anasazi

	Serv.	K-Cal.	Fat	Prot.	Carb.	Flb.	Sod.	FAC
Dried (Arrowhead Mills)	1 Cup	600	2	40	108	36	0	FA

Black

	Serv.	K-Cal.	Fat	Prot.	Carb.	Flb.	Sod.	FAC
Boiled	1 Cup	227	0.9	15	41	15	2	F
Dried	1 Cup	662	2.8	42	121	30	10	FC
Canned (Progresso)	1 Cup	200	2	14	34	14	800	F
Canned (S & W)	1 Cup	140	0	10	34	12	1,040	F
Canned (Westbrae)	1 Cup	220	0	12	44	6	720	F
Organic, Canned (Eden)	1 Cup	200	0	14	36	12	30	F
Prepared From Mix (Fantastic)	1 Cup	320	3	20	58	14	620	F

Black-Eyed Pea—Cowpea

	Serv.	K-Cal.	Fat	Prot.	Carb.	Flb.	Sod.	FAC
Dried	1 Cup	561	2.1	39	100	18	27	FC
Dried, Boiled	1 Cup	160	0.6	5	34	8	7	F
Fresh Young Pods W/Seeds, Boiled	6 Oz	58	0.5	4	12	NV	5	FA
Frozen, Boiled	1 Cup	224	1.1	14	40	11	9	F
Canned, Sun Vista (S & W)	1 Cup	140	0	12	30	8	1,100	F

Cannellini—White Kidney (Also See Bean, Kidney)

	Serv.	K-Cal.	Fat	Prot.	Carb.	Flb.	Sod.	FAC
Dried	1 Cup	613	1.5	43	110	46	44	FC
Canned (Progresso)	1 Cup	200	1	10	36	10	540	F

Cranberry—Borlotti

	Serv.	K-Cal.	Fat	Prot.	Carb.	Flb.	Sod.	FAC
Boiled	1 Cup	241	0.8	17	43	18	2	F
Canned W/Liquids	1 Cup	216	0.7	14	39	16	863	F
Dried	1 Cup	653	2.4	45	117	48	12	FC

Fava—Broad—Horsebean—Jack

	Serv.	K-Cal.	Fat	Prot.	Carb.	Flb.	Sod.	FAC
Dried	1 Cup	512	2.3	39	88	38	20	F
Boiled	1 Cup	187	0.7	13	33	9	9	F
Canned (Progresso)	1 Cup	220	1	12	40	10	500	F

Garbanzo—Chickpea—Cece

	Serv.	K-Cal.	Fat	Prot.	Carb.	Flb.	Sod.	FAC
Boiled	1 Oz	64	2.6	3	8	2	101	
Dried	1 Cup	728	12.1	39	121	35	48	F
Organic (Eden)	1 Cup	220	3	14	38	10	20	F
(Progresso)	1 Cup	220	3	12	36	40	760	F
(Westbrae)	1 Cup	220	4	12	36	10	280	F

Great Northern

	Serv.	K-Cal.	Fat	Prot.	Carb.	Flb.	Sod.	FAC
Boiled	1 Cup	209	0.8	15	37	12	4	F
Dried	1 Cup	620	2.1	40	114	37	26	FC
Canned (Joan of Arc)	1 Cup	200	1	12	36	12	580	F
Canned, Sun Vista (S & W)	1 Cup	140	0	12	34	12	980	F

	Serv.	K-Cal.	Fat	Prot.	Carb.	Fib.	Sod.	FAC
Canned (Westbrae)........	1 Cup	180	0	12	32	8	280	F
Hyacinth								
Dried.................................	1 Cup	722	3.5	50	128	NV	44	FC
Dried, Boiled....................	1 Cup	227	1.1	16	40	NV	14	
Kidney								
Boiled, California Red....	1 Cup	219	0.2	16	40	17	7	F
Boiled, Red.....................	1 Cup	225	0.9	15	40	13	4	F
Boiled, Royal..................	1 Cup	218	0.3	17	39	17	9	F
Dried, California Red.....	1 Cup	607	0.5	45	110	46	20	FC
Dried, Red.......................	1 Cup	620	2.0	42	113	28	22	FC
Dried, Royal Red	1 Cup	605	0.8	47	107	46	24	FC
Canned (Hunt's).............	1 Cup	189	1.1	13	39	10	968	F
Canned (Luck's).............	1 Cup	190	1	12	32	9	400	F
Canned (Van Camp's) ...	1 Cup	180	0	12	40	12	780	F
Red, Canned (Progresso)	1 Cup	220	1	14	40	16	560	F
Lima—Butter								
Boiled, Baby.....................	1 Cup	229	0.7	15	42	14	5	F
Boiled, Large..................	1 Cup	216	0.7	15	39	13	4	F
Dried, Baby	1 Cup	677	1.9	42	127	42	26	F
Dried, Large	1 Cup	602	1.2	38	113	34	32	F
Baby, Frozen (Green Giant)	1 Cup	160	0	8	30	8	260	F
Canned (Joan of Arc)	1 Cup	180	0	12	32	8	900	F
Canned (S & W).............	1 Cup	140	0	12	36	10	880	F
Frozen (Health Valley) ...	1 Cup	50	2	2	8	14	52	F
W/Butter, Frozen (Green Giant)	1 Cup	180	3.8	9	27	9	495	F
W/Pork, Canned (Luck's)	1 Cup	280	6	12	44	10	640	F
Mung								
Sprouted, Raw	1 Cup	31	0.2	3	6	2	6	FA
Boiled..............................	1 Cup	189	1.0	14	33	12	13	F
Dried................................	1 Cup	718	2.4	49	130	34	31	FC
Sprouted, Boiled.............	1 Cup	26	0.1	3	5	1	12	A
Stir Fried..........................	1 Cup	62	0.3	5	13	2	11	FA
Navy								
Boiled..............................	1 Cup	258	1.0	16	48	12	2	F
Dried................................	1 Cup	697	2.7	46	126	51	29	FC
Organic, Canned (Eden)	1 Cup	220	1	14	40	14	30	F
Pink								
Boiled..............................	1 Cup	252	1	15	47	9	4	F
Dried................................	1 Cup	720	2.4	44	135	27	16	FC
Pinto								
Boiled..............................	1 Cup	234	0.9	14	44	15	3	F
Dried................................	1 Cup	656	2.2	40	122	47	19	FAC
Canned (Gebhardt)	1 Cup	184	2.4	13	35	14	1,010	F
Canned (Joan of Arc)	1 Cup	220	1	12	40	10	560	F
Canned, *Sun Vista* (S & W).......................	1 Cup	160	1	6	24	6	1,060	F

	Serv.	K-Cal.	Fat	Prot.	Carb.	Fib.	Sod.	FAC
(Beans cont.)								
White								
Boiled..............................	1 Cup	250	0.6	17	45	11	11	F
Dried................................	1 Cup	722	2.5	45	134	54	26	FC
Canned (S & W)	1 Cup	160	1	14	38	12	880	F
Winged—Goa								
Boiled..............................	1 Cup	252	10	18	26	NV	22	C
Dried................................	1 Cup	744	30	54	76	NV	70	FC

Beans, Baked, Canned (Also See Chili, Canned)

	Serv.	K-Cal.	Fat	Prot.	Carb.	Fib.	Sod.	FAC
(B & M):								
BBQ ....:	1 Cup	380	2	16	76	18	1360	F
LF................................	1 Cup	340	2	16	61	14	440	F
Original........................	1 Cup	360	4	16	66	14	860	F
(Bearitos): FF	1 Cup	260	0	12	52	6	720	F
(Bush): Original	1 Cup	300	2	14	58	14	1100	F
(Campbell's):								
BBQ	1 Cup	210	4	10	43	NV	900	F
Homestyle....................	1 Cup	220	4	11	48	NV	820	F
Old-Fashioned	1 Cup	200	3	10	43	NV	770	F
(Eden):								
Organic, FF.................	1 Cup	300	0	16	54	14	260	F
(Health Valley):								
Honey Baked, FF	1 Cup	220	0	14	48	14	270	FA
(S & W):								
Brick Oven	1 Cup	320	1	14	64	14	1240	FC
Smokey Ranch	1 Cup	220	5	14	44	12	980	F
(Van Camp's):								
FF................................	1 Cup	266	1	13	57	11	1010	F
Original........................	1 Cup	286	2	14	59	11	1070	F
Southern Style	1 Cup	290	2	13	70	16	1110	F

Bean Mix, Canned

	Serv.	K-Cal.	Fat	Prot.	Carb.	Fib.	Sod.	FAC
3 Bean (Green Giant)	1 Cup	140	1	4	36	6	940	F
3 Bean (Joan of Arc)	1 Cup	180	0	6	40	8	980	F

Beans, Refried, Canned

	Serv.	K-Cal.	Fat	Prot.	Carb.	Fib.	Sod.	FAC
(Bearitos):								
Black, LT.....................	1 Cup	240	4	24	42	2	960	F
FF................................	1 Cup	210	0	12	42	6	1050	F
LF, LS	1 Cup	240	6	15	42	6	30	F
Vegetarian, LF	1 Cup	240	6	15	42	6	960	F
(Fantastic):								
Prepared	1 Cup	320	2	18	58	22	640	F
(Gebhardt):								
....	1 Cup	218	5.5	12	40	12	994	F
FF.................................	1 Cup	183	0.9	15	39	12	960	F

	Serv.	K-Cal.	Fat	Prot.	Carb.	Fib.	Sod.	FAC
Jalapeño	1 Cup	210	6	14	38	13	760	F
Vegetarian	1 Cup	236	4.6	15	42	13	1,100	F
(Old El Paso):								
FF	1 Cup	220	0	12	40	12	960	F
(Rosarita):								
Bacon	1 Cup	232	6.2	17	37	16	978	F
FF	1 Cup	246	0.9	14	55	12	1,148	F
Green Chili	1 Cup	220	5.8	12	39	13	990	F
Nacho	1 Cup	274	6.4	16	48	13	1,406	F
Onion	1 Cup	228	5.5	13	42	12	1,016	F
Original	1 Cup	218	5.5	12	40	12	994	F
Spicy	1 Cup	236	5.3	14	43	12	1,148	F
Vegetarian	1 Cup	242	4.1	15	47	13	1,124	F
W/Green Chili, FF	1 Cup	202	0.2	15	44	15	1,130	F

Bearnaise Sauce

	Serv.	K-Cal.	Fat	Prot.	Carb.	Fib.	Sod.	FAC
Prepared (Knorr)	1 Tsp	10	0	0	2	0	100	

Beechnut

	Serv.	K-Cal.	Fat	Prot.	Carb.	Fib.	Sod.	FAC
Dried	1 Oz	164	14.2	2	10	3	11	

Beef
(Beef is choice grade)
(Trimmed = All separable fat removed after cooking)
(Untrimmed = No fat removed after cooking)

	Serv.	K-Cal.	Fat	Prot.	Carb.	Fib.	Sod.	FAC
Brain								
Raw	3 Oz	106	7.8	8	0	0	88	
Cooked, Simmered	3 Oz	136	10.7	9	0	0	102	
Brisket, Whole								
0" Fat, Braised, Trimmed	3 Oz	185	8.6	25	0	0	60	
¼" Fat, Braised, Untrimmed	3 Oz	327	26.8	20	0	0	52	
Chuck Arm								
¼" Fat, Braised, Trimmed	3 Oz	191	7.9	28	0	0	56	
¼" Fat, Braised, Untrimmed	3 Oz	296	21.9	23	0	0	50	
Chuck Blade								
¼" Fat, Braised, Trimmed	3 Oz	224	12.2	26	0	0	60	
¼" Fat, Braised, Untrimmed	3 Oz	309	23.6	22	0	0	54	
Flank								
¼" Fat, Braised, Trimmed	3 Oz	201	11.1	24	0	0	61	
¼" Fat, Braised, Untrimmed	3 Oz	224	14	23	0	0	60	
Liver								
Raw	3 Oz	121	3.3	17	5	0	62	FA
Braised	3 Oz	137	4.2	21	3	0	60	FA

	Serv.	K-Cal.	Fat	Prot.	Carb.	Fib.	Sod.	FAC
(Beef cont.)								
Rib, Large								
¼" Fat, Roasted, Trimmed	3 Oz	212	12.5	23	0	0	62	
¼" Fat, Roasted, Untrimmed	3 Oz	326	27.2	19	0	0	54	
Rib, Small End								
¼" Fat, Roasted, Trimmed	3 Oz	197	11.1	23	0	0	60	
¼" Fat, Roasted, Untrimmed	3 Oz	312	25.7	19	0	0	53	
Round								
¼" Fat, Braised, Trimmed	3 Oz	187	8.0	27	0	0	43	
¼" Fat, Braised, Untrimmed	3 Oz	241	15.2	24	0	0	43	
Round Eye								
¼" Fat, Roasted, Trimmed	3 Oz	149	4.8	25	0	0	53	
¼" Fat, Roasted, Untrimmed	3 Oz	205	12	23	0	0	50	
Round Full								
¼" Fat, Broiled, Trimmed	3 Oz	162	6.2	25	0	0	54	
¼" Fat, Braised, Untrimmed	3 Oz	204	11.6	23	0	0	52	
Round Tip								
¼" Fat, Roasted, Trimmed	3 Oz	160	6.2	24	0	0	55	
¼" Fat, Roasted, Untrimmed	3 Oz	210	12.6	23	0	0	53	
Shank								
¼" Fat, Simmered, Trimmed	3 Oz	171	5.4	29	0	0	54	
¼" Fat, Simmered, Untrimmed	3 Oz	224	12.5	26	0	0	52	
T-Bone								
¼" Fat, Broiled, Trimmed	3 Oz	174	8.5	23	0	0	60	
¼" Fat, Broiled, Untrimmed	3 Oz	263	19.8	20	0	0	54	
Tenderloin								
¼" Fat, Roasted, Trimmed	3 Oz	196	10.6	24	0	0	61	
¼" Fat, Roasted, Untrimmed	3 Oz	288	22.4	20	0	0	55	
Top Loin								
¼" Fat, Broiled, Trimmed	3 Oz	182	8.6	24	0	0	58	
¼" Fat, Broiled,								

	Serv.	K-Cal.	Fat	Prot.	Carb.	Fib.	Sod.	FAC
Untrimmed	3 Oz	253	17.8	22	0	0	54	
Top Sirloin								
¼" Fat, Broiled,								
Trimmed......................	3 Oz	172	6.8	26	0	0	56	
¼" Fat, Broiled,								
Untrimmed	3 Oz	229	14.2	24	0	0	53	
Tongue								
Raw	3 Oz	189	14	13	3	0	60	
Cooked, Simmered	3 Oz	241	17.6	19	0	0	51	

Beef, Corned, Brisket

	Serv.	K-Cal.	Fat	Prot.	Carb.	Fib.	Sod.	FAC
Raw	3 Oz	170	12.7	13	0	0	104	
Cured, Raw	1 Oz	56	4.2	4	0	0	35	
Cooked	3 Oz	213	16.1	15	0	0	964	
Cured, Cooked	1 Oz	71	5.4	5	0	0	321	
(Healthy Choice)	1 Oz	30	0.8	5	0	0	230	
(Hillshire Farm)...............	1 Oz	31	0.2	3	0	0	115	
(Hormel).........................	1 Oz	60	3.5	7	0	0	245	
(Oscar Mayer)	1 Oz	50	4	5	0	0	360	
(Shenson).......................	3 Oz	135	10.5	12	0	0	1,020	

Beef, Corned Hash (See Hash)

Beef Entree, Canned

	Serv.	K-Cal.	Fat	Prot.	Carb.	Fib.	Sod.	FAC
(Chef Boyardee):								
Beefaroni	1 Cup	260	7	10	37	5	870	
Beef-0-Getti.................	1 Cup	250	7	8	37	4	990	
(Dinty Moore): Stew	1 Cup	230	14	11	16	2	950	A
(Hormel):								
Goulash........................	1 Cup	230	11	13	19	3	1,040	
Stew	1 Cup	190	10	11	15	2	990	
(La Choy):								
Chow Mein..................	1 Cup	105	1.7	9	15	3	756	
Pepper Oriental	1 Cup	104	2.7	11	11	3	1,065	
(Libby's):								
Roast Beef W/Gravy ..	1 Cup	210	4.5	39	3	0	1,201	
Stew	1 Cup	290	20	12	19	5	850	A

Beef Entree, Dinner, Frozen
(Serving size given in ounces to reflect weight of 1 serving)

	Serv.	K-Cal.	Fat	Prot.	Carb.	Fib.	Sod.	FAC
Barbecue								
(Healthy Choice)								
Mesquite	11 Oz	310	4	23	45	6	490	
Ribs W/BBQ Sauce ..	11 Oz	330	6	28	40	NV	530	
Meatloaf								
(Healthy Choice)								
Traditional	12 Oz	320	8	16	46	7	460	A

	Serv.	K-Cal.	Fat	Prot.	Carb.	Fib.	Sod.	FAC
(Beef Entree, Dinner, Frozen cont.)								
(Stouffer's):								
W/Macaroni & Cheese								
Lean Cuisine, ...	9.5 Oz	270	10	10	24	4	530	A
W/Whipped Potatoes								
Lean Cuisine, ...	9.5 Oz	250	7	22	25	5	570	
(Swanson) Dinner	11.2 Oz	380	16	16	44	5	1,160	A
Oriental								
(Banquet)........................	9 Oz	200	3	11	32	4	930	
(Healthy Choice):								
Beijing	12 Oz	300	4.5	21	45	6	420	A
W/Peppers Cantonese	11.5 Oz	270	5	16	40	5	560	
(Budget Gourmet Light) .	10 Oz	270	8	16	35	3	1,070	A
(Stouffer's):								
Chop Suey W/Rice.....	12 Oz	300	9	16	38	5	1,170	FA
Lean Cuisine..............	9 Oz	250	8	14	30	4	480	
Szechwan W/Noodles								
Lean Cuisine	9.2 Oz	260	10	20	22	NV	680	A
Pot Pie								
(Stouffer's)	10 Oz	450	26	19	36	3	1,140	A
(Swanson)	7 Oz	400	23	10	39	3	830	A
(Swanson) *Hungry Man*.	14 Oz	710	38	22	71	6	1,440	A
Pot Roast								
(Le Menu) Yankee								
Dinner	10 Oz	330	13	26	27	NV	700	A
(Light & Healthy) *Budget*	10.5 Oz	210	8	23	19	7	440	A
(Right Course)								
Homestyle....................	9.2 Oz	220	7	17	22	NV	550	A
(Stouffer's) *Homestyle,*								
W/Potato	9 Oz	270	10	19	25	4	640	
Steak								
(Banquet) Salisbury........	9.5 Oz	340	19	15	28	4	1,040	
(Budget Gourmet):								
Pepper W/Rice	10 Oz	290	8	18	38	4	1,060	
Sirloin Tip W/Country								
Veg...........................	10 Oz	250	13	14	20	4	1,060	A
(Budget Gourmet Light):								
Sirloin Herb.................	9.5 Oz	260	7	19	30	5	850	F
Sirloin Salisbury..........	11 Oz	260	9	21	28	6	510	A
(Healthy Choice):								
Pepper Steak Oriental	9.5 Oz	250	4	19	34	3	470	
Salisbury, Traditional ..	11.5 Oz	320	6	18	48	7	470	A
Sirloin W/BBQ								
Sauce	11 Oz	280	4	17	44	NV	240	
(Le Menu):								
Pepper	11.5 Oz	370	13	26	36	NV	1,020	A
Salisbury Dinner	10.5 Oz	370	20	20	28	NV	880	A
Sirloin, Chopped.........	12.2 Oz	430	24	25	28	NV	1,010	
Sirloin Tips, Dinner.....	11.5 Oz	400	18	30	29	NV	760	A

	Serv.		K-Cal.	Fat	Prot.	Carb.	Fib.	Sod.	FAC
(Le Menu, Lightstyle):									
Salisbury Dinner	10	Oz	280	9	18	31	NV	400	
(Light & Healthy):									
Sirloin Salisbury	11	Oz	260	9	21	28	6	510	**A**
Sirloin W/Wine Sauce	11	Oz	230	6	17	33	6	570	**FA**
(Stouffer's):									
Green Pepper	10.5	Oz	330	9	17	45	3	650	**A**
Lean Cuisine...............	9.2	Oz	270	9	16	30	NV	950	
(Swanson):									
Salisbury Dinner, *Hungry Man*	17	Oz	590	32	30	45	11	1,610	
Salisbury Entree	10	Oz	310	17	17	23	2	1,070	
Sirloin, Chopped W/Gravy	10.7	Oz	310	9	23	34	5	840	**A**
(Ultra Slim-Fast) Pepper Steak W/Rice	12	Oz	310	5	23	43	2	530	
Stroganoff									
(Budget Gourmet Light) .	8.7	Oz	290	7	20	32	3	580	**A**
(Le Menu) Dinner...........	10	Oz	430	24	26	28	NV	980	
(Stouffer's) W/Noodles ...	9.7	Oz	390	20	23	30	2	1,100	
Swedish Meatballs									
(Healthy Choice)	11	Oz	320	9	22	37	5	600	**A**
(Le Menu Lightstyle)	8	Oz	260	8	18	30	NV	700	
(Stouffer's).......................	9.2	Oz	440	23	23	36	3	840	
(Wt Watchers)	9	Oz	280	8	18	34	3	510	
Teriyaki									
(Light and Elegant)	8	Oz	240	3	18	37	NV	625	
(Stouffer's) W/Rice/ Vegetables	9.7	Oz	290	8	22	33	1	1,450	**A**

Beef Entree, Vegetarian Alternative

(Serving size given in ounces to reflect weight of 1 serving)

	Serv.		K-Cal.	Fat	Prot.	Carb.	Fib.	Sod.	FAC
Roast Beef, *Meat of Wheat* (Ivy Foods)......	3.5	Oz	205	6	38	12	5	380	
Canned									
(Loma Linda) Stake, Swiss W/Gravy	3.2	Oz	120	5.6	9	8	4	433	
(Worthington):									
Cutlet, Multigrain.........	1.6	Oz	49	0.9	8	3	2	192	
Cutlets	2	Oz	66	1.1	11	3	2	340	
Stake, Prime.................	3.2	Oz	136	9.3	9	4	4	445	
Frozen									
(Amy's Kitchen) Salisbury, Vegetarian	11	Oz	480	19	12	48	4	760	
(Loma Linda):									
Griddle	2	Oz	129	7	13	4	4	410	
Sizzle Burger	2.5	Oz	200	12	13	10	6	538	
(Worthington):									
Beef Style	2	Oz	113	6.8	9	4	3	624	

	Serv.	K-Cal.	Fat	Prot.	Carb.	Fib.	Sod.	FAC
(Beef Entree, Vegetarian Alternative cont.)								
Stakelets	2.5 Oz	144	8	12	6	2	484	

Beef, Ground
Extra Lean, Raw	3 Oz	198	14.5	16	0	0	57	
Lean, Raw	3 Oz	225	17.7	15	0	0	60	
Medium, Raw	3 Oz	225	17.6	15	0	0	60	
Regular, Raw	3 Oz	264	22.6	14	0	0	60	
Extra Lean, Broiled, Well	3 Oz	225	13.4	24	0	0	70	
Lean, Broiled, Well	3 Oz	238	15	24	0	0	76	
Medium, Broiled	3 Oz	231	15.7	21	0	0	66	
Regular, Broiled, Well	3 Oz	248	16.5	23	0	0	79	

Beef Jerky (See Jerky)

Beef, Roast, Luncheon Meat
(Columbus)	2 Oz	80	3	12	0	0	270	
(Healthy Choice)	2 Slices	50	1	8	0	0	360	
(Hormel)	2 Oz	70	3	10	0	0	630	

Beef Stew (See Beef Entree, Canned)

Beef Tallow
	1 Tbsp	116	13	0	0	0	0	

Beet
Fresh
Raw	1 Cup	60	0.2	2	13	4	106	FA
Boiled	1 Cup	77	0.1	3	17	5	121	FA
Canned								
Julienne (S & W)	1 Cup	60	0	2	14	2	460	F
Pickled (Del Monte)	1 Cup	160	0	2	38	4	760	F
Sliced (S & W)	1 Cup	60	0	2	14	2	460	F
Sliced, LS (Green Giant)	1 Cup	70	0	2	16	4	120	F
Whole (Del Monte)	1 Cup	70	0	2	16	4	580	F

Beet Greens
Raw	1 Lb	49	0.2	5	10	3	510	A
Boiled	1 Cup	39	0.3	4	8	4	347	A
Boiled	2 Cups	78	0.6	7	16	8	694	FAC

Berry Juice
(Hawaiian Punch) Very Berry	1 Cup	120	0	0	29	0	45	
(Libby's) Berry	1 Cup	130	0	1	31	0	15	
(Odwalla) Fruitshake, Blackberry	1 Cup	160	0	1	39	3	50	A
(R. W. Knudsen) Blue Nectar	1 Cup	130	0	0	33	NV	35	

	Serv.	K-Cal.	Fat	Prot.	Carb.	Fib.	Sod.	FAC
(Santa Cruz Orchards)								
Berry Nectar, Organic	1 Cup	90	0	0	22	NV	NV	
(Tropicana) Berries &								
Berries..................	1 Cup	125	0	0	18	0	16	

Betel Leaves
Fresh	1 Oz	17	0	2	2	NV	2	**A**

Beverages (See individual listings)

Biscuit, Mix
Dry Mix
(Arrowhead Mills)	¼ Cup	120	1	5	23	3	200	
(Bisquick):......................	⅓ Cup	170	6	3	25	<1	490	
RF	⅓ Cup	150	2.5	3	27	<1	460	
(Jiffy):								
....	¼ Cup	130	4.5	2	22	1	320	
Banana Nut................	¼ Cup	160	5	2	25	2	300	
Blueberry.....................	¼ Cup	160	5	2	28	1	270	
Buttermilk	⅓ Cup	160	4	3	29	1	380	
Corn	¼ Cup	160	4	2	28	1	320	

Prepared From Mix
(Bob's Red Mill)								
Buttermilk	1 Item	103	4	2	13	0	172	
Wheat-Free	1 Item	180	9	4	22	1	550	
(General Mills) Gold								
Medal	2 Items	180	7	4	27	<1	490	
(Krusteaz)	2 Items	180	6	4	27	NV	460	

Biscuit, Refrigerated, Prepared
(1869):								
Baking Powder	1 Item	100	5	2	12	0	300	
Butter Tastin	1 Item	100	5	2	12	0	300	
(Ballard):								
Buttermilk, ...	1 Item	50	0.7	1	10	0	163	
Oven-Ready,...............	1 Item	50	0.7	1	10	0	163	
(Hungry Jack):								
Butter	1 Item	85	3.5	2	12	0	290	
Buttermilk	1 Item	85	3.5	2	12	0	300	
Buttermilk, Extra	1 Item	50	1	1	9	0	180	
Fluffy	1 Item	90	4	2	12	0	285	
(Pillsbury):								
Big Country.................	1 Item	100	4	2	13	0	300	
Buttermilk, *Big*								
Country.....................	1 Item	100	4	2	14	0	300	
Buttermilk, *Heat 'N Eat*	1 Item	85	2.5	2	14	NV	265	
Good 'N Buttery, Fluffy	1 Item	90	5	1	11	0	270	

	Serv.	K-Cal.	Fat	Prot.	Carb.	Fib.	Sod.	FAC
(Biscuit, Refrigerated, Prepared cont.)								
Heat 'N Eat, Big								
Premium.....................	1 Item	140	7.5	3	16	3	305	
(Roman Meal) Honey								
Nut/Oat Bran..............	1 Item	130	5	2	20	1	280	

Bitter Melon—Balsam Pear

Cooked	1 Cup	23	0.2	1	5	2	294	FA
Leafy Tips, Boiled	1 Cup	20	0.1	2	4	1	8	FA
Pods, Boiled	1 Cup	24	0.2	1	5	2	7	FA

Black Bean (See Bean, Black)

Blackberry

Raw (5 Oz)....................	1 Cup	75	0.6	1	18	8	46	FA
Frozen, Unsweetened	1 Cup	97	0.7	2	24	8	2	FA
Canned, LT Syrup,								
(Oregon).....................	1 Cup	260	0	2	58	12	20	FA

Blackberry Syrup

(Knott's Berry Farm)	1 Oz	120	0	0	30	0	0	

Black-Eyed Pea—Cowpea (See Bean, Black-Eyed Pea)

Blintz

Cheese-filled..................	1 Item	138	6.1	7	14	0	295	
Fruit Filling....................	1 Item	124	4.5	4	17	0	151	
(Empire):								
Apple............................	1 Item	110	0.8	3	18	3	130	
Blueberry......................	1 Item	80	2	2	18	1	130	
Cheese.........................	1 Item	100	3	6	15	2	15	
Cherry	1 Item	100	2	3	19	2	140	
Potato..........................	1 Item	95	3	3	16	2	265	

Blueberry
Fresh

Raw (5 Oz)....................	1 Cup	81	0.6	1	21	4	9	A
Raw	1 Oz	14	0.1	0	3	1	0	
Canned W/								
Heavy Syrup (S & W)....	1 Cup	210	0	0	48	18	0	
LT Syrup (Oregon).........	1 Cup	220	0	1	54	4	10	
Frozen								
Unsweetened..................	1 Cup	70	0	1	16	4	10	
Sweetened.....................	1 Cup	186	0.3	1	51	5	2	
(Cascadian Farms).........	1 Cup	90	.5	1	22	2	10	A
Topping (Flav R Pac)	1 Tbsp	20	0	0	5	1	3	

Blueberry Syrup

(Knott's Berry Farm)	1 Oz	120	0	0	30	0	0	

	Serv.	K-Cal.	Fat	Prot.	Carb.	Fib.	Sod.	FAC
(Knott's Berry Farm)								
LT	1 Oz	50	0	0	12	0	0	
(R.W. Knudsen)	1 Oz	75	0	0	19	0	NV	
(S & W) 70% Calorie-								
Reduced	1 Oz	28	0	0	7	0	50	
Bluefish								
Raw	3 Oz	105	3.6	17	0	0	51	
Broiled	3 Oz	135	4.6	22	0	0	65	

Bockwurst (See Sausage, Bratwurst)

Bok Choy—Chinese White Cabbage—Pak Choi

	Serv.	K-Cal.	Fat	Prot.	Carb.	Fib.	Sod.	FAC
Raw	1 Oz	5	0.1	1	0	0	5	
Raw	1 Cup	10	0.2	2	2	1	46	
Raw	1 Lb	52	0.8	6	9	4	257	A
Boiled	1 Cup	20	0.2	3	3	3	60	A

Bologna
(Average slice weighs approximately 1 Oz)
Beef

	Serv.	K-Cal.	Fat	Prot.	Carb.	Fib.	Sod.	FAC
(Healthy Choice)	1 Oz	35	1	4	3	0	240	
(Oscar Mayer)	1 Oz	90	8	3	1	0	300	
LT	1 Oz	60	4	3	2	0	310	
Chicken								
(Foster Farms)	1 Oz	60	5	4	0	0	200	
(Tyson)	1 Oz	70	5.5	4	1	0	330	
Mixed Meats								
(Healthy Choice)	1 Oz	30	1	4	2	0	240	
(Hillshire Farm)								
Specialty	1 Oz	90	8	3	1	0	260	
(Oscar Mayer):								
	1 Oz	90	8	3	1	0	270	
FF	1 Oz	20	0	4	2	0	280	
LT	1 Oz	60	4	3	2	0	310	
Wisconsin Ring	1 Oz	90	8	3	1	0	230	
(Smok-A-Roma)	1.6 Oz	150	14	4	2	0	520	
Turkey								
(Louis Rich)	1 Oz	50	4	3	1	0	270	
(Mr. Turkey)	1 Oz	67	5.6	3	1	0	377	

Bologna, Alternative
(Light Life) Foney

	Serv.	K-Cal.	Fat	Prot.	Carb.	Fib.	Sod.	FAC
Baloney	3 Slices	60	2.5	8	2	0	240	
(Worthington) Bolono	3 Slices	80	3.5	10	2	2	720	

Borage

	Serv.	K-Cal.	Fat	Prot.	Carb.	Fib.	Sod.	FAC
Raw	1 Cup	18	0.6	2	3	1	70	A

	Serv.	K-Cal.	Fat	Prot.	Carb.	Fib.	Sod.	FAC

Borecole (See Kale)

Borlotti (See Bean, Cranberry)

Bouillon (See Soup, Bouillon)

Bourbon (See Alcoholic Beverage, Liqueur)

Boysenberry

	Serv.	K-Cal.	Fat	Prot.	Carb.	Fib.	Sod.	FAC
Canned, Heavy Syrup....	1 Cup	225	0.3	3	57	7	8	FA
Frozen, Unsweetened....	1 Cup	66	0.3	1	16	5	1	F

Boysenberry Juice
(R.W. Knudsen):

	Serv.	K-Cal.	Fat	Prot.	Carb.	Fib.	Sod.	FAC
Nectar	1 Cup	130	0	0	33	NV	35	
Spritzer.......................	1 Cup	107	0	0	28	0	17	
W/Apple	1 Cup	120	0	0	30	0	25	

Boysenberry Syrup

	Serv.	K-Cal.	Fat	Prot.	Carb.	Fib.	Sod.	FAC
(Knott's Berry Farm)	1 Oz	120	0	0	30	0	0	
(Knott's Berry Farm) LT.	1 Oz	50	0	0	12	0	0	

Bran (See individual listings)

Brandy (See Alcoholic Beverage, Liqueur)

Bratwurst (See Sausage, Bratwurst)

Braunschweiger (See Liverwurst)

Brazil Nut—Butternut

	Serv.	K-Cal.	Fat	Prot.	Carb.	Fib.	Sod.	FAC
Dried...............................	1 Oz	174	16.2	7	3	1	0	
Dried, Shelled (5 Oz).....	1 Cup	918	92.7	20	18	8	3	AC

Bread
(Also See Bagel; Biscuit; Bun; Cornbread; Muffin, Ready-to-Serve; Muffin, Mix; Pastry; Roll)

Apple

	Serv.	K-Cal.	Fat	Prot.	Carb.	Fib.	Sod.	FAC
(Arnold) W/Walnut..........	1 Slice	64	1.3	2	13	1	103	
(Elfin) W/Cinnamon........	1 Slice	180	4.5	3	31	1	260	

Bran

	Serv.	K-Cal.	Fat	Prot.	Carb.	Fib.	Sod.	FAC
(Arnold) *Bran'nola*	1 Slice	85	1.4	4	18	3	137	
(Oroweat) *Bran'nola*	1 Slice	100	1	4	19	2	160	
(Wonder) LT, W/Honey..	1 Slice	40	0.3	3	9	3	95	

Brown Bread

	Serv.	K-Cal.	Fat	Prot.	Carb.	Fib.	Sod.	FAC
(S & W) (3 Oz)	1 Slice	180	2	6	42	4	440	

Egg

	Serv.	K-Cal.	Fat	Prot.	Carb.	Fib.	Sod.	FAC
Challah	1 Slice	115	2.4	4	19	1	197	

French

	Serv.	K-Cal.	Fat	Prot.	Carb.	Fib.	Sod.	FAC
(Bread Du Jour)	2 Oz	130	1	6	26	1	300	

	Serv.	K-Cal.	Fat	Prot.	Carb.	Fib.	Sod.	FAC
(Colombo):								
Extra Sour	2 Oz	150	1.3	8	27	NV	311	
Sweet	2 Oz	140	1.5	4	27	1	320	
(Dicarlo) Parisian	1 Slice	75	1	3	14	1	160	
(Pepperidge Farm)								
Enriched	1 Slice	130	1.5	4	25	1	280	
(Pillsbury)	1 Loaf	750	5	30	140	3	1,850	F
(Wonder)	1 Slice	80	1.5	3	15	<1	160	
Health								
(Natural Ovens)	1 Slice	80	0.5	5	19	2	70	F
High Calcium								
(Wonder)								
Wheat, LT	1 Slice	40	0.3	3	9	3	120	C
White, LT	1 Slice	40	0.5	3	9	3	130	C
Italian								
(Arnold) *Francisco*								
International	1 Slice	66	0.8	2	14	1	111	
(Pepperidge Farm)								
Brown & Serve	1 Slice	130	2	4	24	1	260	
(Wonder)	1 Slice	70	1	2	13	1	160	
Oat								
(Kilpatrick) *Family*								
Recipe	1 Slice	70	1	3	13	0	140	
(Oroweat) LT	1 Slice	40	0	2	10	2	135	
(Pepperidge Farm)								
Hearty Crunchy	1 Slice	100	2	4	17	2	180	
Oat Bran								
(Awrey)	1 Slice	50	0	2	10	1	130	
(Elfin)	1 Slice	170	6	4	30	5	160	F
(Monterey Baking Co.)	1 Slice	100	1.5	3	18	3	160	
(Roman Meal) W/Honey	1 Slice	71	1.2	3	13	1	130	
(Wt Watchers)	1 Slice	40	1	1	10	NV	100	
Oatmeal								
(Oatmeal Goodness):								
W/Bran	1 Slice	90	2	4	15	1	140	
W/Cinnamon	1 Slice	90	2	4	15	1	140	
(Pepperidge Farm):								
	1 Slice	90	1	3	17	1	200	
Crunchy	1 Slice	95	2	4	17	2	170	
LT	1 Slice	45	0	2	9	1	95	
(Pillsbury) *Hearty Grain*	1 Slice	90	2	2	16	1	210	
(Wonder) LT	1 Slice	45	0.5	3	9	2	115	
Pita								
(Thomas):								
Sahara, Oat Bran	1 Item	130	1	6	30	3	300	
Sahara, White	1 Item	150	1	6	31	1	290	
Sahara, WW	1 Item	130	1	7	28	5	310	
(Western Sierra):								
Onion	1 Item	140	0.5	5	29	5	195	

	Serv.	K-Cal.	Fat	Prot.	Carb.	Fib.	Sod.	FAC
(Bread cont.)								
White	1 Item	140	0.5	4	30	1	195	
WW	1 Item	140	0.5	5	29	5	195	
Protein								
Gluten	1 Slice	47	0.4	2	8	1	104	
Pumpernickel								
(Arnold)	1 Slice	70	1	3	15	1	198	
(Beefsteak)	1 Slice	70	1	3	13	1	180	
(Pepperidge Farm):								
Family	1 Slice	80	1	3	15	2	230	
Seedless	1 Slice	80	1	3	16	2	210	
Raisin								
(Arnold) W/Cinnamon	1 Slice	67	1.4	2	13	1	86	
(Brownberry) W/Walnut	1 Slice	68	1	1	16	NV	90	
(Ener-G) Egg & Gluten-Free	1 Slice	116	2.7	1	20	1	139	
(Pepperidge Farm) W/ Cinnamon	1 Slice	90	2	2	16	1	100	
(Sun-Maid) W/Cinnamon	1 Slice	80	1.5	3	14	1	110	
Rice Bran								
(Roman Meal)	1 Slice	71	1.6	3	13	1	127	
Rye								
(Beefsteak) Hearty	1 Slice	70	1	3	13	1	170	
(Earth Grains) LT	1 Slice	70	1	3	14	NV	230	
(Levy's) Jewish, Seeded	1 Slice	76	0.9	3	16	1	181	
(Natural Ovens)	1 Slice	65	0.5	4	17	1	70	F
(Pepperidge Farm):								
Dijon	1 Slice	50	1	2	9	1	170	
Seedless	1 Slice	80	1	3	16	2	210	
(Ryemeal)	1 Slice	73	0.5	3	14	15	113	
(Wt Watchers)	1 Slice	40	<1	2	10	NV	100	
Sourdough								
(Earth Grains) LT	1 Slice	40	1	2	9	NV	115	
(Sara Lee):								
Garlic	⅙ Loaf	170	6	5	24	1	290	
Garlic, RF	⅙ Loaf	150	3	5	24	1	290	
(Wonder)	1 Slice	90	1.5	3	17	<1	180	
Wheat								
(Beefsteak) Soft	1 Slice	70	1	5	13	<1	150	
(Brownberry)	1 Slice	80	1.3	3	17	2	183	
(Earth Grains) Cracked	1 Slice	70	1	2	12	NV	180	
(Homepride):								
	1 Slice	70	1	3	13	1	160	
LT	1 Slice	37	0.5	2	8	2	100	
W/Honey	1 Slice	70	1	3	13	1	150	
(Natural Ovens) 7-Grain	1 Slice	70	0.5	4	15	2	70	F
(Pepperidge Farm) Cracked	1 Slice	70	1	2	13	1	140	
(Pillsbury) *Pipin Hot* Loaf	1 Slice	70	2	2	12	1	170	

	Serv.	K-Cal.	Fat	Prot.	Carb.	Flb.	Sod.	FAC
(Wt Watchers)	1 Slice	40	<1	2	14	1	120	
(Wonder) Cracked..........	1 Slice	70	1	3	13	1	180	
White								
(Arnold):								
Brick Oven..................	1 Slice	61	1.2	2	11	1	134	
High Fiber....................	1 Slice	55	1	2	12	2	95	
(Beefsteak) Robust	1 Slice	70	1	3	13	<1	140	
(Brownberry) Natural......	1 Slice	59	1.1	2	11	1	136	
(Earth Grains) Thin	1 Slice	80	1	2	14	NV	160	
(Homepride):								
....	1 Slice	70	1	2	13	0	160	
LT..............................	1 Slice	37	0.5	2	8	2	105	
(Pepperidge Farm)								
Hearty Country	1 Slice	95	1	4	19	1	170	
(Wt Watchers)	1 Slice	40	<1	2	10	NV	100	
(Wonder):								
....	1 Slice	70	1	3	13	1	140	
High Fiber...................	1 Slice	40	0	2	6	3	80	
Whole Wheat								
(Arnold) Stoneground.....	1 Slice	48	1	2	10	2	97	
(Earth Grains)................	1 Slice	70	1	3	11	NV	150	
(Homepride)...................	1 Slice	90	1.5	5	18	3	250	
(Natural Ovens) 100%								
Whole Grain...............	1 Slice	70	0.5	5	17	3	70	F
(Pepperidge Farm) Thin.	1 Slice	60	1	2	12	2	110	
(Wonder) *Family*.............	1Slice	70	1	3	13	1	140	
Bread, Machine Mix								
(Fleischmann's):								
Italian Herb	⅛ Loaf	150	2	5	28	1	220	
Sourdough	⅛ Loaf	150	0.5	5	30	1	240	
(Krusteaz):								
Cinnamon Raisin	1/12 Loaf	180	2.5	5	35	2	250	
Cracked Wheat...........	1/10 Loaf	150	2	5	28	5	270	
Dill Rye	1/10 Loaf	150	2	5	29	2	170	
Homestyle	1/10 Loaf	150	2	0	28	1	280	
Honey Wheat Berry....	1/10 Loaf	150	2	4	28	1	260	
Italian Herb	1/10 Loaf	150	2	5	28	1	250	
Sourdough	1/10 Loaf	150	2	5	28	1	280	
(Pillsbury):								
Cracked Wheat...........	1/12 Loaf	130	2	4	25	2	260	
Crusty White	1/12 Loaf	130	2	4	25	<1	250	
Bread, Quick Mix								
(Dromedary) Ginger	1/12 Loaf	130	2	2	26	2	210	
(Pillsbury):								
Apple/Cinnamon	1/12 Loaf	141	1.5	2	30	1	171	
Banana.......................	1/12 Loaf	120	1.5	2	26	1	191	
Blueberry....................	1/12 Loaf	141	1.5	2	30	1	161	

	Serv.	K-Cal.	Fat	Prot.	Carb.	Fib.	Sod.	FAC
(Bread, Quick Mix, cont.)								
Cranberry	¹⁄₁₂ Loaf	141	1.5	2	30	1	151	
Date	¹⁄₁₂ Loaf	151	1.5	2	32	1	151	
Nut	¹⁄₁₂ Loaf	151	3.5	3	27	1	181	
Oatmeal/Raisin	¹⁄₁₂ Loaf	140	2	3	30	0	170	

Bread Crumbs

	Serv.	K-Cal.	Fat	Prot.	Carb.	Fib.	Sod.	FAC
(Contadina)	1 Cup	300	4.5	9	57	3	2,102	
(Progresso):								
	1 Cup	440	6	16	76	16	840	
Italian	1 Cup	440	8	16	80	16	1,720	
Tomato Basil	1 Cup	480	6	16	28	32	3,000	C

Breadfruit

	Serv.	K-Cal.	Fat	Prot.	Carb.	Fib.	Sod.	FAC
Raw	3 Oz	88	0.2	1	23	4	2	C

Breadfruit Seeds

	Serv.	K-Cal.	Fat	Prot.	Carb.	Fib.	Sod.	FAC
Roasted	1 Oz	59	0.8	2	11	NV	8	

Breadsticks

	Serv.	K-Cal.	Fat	Prot.	Carb.	Fib.	Sod.	FAC
Plain	1 Item	25	0.6	1	4	0	39	
Vienna Type	1 Item	106	1.1	3	20	1	548	
(Barbara's):								
WW, Italian	1 Item	15	0.4	1	2	NV	21	
WW, Plain	1 Item	15	0.4	1	2	NV	21	
(Bread Du Jour):								
Italian	1 Item	130	1	5	25	1	280	
Sourdough	1 Item	130	1	5	25	1	280	
(Keebler):								
Garlic	1 Item	15	0.3	0	3	0	30	
Onion	1 Item	15	0.5	0	3	0	30	
Plain	1 Item	13	0	0	2	0	28	
Sesame	1 Item	13	0.4	0	2	0	25	
(Pillsbury) Soft	1 Item	110	2.5	3	18	1	290	
(Stella D'oro):								
Plain	1 Item	40	1	1	7	0	40	
Plain, FF	1 Item	20	0	1	4	NV	40	

Breakfast Bar

(Also see Diet Bar; Snack Bar; Sport Bar)

	Serv.	K-Cal.	Fat	Prot.	Carb.	Fib.	Sod.	FAC
(Carnation):								
Chocolate Chip	1 Item	150	6	2	24	0	80	FAC
Chocolate Granola	1 Item	130	2.5	2	26	1	40	FAC
Honey Oat Granola	1 Item	130	2.5	2	23	1	45	FAC
Peanut Chocolate	1 Item	150	5	3	22	1	85	FAC
(Fibar):								
Apple, *A.M.*	1 Item	150	3	3	27	5	25	F
Banana, *A.M.*	1 Item	150	4	2	26	5	20	F
Strawberry, *A.M.*	1 Item	150	4	3	24	5	30	F

	Serv.	K-Cal.	Fat	Prot.	Carb.	Flb.	Sod.	FAC
(Health Valley):								
Apple, FF	1 Item	110	0	2	26	3	25	
Apricot, FF	1 Item	110	0	2	26	3	25	
Blueberry, FF..............	1 Item	110	0	2	26	3	25	
Cherry, FF	1 Item	110	0	2	26	3	25	
Chocolate, FF.............	1 Item	110	0	3	26	4	30	
Raspberry, FF.............	1 Item	110	0	2	24	3	65	
Strawberry, FF............	1 Item	100	0	2	28	3	25	

Breakfast Drink
Mix
(Carnation):								
Chocolate Malt............	1 Pouch	130	1.5	5	26	1	130	FAC
Chocolate, NSA	1 Pouch	70	1	5	12	1	95	FAC
Malt, NSA	1 Pouch	70	1.5	5	11	1	115	FAC
Strawberry..................	1 Pouch	130	0	5	28	0	160	FAC
Strawberry, NSA.........	1 Pouch	70	0	5	12	0	95	FAC
Vanilla	1 Pouch	130	0	5	27	0	95	FAC
Vanilla, NSA	1 Pouch	70	0	5	12	0	95	FAC

Ready-to-Serve
(Carnation) Chocolate....	6 Fl Oz	132	1.5	7	22	1	138	FAC
Malt, Skim Milk	6 Fl Oz	103	1.3	9	15	1	160	FAC

Broad Bean (See Bean, Fava)

Broccoflower
Raw	1 Cup	21	0.2	2	4	2	15	A

Broccoli
Fresh
Raw, Chopped (3 Oz)....	1 Cup	25	0.3	3	5	3	24	FA
Raw, Stalk, Medium.......	5 Oz	45	0.5	4	4	NV	55	FA
Boiled, Chopped (6 Oz).	1 Cup	44	0.6	5	8	5	41	FA

Frozen
(Flav R Pac):								
Chopped	1 Cup	40	0	3	7	4	7	A
Cut	1 Cup	25	0	2	4	2	20	A
Florets	1 Item	6	0	1	1	1	5	
Spears........................	1 Cup	25	0	2	4	2	20	A
(Green Giant) Cut	1 Cup	38	0	3	6	3	225	A
Spears........................	1 Oz	7	0	1	1	11	36	A
(Health Valley) Boiled	1 Cup	50	2	6	10	4	44	A

Frozen—Dish
(Flav R Pac) Broccoli								
Normandy	1 Cup	33	0	3	5	3	40	A
(Green Giant):								
Spears W/Butter	1 Oz	13	0.4	1	2	10	83	A
W/Butter	4.5 Oz	45	2	3	7	3	420	A
W/Cheese Sauce........	1 Cup	105	3.8	5	14	3	780	A

	Serv.	K-Cal.	Fat	Prot.	Carb.	Fib.	Sod.	FAC
(*Broccoli cont.*)								
(Seneca) Broccoli Normandy W/Cheese	1 Cup	90	4	6	12	4	420	**A**

Broccoli, Chinese—Chinese Kale

Raw	1 Oz	12	0.1	1	2	0	5	**A**

Broth (See Soup, Canned)

Brownie

(Serving size given in Oz to reflect weight of 1 serving)

	Serv.	K-Cal.	Fat	Prot.	Carb.	Fib.	Sod.	FAC
(Auburn Farms): *Jammer* Butterscotch, FF..............................	1 Oz	100	0	2	22	2	90	
Cappuccino Fudge, FF..............................	1 Oz	90	0	2	22	2	90	
Raspberry Fudge, FF	1 Oz	90	0	2	22	2	100	
(Ener-G) Gluten-Free	1 Oz	108	4.1	2	16	2	178	
(Entenmann's) Chocolate, FF....................................	1 Oz	92	0	1	22	1	103	
(Hostess) LT....................	1.4 Oz	140	2.5	2	29	1	95	
(Little Debbie):								
Brownie LT	2 Oz	190	3	3	39	1	200	
Fudge..........................	2 Oz	270	13	2	39	1	170	
(Pepperidge Farm) Fudge, *Newport*..........	3.2 Oz	400	20	4	50	NV	160	
(Pillsbury) Fudge Bake, *Lovin Lites*	1.6 Oz	160	3.5	2	29	0	125	
(Wt Watchers):								
Brownie A La Mode ...	3 Oz	190	4	5	34	2	170	
Chocolate, Frosted	1.3 Oz	100	2.5	2	22	3	135	
Mint, Frosted...............	1.2 Oz	100	2	2	22	3	130	
Peanut Butter Fudge..	1.2 Oz	110	2.5	2	21	3	140	
Swiss Mocha Fudge...	1.2 Oz	90	2	2	18	2	140	

Brownie, Mix, Prepared

(Serving size given in Oz to reflect weight of 1 serving)
(Prepared as indicated on box)

	Serv.	K-Cal.	Fat	Prot.	Carb.	Fib.	Sod.	FAC
(Arrowhead Mills):								
....	1 Oz	110	0	2	27	2	100	
FF...................................	1 Oz	120	0	2	28	2	110	
Wheat-Free	1 Oz	120	2	3	26	2	110	
(Betty Crocker):								
Caramel	1.5 Oz	190	9	2	27	0	150	
Chocolate Chip	1.5 Oz	200	10	2	26	0	100	
Fudge, Family.............	1.5 Oz	200	9	2	28	1	125	
Fudge, LF	1.2 Oz	130	2.5	2	26	1	110	

	Serv.	K-Cal.	Fat	Prot.	Carb.	Flb.	Sod.	FAC
Original......................	1.5 Oz	200	9	2	29	1	120	
Walnut......................	1.4 Oz	200	11	2	24	1	105	
(Duncan Hines):								
Blonde W/Walnut........	1.3 Oz	160	8	2	22	0	100	
Dark Chocolate								
Fudge	1.4 Oz	170	8	2	25	1	110	
Double Fudge.............	1.5 Oz	170	7	2	29	1	130	
Fudge, Chewy	1.4 Oz	160	7	2	25	1	120	
Milk Chocolate								
Chunk.....................	1.4 Oz	170	7	2	26	1	120	
Mississippi Mud	1.4 Oz	160	6	1	26	0	100	
Peanut Butter..............	1.4 Oz	160	8	2	23	1	120	
Turtle.......................	1.4 Oz	160	6	2	26	1	110	
Walnut......................	1.4 Oz	170	8	2	24	0	105	
(Hostess) LT.................	1.4 Oz	140	2.5	2	29	1	95	
(Pillsbury) Fudge,								
Microwave.................	1.2 Oz	130	3	2	25	NV	110	
Walnut, Microwave	1.4 Oz	160	5	3	26	1	110	

Brussels Sprout
Fresh

	Serv.	K-Cal.	Fat	Prot.	Carb.	Flb.	Sod.	FAC
Raw	1 Cup	87	0.6	7	18	8	51	FA
Raw	1 Lb	195	1.4	15	41	19	113	FAC
Boiled......................	1 Cup	61	0.8	4	14	4	33	FA

Frozen

	Serv.	K-Cal.	Fat	Prot.	Carb.	Flb.	Sod.	FAC
Boiled......................	1 Cup	65	0.6	6	13	6	36	FA
Butter Sauce								
(Flav R Pac)	1 Item	6	0	1	1	1	4	
(Green Giant).............	1 Cup	90	2.3	5	14	6	405	FA

Buckwheat Flour

	Serv.	K-Cal.	Fat	Prot.	Carb.	Flb.	Sod.	FAC
Whole Groat..................	1 Oz	95	0.9	4	20	3	3	
Whole Groat	1 Cup	402	3.7	15	85	12	13	
(Arrowhead Mills)	1 Cup	400	4	12	84	12	0	

Buckwheat Groats—Kasha

	Serv.	K-Cal.	Fat	Prot.	Carb.	Flb.	Sod.	FAC
Dry, Brown (Arrowhead								
Mills).....................	1 Cup	560	4	20	120	12	0	F
Dry, Whole	1 Cup	583	5.8	23	122	17	2	F
Roasted, Cooked	1 Cup	182	1.2	7	40	5	8	
Roasted, Dry	1 Cup	567	4.4	19	123	17	18	F

Buffalo

	Serv.	K-Cal.	Fat	Prot.	Carb.	Flb.	Sod.	FAC
Raw	3 Oz	84	1.2	17	0	0	45	
Roasted	3 Oz	111	1.5	23	0	0	48	

Bulgur (Also See Tabouli)

	Serv.	K-Cal.	Fat	Prot.	Carb.	Flb.	Sod.	FAC
Dry......................................	1 Cup	479	1.9	17	106	26	24	F
Cooked	1 Cup	151	0.4	6	34	8	9	

	Serv.	K-Cal.	Fat	Prot.	Carb.	Flb.	Sod.	FAC
Bun (Also See Bread; Pastry; Bun, Roll)								
Hamburger								
(Colombo) W/Onion	1 Item	240	3	8	48	3	300	
(Ener-G) Brown Rice, Gluten-Free	1 Item	258	9.8	3	41	1	10	
(Pepperidge Farm)	1 Item	130	2	5	22	1	240	
Whole Grain (Roman Meal)	1 Item	130	3	4	20	NV	230	
(Wonder):								
	1 Item	120	2	4	21	1	230	
LT	1 Item	80	1.5	5	13	5	210	
Wheat	1 Item	170	2.5	6	31	1	370	
Hot Dog								
(Ener-G) Tapioca, Gluten-Free	1 Item	339	14.3	2	46	9	419	
(Pepperidge Farm):								
Dijon	1 Item	160	5	5	23	2	230	
Enriched	1 Item	140	3	5	24	1	270	
(Roman Meal)	1 Item	104	2	4	20	2	210	
(Wonder)	1 Item	80	1	2	14	1	150	
Burdock Root—Gobo								
Boiled (6 Oz)	1 Item	146	0.2	3	35	3	7	F
Burrito, Fast Food								
(Carl's Jr) Breakfast	1 Item	430	26	22	29	1	810	AC
(Del Taco):								
Breakfast	1 Item	256	11	9	30	NV	409	
Chicken	1 Item	264	10	13	32	NV	771	
Chicken Deluxe	1 Item	549	34	21	40	NV	978	
Chicken, Spicy	1 Item	392	11	16	59	NV	1,243	
Combination	1 Item	413	17	21	46	NV	1,035	
Del Beef	1 Item	440	20	23	43	NV	878	
Del Beef, Deluxe	1 Item	479	23	25	45	NV	890	
Deluxe Combo	1 Item	453	20	22	49	NV	1,047	
Green	1 Item	229	8	9	32	NV	714	
The Works	1 Item	448	18	15	60	NV	1,248	
(Mighty Taco):								
Bean & Cheese	1 Item	408	14	14	59	12	1,138	
Beef, Bean, & Cheese	1 Item	448	19	21	50	9	1,188	
Beef & Cheese	1 Item	488	24	29	41	6	1,238	
Vegetarian	1 Item	503	29	24	38	2	1,480	
(Taco Bell):								
Bean, LT	1 Item	330	6	14	55	8	1,340	A
Burrito Supreme	1 Item	439	17.5	19	50	8	1,229	A
Chicken, LT	1 Item	288	8.1	16	39	3	802	A
Chicken Supreme, LT	1 Item	418	13.8	25	51	3	1,147	A
Supreme, LT	1 Item	350	8	20	50	4	1,300	A

	Serv.	K-Cal.	Fat	Prot.	Carb.	Fib.	Sod.	FAC
(Taco Time):								
Bean, Crisp	1 Item	391	17	14	46	NV	530	
Bean, Soft	1 Item	547	21	22	68	NV	1,027	
Casita	1 Item	602	32	31	51	NV	1,428	
Combo, Soft	1 Item	550	24	30	55	NV	1,227	
Confetti Chicken	1 Item	540	12.7	31	67	14	1,041	
Meat, Crisp	1 Item	393	20	23	30	NV	752	
Meat, Soft	1 Item	552	26	37	43	NV	1,427	
Veggie	1 Item	535	20	21	71	NV	890	

Burrito, Frozen
Bean

	Serv.	K-Cal.	Fat	Prot.	Carb.	Fib.	Sod.	FAC
W/Cheese (Don Miguel)	1 Item	450	13	17	67	8	970	AC
W/Cheese (Old El Paso)	1 Item	300	9	12	44	3	840	
W/Cheese (Tina's)	1 Item	340	9	12	52	8	600	
W/Cheese, Lean (Don Miguel)	1 Item	350	4	14	73	13	630	A
W/Rice (Amy's Kitchen)	1 Item	250	5	9	44	6	450	
W/Rice/Cheese (Amy's Kitchen)	1 Item	280	8	10	43	6	460	

Beef

	Serv.	K-Cal.	Fat	Prot.	Carb.	Fib.	Sod.	FAC
Ranchero (Healthy Choice)	1 Item	290	7	13	44	6	500	
(Tina's)	1 Item	380	15	12	49	6	630	
W/Beans (Don Miguel)	1 Item	390	8	18	61	5	900	A
W/Beans (Old El Paso)	1 Item	320	9	12	48	4	690	
W/Cheese (Prima Rosa)	1 Item	330	10	20	39	2	730	
W/Cheese/Chili (Don Miguel)	1 Item	720	36	20	90	14	1,220	A

Chicken

	Serv.	K-Cal.	Fat	Prot.	Carb.	Fib.	Sod.	FAC
(Don Miguel):								
	1 Item	390	8	18	60	5	840	A
W/Bean/Rice, Lean	1 Item	360	4	18	67	7	380	A
W/Cheese/Chile	1 Item	420	12	19	59	3	880	A
(Healthy Choice) Con Queso	1 Item	360	3	16	66	8	590	A
(Patio)	1 Item	250	4	12	44	3	740	
(Tina's)	1 Item	250	4	9	45	3	660	

Butter
(2 Tbsp weigh approximately 1 Oz)
Clarified—Ghee

	Serv.	K-Cal.	Fat	Prot.	Carb.	Fib.	Sod.	FAC
	1 Oz	250	27.7	0	0	0	9	

Salted

	Serv.	K-Cal.	Fat	Prot.	Carb.	Fib.	Sod.	FAC
Pat	1 Item	36	4.1	0	0	0	41	
Stick	4 Oz	813	92	1	0	0	937	A
Stick (8 Oz)	1 Cup	1,627	184	2	0	0	1,876	A

	Serv.	K-Cal.	Fat	Prot.	Carb.	Flb.	Sod.	FAC
(Butter cont.)								
Stick, Whipped	2.6 Oz	542	61.3	1	0	0	625	
(Land O Lakes):								
....	1 Tbsp	100	11	0	0	0	85	
LT..................................	1 Tbsp	50	6	0	0	0	70	
Sweet Cream..............	1 Tbsp	90	10	0	0	0	95	
Whipped, LT	1 Tbsp	35	4	0	0	0	45	
(Nucoa) Heart Beat........	1 Tbsp	25	3	0	0	0	110	
Unsalted								
Whipped	1 Tsp	27	3.1	0	0	0	0	
(Challenge)	1 Tbsp	100	11	0	0	0	2	
(Challenge) Sweet..........	1 Tbsp	100	11	0	0	0	2	
(Land O Lakes) LT	1 Tbsp	50	6	0	0	0	5	
Sweet Cream..............	1 Tbsp	90	10	0	0	0	0	
Butter, Alternative								
(Butter Buds) Granules..	1 Tsp	8	0	0	2	0	70	
(Butter Buds) Sprinkles..	1 Tsp	5	0	0	2	NV	120	
(Molly McButter)	1 Tsp	5	0	0	1	NV	180	

Butter Bean (See Bean, Lima)

Butterfish

	Serv.	K-Cal.	Fat	Prot.	Carb.	Flb.	Sod.	FAC
Raw	3 Oz	124	6.8	15	0	0	76	
Broiled	3 Oz	159	8.7	19	0	0	97	

Butter Lettuce (See Lettuce)

Buttermilk (See Milk, Cow)

Butternut (See Brazil Nut)

Butternut Squash (See Squash, Winter)

Butterscotch Topping

	Serv.	K-Cal.	Fat	Prot.	Carb.	Flb.	Sod.	FAC
(Baskin Robbins).............	1 Tbsp	50	0.5	1	12	0	40	
(Mrs. Richardson's)								
Caramel	1 Tbsp	65	1	1	14	0	45	
(Smucker's)	1 Tbsp	70	0.7	0	16	0	37	

(

	Serv.	K-Cal.	Fat	Prot.	Carb.	Fib.	Sod.	FAC
Cabbage								
Danish, Boiled W/Salt,								
Drained	1 Cup	33	0.7	2	7	4	382	**A**
Green.................................	1 Cup	49	0.4	2	11	3	36	**FA**
Green, Head.....................	2 Lb	227	2.5	13	49	21	163	**FAC**
Green, Shredded.............	2.5 Oz	18	0.2	1	4	2	13	**A**
Green, Boiled, Drained ..	5 Oz	33	0.7	2	7	3	12	**A**
Napa, Shredded.............	1 Cup	10	0.2	1	2	1	46	**FA**
Red, Shredded	1 Cup	19	0.2	1	4	1	8	**A**
Savoy, Raw, Shredded..	1 Cup	19	0.1	1	4	2	20	**FA**
Cabbage, Chinese (See Bok Choy)								
Cactus—Nopal								
Raw	1 Cup	48	0.6	1	11	4	6	**A**
Cooked W/Salt	1 Cup	61	0.8	1	14	5	352	**A**
Cactus Pear—Prickly Pear								
Raw	1 Item	42	0.5	1	10	4	5	**A**
Cake								
(Prepared as indicated on the package)								
Angel Food								
(Betty Crocker):								
One Step	¹⁄₁₂ Cake	140	0	3	32	0	280	
Traditional	¹⁄₁₂ Cake	130	0	3	30	0	160	
(Duncan Hines)	¹⁄₁₂ Cake	140	0	3	31	NV	310	
Banana								
(Duncan Hines)								
Supreme	¹⁄₁₂ Cake	250	11	3	36	0	270	
(Pillsbury) *Plus*	¹⁄₁₂ Cake	260	11	3	36	0	280	
Butter								
(Betty Crocker):								
Chocolate....................	¹⁄₁₂ Cake	270	13	4	34	1	380	
Yellow	¹⁄₁₂ Cake	260	11	3	37	0	330	
(Duncan Hines)	¹⁄₁₂ Cake	320	16	3	42	2	190	

	Serv.	K-Cal.	Fat	Prot.	Carb.	Fib.	Sod.	FAC
(*Cake cont.*)								
(Pillsbury):								
Chocolate....................	¹⁄₁₂ Cake	270	13	4	33	1	420	
Plus.............................	¹⁄₁₂ Cake	260	12	3	36	0	370	
Carrot								
(Betty Crocker)								
Supermoist................	¹⁄₁₀ Cake	300	13	4	41	0	340	
(Pillsbury)	¹⁄₁₂ Cake	260	12	3	35	1	290	
Cheesecake								
(Jell-O):								
Homestyle, No Bake ..	⅛ Cake	165	3	4	31	1	321	
New York....................	⅛ Cake	175	3	4	33	0	320	
Chocolate								
(Betty Crocker):								
Supermoist, Chip........	¹⁄₁₂ Cake	260	12	3	33	1	380	
Supermoist, Fudge	¹⁄₁₂ Cake	250	11	3	34	1	430	
Supermoist, Milk								
Chocolate	¹⁄₁₂ Cake	250	12	3	33	1	320	
(Pillsbury):								
Plus.............................	¹⁄₁₂ Cake	260	12	3	34	1	330	
Plus, Dark...................	¹⁄₁₂ Cake	250	2	3	33	1	340	
(Duncan Hines) Swiss ...	¹⁄₁₂ Cake	290	15	4	34	1	390	
Devil's Food								
(Betty Crocker)								
Supermoist..................	¹⁄₁₀ Cake	230	4.5	4	42	2	400	
(Duncan Hines):								
Delight.........................	¹⁄₁₂ Cake	220	6	3	41	1	420	
Moist Deluxe...............	¹⁄₁₂ Cake	290	15	4	34	0	360	
(Pillsbury) *Plus*	¹⁄₁₂ Cake	270	14	4	33	1	340	
(Robin Hood)..................	⅕ Cake	310	17	4	36	1	430	
Fudge								
(Betty Crocker)								
Supermoist, Marble	¹⁄₁₂ Cake	250	11	3	35	0	270	
(Duncan Hines):								
Dutch Dark.................	¹⁄₁₂ Cake	290	15	4	34	1	390	
Marble	¹⁄₁₂ Cake	250	11	3	36	0	270	
(Pillsbury) *Plus*, Swirl	¹⁄₁₂ Cake	250	10	3	37	1	290	
German Chocolate								
(Betty Crocker)								
Supermoist..................	¹⁄₁₂ Cake	250	11	3	34	1	390	
(Pillsbury)	¹⁄₁₂ Cake	250	11	3	34	1	280	
Gingerbread								
(Betty Crocker)	⅛ Cake	230	7	3	37	0	370	
(Dromedary)	¹⁄₁₀ Cake	170	3	2	33	NV	330	
Key Lime								
(Duncan Hines)	¹⁄₁₂ Cake	250	11	3	36	0	270	
Lemon								
(Betty Crocker):								
Chiffon........................	¹⁄₁₆ Cake	140	3	3	26	0	140	

	Serv.	K-Cal.	Fat	Prot.	Carb.	Fib.	Sod.	FAC
Pudding	⅛ Cake	180	4	2	33	0	210	
Supermoist	¹⁄₁₂ Cake	250	11	3	36	0	260	
(Duncan Hines)								
Supreme	¹⁄₁₂ Cake	250	11	3	36	0	270	
(Pillsbury) *Plus*	¹⁄₁₀ Cake	310	13	4	43	1	340	
Pineapple								
(Betty Crocker) *Classic*	⅙ Cake	400	15	3	63	1	350	
(Duncan Hines)								
Supreme	¹⁄₁₂ Cake	250	11	3	36	0	270	
Pound								
(Betty Crocker)								
Classic	⅛ Cake	290	13	4	41	0	240	
Spice								
(Betty Crocker)								
Supermoist	¹⁄₁₂ Cake	250	11	3	35	0	310	
(Duncan Hines) *Moist*								
Deluxe	¹⁄₁₂ Cake	250	11	3	36	0	270	
Strawberry								
(Betty Crocker)								
Supermoist	¹⁄₁₀ Cake	300	12	4	43	0	360	
(Duncan Hines)								
Supreme	¹⁄₁₂ Cake	250	11	3	36	0	270	
(Pillsbury) *Plus*	¹⁄₁₂ Cake	260	11	3	36	0	310	
Vanilla								
(Betty Crocker):								
Supermoist, French	¹⁄₁₂ Cake	250	11	3	34	0	300	
Supermoist, Golden	¹⁄₁₂ Cake	280	14	3	35	0	260	
(Duncan Hines) French	¹⁄₁₂ Cake	250	11	3	36	0	270	
White								
(Betty Crocker):								
Supermoist	¹⁄₁₂ Cake	240	10	3	34	0	310	
Supermoist, LT	¹⁄₁₀ Cake	210	3.5	3	43	0	390	
(Duncan Hines) *Moist*								
Deluxe	¹⁄₁₂ Cake	190	6	3	34	NV	300	
(Nabisco) *Snackwell's*	⅙ Cake	210	4.5	3	39	1	320	
(Pillsbury) *Plus*	¹⁄₁₀ Cake	280	11	3	41	1	350	
Yellow								
(Betty Crocker):								
Supermoist	¹⁄₁₂ Cake	250	10	3	36	0	300	
Supermoist LT	¹⁄₁₀ Cake	230	4.5	4	43	0	350	
(Duncan Hines):								
Delights	¹⁄₁₂ Cake	220	4.5	3	44	0	320	
Moist Deluxe	¹⁄₁₂ Cake	250	11	3	36	0	270	
(Nabisco) *Snackwells*	⅙ Cake	210	4.5	3	39	4	320	
(Pillsbury):								
Lovin Lites	¹⁄₁₂ Cake	230	5	3	43	1	380	
Plus	¹⁄₁₂ Cake	250	11	3	35	1	300	
(Robin Hood)	⅕ Cake	280	13	3	37	0	310	

	Serv.		K-Cal.	Fat	Prot.	Carb.	Fib.	Sod.	FAC

Cake, Ready-to-Serve
Angel
(Hostess)	⅙	Cake	150	3	2	29	0	220	

Banana
(Entenmann's):
Crunch FF	⅛	Cake	140	0	2	33	2	150	
Loaf FF	⅛	Cake	150	0	2	34	1	190	
(Sara Lee)	⅛	Cake	170	6	1	28	NV	160	

Carrot
(Entenmann's):
	⅙	Cake	340	19	3	42	1	290	A
FF	⅛	Cake	170	0	3	40	1	230	A
(Oregon Farms)	⅙	Cake	180	15	4	38	3	370	
(Sara Lee)	⅙	Cake	290	12	4	40	1	210	

Cheesecake
(Sara Lee):
Chocolate	¼	Cake	410	21	8	47	2	300	
French	⅕	Cake	410	25	6	41	1	330	
Original	¼	Cake	350	18	7	39	1	320	

(Wt Watchers):
Brownie	1	Item	200	6	9	33	4	220	
New York	1	Item	150	5	6	21	0	140	
Strawberry	1	Item	180	5	7	28	2	230	

Chocolate
(Entenmann's):
Chip Loaf, FF	1/16	Cake	80	0	2	18	NV	85	
Crunch, FF	⅛	Cake	130	0	2	32	2	170	
Fudge Icing, FF	⅙	Cake	210	0	3	51	2	210	
Loaf, FF	⅙	Cake	173	0	4	40	1	333	
(Sara Lee) Free & Light	⅛	Cake	110	0	2	26	2	140	
Layer, Double	2	Oz	260	13	3	33	2	180	

(Pepperidge Farm):
Layer, German	1/12	Cake	180	10	1	22	NV	170	
Mousse	2.6	Oz	250	10	2	35	2	120	
Supreme	2⅞	Oz	300	16	3	37	NV	140	

(Wt Watchers) Irish
Cream	2	Oz	170	5	4	26	3	240	

Coconut
(Pepperidge Farm):
Classic	2.25	Oz	230	11	2	31	NV	160	
Layer	1/12	Cake	180	8	1	24	0	120	
Lemon	3	Oz	280	13	3	38	NV	220	

Coffee
(Entenmann's):
Apple Spice Crumb,
FF	⅛	Cake	130	0	2	30	2	140	
Cinnamon/Apple, FF	⅑	Cake	130	0	2	29	2	110	

(Sara Lee):
Butter Streusel	⅙	Cake	220	12	4	25	0	240	

	Serv.		K-Cal.	Fat	Prot.	Carb.	Flb.	Sod.	FAC
Crumb	1/8	Cake	220	9	3	32	0	210	
Pecan	1/8	Cake	230	12	4	24	0	170	
(Wt Watchers)									
Cinnamon Streusel	2.3	Oz	190	3.5	4	35	2	190	
Devil's Food									
(Nabisco)*Snackwell's*	1/8	Cake	190	3.5	2	13	3	380	
(Pepperidge Farm)									
Layer	3	Oz	290	14	2	40	2	220	
Fudge									
(Wt Watchers) Double	1	Item	190	4.5	4	36	2	200	
Golden									
(Entenmann's):									
Choc Chip, FF	1/8	Cake	130	0	3	31	1	220	
French Crumb, FF	1/8	Cake	140	0	2	35	2	150	
Fudge Iced, FF	1/6	Cake	220	0	3	52	2	200	
Loaf, FF	1/8	Loaf	120	0	2	28	<1	160	
(Little Debbie) Cremes	1.5	Oz	170	7	2	25	0	180	
(Pepperidge Farms)									
Layer	3	Oz	290	14	3	38	1	230	
Lemon									
(Pepperidge Farm)									
Supreme LT	1/12	Cake	170	5	4	26	NV	100	
Pound									
(Hostess)	1/5	Cake	350	16	5	48	1	360	
(Sara Lee):									
	1/4	Cake	320	16	4	38	0	280	
Free & Light	1/10	Cake	70	0	1	17	0	105	
Vanilla									
(Hostess) *Lights*	1.5	Oz	140	1	2	30	NV	160	
(Pepperidge Farm):									
Classic Fudge	1/12	Cake	250	11	2	33	NV	160	
Layer	1/12	Cake	290	13	2	41	1	190	

Cake, Snack
(Individual Servings)
(Hostess):

	Serv.		K-Cal.	Fat	Prot.	Carb.	Flb.	Sod.	FAC
Apple Pie	1	Item	230	10	2	34	1	190	
Cherry Pie	1	Item	235	11	2	37	1	230	
Ding Dong	1	Item	180	9	2	22	1	115	
Ho-Ho-Ho	1	Item	55	6	1	17	0	75	
Suzy-Q	1	Item	230	9	2	35	1	270	
Twinkies	1	Item	150	5	1	25	0	190	
(Little Debble):									
Banana Twin	1	Item	250	10	2	39	0	170	
Be My Valentine	1	Item	280	14	1	38	0	170	
Chocolate Twins	1	Item	240	8	2	42	1	240	
Coffee–Apple Streusel	1	Item	230	7	2	39	1	190	
Devil Cremes	1	Item	190	8	1	29	0	170	
Devil Squares	1	Item	270	13	2	39	1	180	

	Serv.	K-Cal.	Fat	Prot.	Carb.	Fib.	Sod.	FAC
(Cake, Snack cont.)								
Fudge Rounds.............	1 Item	140	6	1	23	1	85	
Golden Cremes	1 Item	170	7	2	25	0	180	
Honey.........................	1 Item	210	13	3	22	1	180	
Swiss Roll...................	1 Item	260	12	1	39	1	180	
Tiger..........................	1 Item	310	15	2	44	1	190	

Calamari (See Squid)

Canadian Bacon (See Bacon, Canadian)

Candy
Almond
Delights (Russell

	Serv.	K-Cal.	Fat	Prot.	Carb.	Fib.	Sod.	FAC
Stover) (1 Oz)............	1 Item	210	12	3	22	1	55	
(Hershey's):								
Golden Solitaires (3 Oz)	1 Item	484	31.5	10	40	4	44	
Hugs.............................	1 Item	24	1.5	0	2	0	3	
Kisses	1 Item	27	1.7	1	2	0	3	
Bar								
(Auburn Farms):								
A-Ok (1 Oz)	1 Item	137	6.9	5	14	1	51	
Nut Wit (1 Oz)	1 Item	137	7.4	4	14	1	49	
Nuttin Like't Crunchy								
(1 Oz)	1 Item	180	11	6	18	1	100	
Bit-O-Honey (1 Oz)........	1 Item	28	0.5	0	6	0	3	
Golden III (3 Oz)............	1 Item	471	30	6	51	5	79	
(Hershey's):								
Almond Joy (2 Oz)	1 Item	246	13.8	2	28	2	68	
5th Avenue (2 Oz)......	1 Item	295	12.8	5	40	1	99	
Krackel (3 Oz)	1 Item	393	21.2	5	46	2	102	
Milk Chocolate (2 Oz)	1 Item	238	13.7	3	25	1	36	
Mounds (2 Oz)	1 Item	258	13.6	2	32	3	72	
Mr. GoodBar (3 Oz) ...	1 Item	449	28.8	11	37	3	36	F
Symphony (2 Oz)	1 Item	375	22	5	39	1	56	
(M & M/Mars):								
Chocolate Chunk,								
Kudos (0.7 Oz)	1 Item	90	3	1	13	1	60	C
Dove Milk Chocolate,								
(1 Oz)	1 Item	200	12	2	22	1	25	
M & M's......................	1 Item	200	11	3	21	2	15	A
Milky Way	1 Item	280	11	2	43	1	100	
Snickers	1 Item	280	14	5	35	1	160	
Three Musketeers								
(2 Oz)	1 Item	260	8	2	46	1	110	
Twix Caramel (1 Oz)..	1 Item	140	7	2	19	1	58	
Twix Peanut Butter								
(1 Oz)......................	1 Item	130	8	3	13	1	70	
(Nestlé):								
Baby Ruth (2 Oz)	1 Item	280	12	4	38	2	135	

	Serv.		K-Cal.	Fat	Prot.	Carb.	Fib.	Sod.	FAC
Butterfinger (2 Oz)	1	Item	280	11	4	41	1	120	
Chunky (1 Oz)	1	Item	200	11	3	22	2	20	
Crunch (2 Oz)	1	Item	230	12	3	28	1	60	
Milk Chocolate (0.5 Oz)	1	Item	220	13	4	23	2	30	
Oh Henry (2 Oz)	1	Item	230	9	6	32	2	125	
Tootsie Roll (1 Oz)	1	Item	112	2.5	1	23	0	8	
Caramel									
Pom Poms	1	Oz	100	3	1	15	NV	70	
(Cadbury) *Caramello* (5 Oz)	1	Item	672	30.8	9	90	2	192	C
(Hershey's) *Rolos*	2	Oz	266	12.5	2	36	1	96	
(Kraft)	1	Item	30	1	0	6	0	25	
(Nabisco) *Sugar Babies* (2 Oz)	1	Item	180	2	1	40	NV	85	
(Pearson) *Nips*	1	Item	30	0.8	0	6	0	20	
Carob									
Chips	1	Oz	151	9.4	4	14	2	0	
(Natural Touch) Milk									
Bar	1	Item	150	9	4	13	NV	55	
Milk Free (1 Oz)	1	Item	160	11	4	11	NV	25	
(Tiger's Milk) Peanut									
Butter (1 Oz)	1	Item	140	5	6	18	1	75	C
Protein-Rich (1 Oz)	1	Item	145	5	7	18	1	70	C
Chocolate									
(Ghirardelli):									
Bittersweet	3	Oz	488	34.8	6	56	8	7	
Dark	3	Oz	504	33.6	4	60	5	5	
Dark W/Almonds	3	Oz	520	37.2	7	53	7	6	
Dark W/Raspberries	3	Oz	498	32.5	4	61	6	5	
Milk	3.3	Oz	523	32	7	59	2	76	
Milk/Almonds	3.3	Oz	536	36	9	52	4	63	
Milk/Macadamia Nut	3.3	Oz	543	36.5	7	54	3	69	
Milk W/Pecans	3.3	Oz	550	38.5	7	51	3	61	
Milk W/Toffee	3.3	Oz	520	31	6	61	2	109	
Mint	3.3	Oz	520	32.5	4	61	3	32	
Raspberry & Cream	3.3	Oz	547	33.8	5	59	1	94	
White Confection	3.3	Oz	555	35	5	58	0	98	
(Hershey's) *Kisses*	1	Item	26	1.5	0	3	0	4	
M & M's (2 Oz) (M & M/Mars)	1	Item	240	10	2	34	1	30	
Mexican	3	Oz	396	25.6	5	51	7	7	
Coffee									
Cappucino Almond (Nectar Nuggets)	1	Item	110	5	2	14	5	30	
Nips (Pearson)	1	Item	30	0.8	0	6	0	23	

	Serv.		K-Cal.	Fat	Prot.	Carb.	Fib.	Sod.	FAC
(Candy cont.)									
Fruit									
Bonkers	1	Item	20	0	0	5	NV	NV	
Jujyfruits (Heide)	11	Items	100	<1	<1	25	0	0	
Skittles, Bite Size									
(M & M/Mars)	2	Oz	250	3	0	55	0	10	A
Starburst (M & M/									
Mars)	2	Oz	240	5	0	48	NV	30	
Sweetarts (Nestlé)	1	Oz	113	1	0	25	NV	NV	
Twizzlers, (Hershey's)	5	Oz	484	2.7	5	110	2	337	
Fudge									
Chocolate, Plain	1	Oz	102	2.3	0	22	0	17	
W/Marshmallow	1	Oz	120	4.8	1	20	0	29	
W/Marshmallow W/									
Nuts	1	Oz	125	5.6	1	20	0	27	
W/Peanut Butter	1	Oz	107	1.9	1	23	0	21	
W/Nuts	1	Oz	111	2.8	1	22	0	27	
Gum									
All Flavors (Dentyne)	1	Item	6	0	2	0	0	0	
All Flavors (Wrigley's)	1	Item	10	0	0	2	0	0	
Sugarless (Care*Free)	1	Item	10	0	0	2	0	0	
Sugarless (Dentyne)	1	Item	5	0	1	0	0	0	
Halvah									
Plain	1	Oz	143	8.3	3	16	0	5	
Hard									
Butterscotch, *Life*									
Savers (Nabisco)	1	Item	8	0	0	2	0	0	
Cherry (Jolly Rancher)	1	Item	23	0	0	6	0	3	
Cherry Nib (Hershey's)	1	Oz	98	0.7	1	22	0	2	
Lemon Drops (Brach's)	1	Oz	110	0	0	27	0	5	
Peppermint (Breath									
Savers)	1	Item	8	0	0	2	0	0	
Jelly									
Gum Drops	1	Item	14	0	0	3	0	0	
Gummy Bears	1	Item	8	0	0	2	0	3	
Jelly Beans	1	Item	7	0	0	3	0	0	
Licorice									
Bears (Bearito)	1	Item	7	0.1	0	2	0	6	
Good & Plenty									
(Hershey's)	1	Oz	106	<0.1	1	26	0	52	
Licorice	1	Cup	807	1.1	0	205	0	55	
Nips (Pearson)	1	Oz	120	3	1	23	0	70	
Twists (Bearitos)	1	Item	28	0.2	0	6	0	22	
Twists (Brach's)	1	Oz	100	1	2	22	0	50	
Lollipop									
Dum Dums (Spangler)	1	Item	25	0	0	6	0	0	
Fruit Juicers	1	Item	40	0	0	10	0	0	
Life Savers (Nabisco)	1	Item	45	0	0	11	0	10	

	Serv.		K-Cal.	Fat	Prot.	Carb.	Fib.	Sod.	FAC
Maltball									
(Brach's)	1	Oz	130	5	1	21	NV	40	
(Sunspire)	1	Item	21	1	0	3	0	7	
Whoppers (Hershey's)	1	Oz	136	6	1	20	NV	NV	
Mint									
After Eight (Rowntree)	1	Item	14	0.6	0	3	0	0	
Chocolate Mint, *Nips*									
(Pearson)	1	Item	30	0.8	0	6	0	20	
Junior Mints									
(1 Oz)	12	Items	120	3	1	24	0	46	
Peppermint Patty									
(York)	1	Item	177	4.2	1	33	1	13	
Peanut									
Goobers Pkg	1	Oz	210	13	5	19	3	20	
M & M's Pkg									
(M & M/Mars)	2	Oz	250	13	5	30	2	25	
Parfait Nip (Pearson)	1	Item	30	1	0	6	0	20	
Peanut Brittle	1	Oz	123	4.4	2	20	1	11	
Peanut Butter									
(Hershey's):									
Bar None	1.5	Oz	240	14	4	23	NV	50	
Reese's PB Cup									
Miniatures	1	Item	92	5.3	2	9	1	55	
Reese's PB Cup	2	Oz	247	15.9	6	24	2	148	
Kudos (M & M/Mars)	1	Item	130	5	2	18	1	85	C
Raisin									
Milk-Chocolate-									
Covered (Sunspire)	1	Item	6	0.2	0	1	0	1	
Raisinets (Nestlé)	10	Items	41	1.6	0.5	7	0	4	
Raisinets Pkg (Nestlé)	1	Oz	180	6	2	28	NV	10	
Yogurt-Covered									
(Sunspire)	1	Item	6	0.2	0	1	0	1	
Cane Syrup									
Table Blend	1	Tbsp	51	0	0	13	0	1	
Table Blend	1	Oz	101	0	0	26	0	2	

Cannellini Bean—White Kidney (See Bean, Cannellini)

Canola Oil									
Organic (Spectrum)	1	Tbsp	120	14	0	0	0	0	A
Smart Beat (Nucoa)	1	Tbsp	120	14	0	0	0	10	A
Blend									
W/Corn (Crisco)	1	Tbsp	120	14	0	0	0	0	A
W/Corn (Mazola)	1	Tbsp	120	14	0	0	0	0	A
W/Olive (Spectrum)	1	Tbsp	120	14	0	0	0	0	A

	Serv.	K-Cal.	Fat	Prot.	Carb.	Fib.	Sod.	FAC
Cantaloupe—Muskmelon								
Raw (6 Oz)	1 Cup	55	0.4	1	13	1	14	A
Raw	1 Lb	158	1.2	4	38	3	41	FA
Balls, Frozen	1 Cup	53	0	1	13	0	21	A
Cape Gooseberry—Ground-Cherry—Physalis								
Raw (5 Oz)	1 Cup	74	1	3	16	NV	NV	A
Raw	1 Lb	240	3.2	9	51	NV	NV	A
Capers								
(Crosse & Blackwell)	1 Tbsp	5	0	0	1	0	350	
Cappuccino (See Coffee, Cappuccino)								
Carambola—Star Fruit—Chinese Star Fruit								
Raw (5 Oz)	1 Item	42	0.5	1	10	3	3	A
Raw	1 Oz	7	0	0	1	1	2	
Caramel Topping								
(Hershey's)	1 Tbsp	50	0	0	13	NV	47	
(Kraft)	1 Tbsp	60	0	1	14	0	45	
(Smucker's)	1 Tbsp	75	2	.5	14	0	36	
Caraway Seed								
Ground	1 Tsp	14	0.8	1	1	1	0	
Whole	1 Tsp	7	0.3	0	1	1	0	
Cardamon Seed								
Ground	1 Tsp	7	0	0	2	1	0	
Cardoon—Cardini—Cardi								
Raw, Shredded	1 Cup	36	0.2	1	9	3	303	FA
Carob Flour								
	1 Cup	185	0.7	5	92	41	36	C
Carob Powder								
	1 Oz	51	0.4	1	21	2	90	
Carp								
Raw	3 Oz	108	4.8	15	0	0	42	
Broiled	3 Oz	138	6.1	19	0	0	54	
Carrot								
Fresh								
Raw, Grated	1 Cup	90	0.4	2	22	5	73	A
Baby, 2¾"	1 Med	4	0.1	0	1	0	4	
Whole, Peeled (3 Oz)	1 Med	31	0.1	1	7	2	25	A
Boiled, Slice	1 Cup	70	0.3	2	16	5	104	A

	Serv.	K-Cal.	Fat	Prot.	Carb.	Fib.	Sod.	FAC
Canned								
(Del Monte) Sliced	1 Cup	70	0	0	16	6	600	A
(Lesueur) Baby, Whole ..	1 Cup	70	0	1	6	6	820	A
(S&W)	1 Cup	50	1	2	12	4	500	A
(Seneca)	1 Cup	50	0	1	12	4	500	A
Frozen								
Baby (Green Giant)	1 Cup	30	0	0	8	3	105	A
(Seneca)	1 Cup	50	0	2	12	4	50	A
Carrot Juice								
Canned (Hollywood)	1 Cup	80	0.6	1	18	1	167	A
Fresh (Odwalla)	1 Cup	80	0	2	18	2	200	A
Casaba Melon								
Sliced (6 Oz)	1 Cup	44	0.2	2	10.5	1	20	A
Cashew								
(1 cup weighs approximately 4 oz)								
Dry-Roasted								
Unsalted, Whole	1 Oz	164	13.2	6	5	2	6	
Salted, Whole	1 Oz	164	13.2	4	11	1	183	
Halves (Fisher)	1 Oz	170	15	5	8	1	10	
Halves (Fisher)	1 Cup	680	60	20	32	2	40	F
Honey-Roasted								
Whole (Fisher)	1 Oz	150	13	4	7	NV	90	
Oil-Roasted								
Salted	1 Oz	190	15.6	5	9	1	204	
Salted, Halves	1 Oz	170	15	5	8	1	130	
Salted, Whole								
(Fisher)	1 Oz	170	15	5	8	1	130	
Cashew Butter								
Raw								
(Bearitos)	1 Tbsp	150	14	3	4	NV	0	
(Hain)	1 Tbsp	80	7.5	3	4	NV	0	
Roasted								
(Bearitos)	1 Tbsp	95	8.5	3	4	NV	0	
(Hain)	1 Tbsp	105	8.5	4	4	NV	7	
(Maranatha)	1 Tbsp	80	7	3	5	NV	5	
Cassava-Yuca								
Raw	1 Lb	544	1.8	14	122	NV	36	FC
Raw	1 Oz	34	0.1	1	8	NV	2	
Catfish								
Raw	3 Oz	115	6.4	13	0	0	45	
Broiled	3 Oz	129	6.8	16	0	0	68	

	Serv.	K-Cal.	Fat	Prot.	Carb.	Fib.	Sod.	FAC
Catsup (See Ketchup)								
Cauliflower								
Fresh								
Raw	1 Oz	7	0.1	1	1	1	4	**A**
Raw, Chopped	1 Cup	26	0.2	2.0	5	3	30	**FA**
Head	2 Lbs	147	2.1	19	24	23	290	**FA**
Boiled, Drained	1 Cup	29	0.6	2	5	3	19	**FA**
Frozen								
(Frosty Acres)	1 Cup	20	0	2	3	2	25	**FA**
(Green Giant)	1 Cup	25	0	2	4	8	25	**FA**
Caviar								
Black Lumpfish								
(Romanoff)	1 Tbsp	15	1	1	0	0	380	
Lumpfish (Roland)	1 Tbsp	15	0.5	2	0	0	420	
Sturgeon, Granular	1 Tbsp	40	2.9	4	1	0	240	
Cayenne Pepper (See Pepper, Dried)								
Cece Bean (See Bean, Garbanzo)								
Celeriac—Celery Root								
Raw	1 Cup	60	0.4	2	14	3	156	**A**
Celery								
Stalk	1 Med	6	0.1	0	1	1	35	
Boiled	1 Cup	42	0.4	2	9	4	210	**FA**
Chopped	1 Oz	3	0	0	1	1	11	
Diced	1 Cup	34	0.3	2	7.8	4	185	**FA**
Celery Root (See Celeriac)								
Celery Seed								
(McCormick)	1 Tsp	7	0.4	0	1	1	3	
Cellophane Noodles (See Noodle, Chinese)								
Cereal, Ready-to-Serve								
Bran								
(General Mills):								
Bran Flakes	1 Cup	159	0.7	6	39	7	456	**FA**
Fiber One	1 Cup	120	2	4	48	26	250	**FA**
Raisin Nut Bran	1 Cup	280	6	7	55	7	347	**FA**
(Health Valley):								
100% Organic Bran/								
Raisin	1 Cup	212	0	7	52	8	13	**F**
Fiber 7 Flakes	1 Cup	133	0	4	32	5	20	

	Serv.	K-Cal.	Fat	Prot.	Carb.	Fib.	Sod.	FAC
Organic Oat Bran								
Flakes	1 Cup	133	0	4	32	5	20	
Organic Oat Bran O's	1 Cup	133	0	4	31	4	120	
Real Oat Bran, Raisin	1 Cup	400	6	12	68	10	180	**F**
(Kellogg's):								
All Bran......................	½ Cup	80	1	4	22	10	280	**FA**
All Bran Extra								
Fiber.........................	½ Cup	50	1	4	22	15	150	**FA**
Bran Buds..................	½ Cup	105	1.5	5	36	15	315	**FA**
Bran Flakes	1 Cup	133	0.7	4	33	7	307	**FA**
Cracklin' Oat Bran......	1 Cup	307	10.7	5	53	8	240	**FA**
40% Bran Flakes........	1 Cup	127	0.7	5	31	8	363	**FA**
Frosted Bran..............	1 Cup	133	0	3	35	4	267	**FA**
Fruitful Bran...............	1 Cup	136	0.8	3	35	5	264	**F**
Kenmei Rice Bran......	1 Cup	147	1.3	3	33	1	333	**FA**
Oat Bran, *Common*								
Sense.....................	1 Cup	147	1.3	5	31	5	360	**FA**
Raisin Bran................	1 Cup	170	1	5	43	7	310	**FA**
(Mother's) *Oat Bran*	1 Cup	300	6	16	48	12	0	
(Nabisco) *100% Bran*.....	½ Cup	120	0.8	6	35	12	1	**FA**
(Nature Valley) *Fruit &*								
Nut	1 Cup	375	16.5	9	51	5	112	**FA**
(Post):								
Bran Flakes	1 Cup	270	1.5	9	66	18	631	**FA**
Bran'nola, Original	1 Cup	400	6	8	86	10	480	**FA**
40% Bran Flakes........	1 Cup	152	0.8	5	37	9	431	**FA**
Peach/Raisin/Almond								
Fruit & Fibre	1 Cup	210	3	4	46	6	270	**FA**
(Quaker) *Oat Bran*	1 Cup	300	6	16	48	12	0	**A**
Ralston Purina:								
Multibran Chex	1 Cup	176	0.8	4	38	6	240	**F**
Raisin Bran.................	1 Cup	178	0.3	4	47	8	486	**FA**
Corn								
(Barbara's Bakery) *Corn*								
Flakes	1 Cup	110	0	2	26	2	130	**A**
(General Mills) *Country*								
Corn Flakes	1 Cup	120	0.5	2	26	0	290	**FA**
(Health Valley):								
Honey Puffed Corn.....	1 Cup	80	0	2	20	2	0	**FA**
Organic Blue Corn								
Flakes......................	1 Cup	133	0	4	32	4	13	
(Kellogg's):								
Corn Flakes...............	1 Cup	110	0	2	26	1	330	**FA**
Corn Flakes, LS	1 Cup	110	0.1	2	22	1	3	
Corn Pops..................	1 Cup	110	0	1	27	1	95	**FA**
Nutri-Grain, Corn	1 Cup	160	1	3	36	2	276	**FA**
Ralston Purina:								
Corn Chex	1 Cup	88	0	2	21	1	224	**F**
Corn Flakes.................	1 Cup	98	0.1	2	22	0	239	

	Serv.	K-Cal.	Fat	Prot.	Carb.	Fib.	Sod.	FAC
(Cereal, Ready-to-Serve cont.)								
Multigrain								
(General Mills):								
Basic Four	1 Cup	168	2.4	3	34	2	256	**FAC**
Cocoa Puffs	1 Cup	120	1	1	27	0	190	**FA**
Total Corn Flakes	1 Cup	83	0.4	2	19	0	158	**FA**
Total Whole Grain	1 Cup	147	1.3	3	32	4	267	**FAC**
Trix	1 Cup	120	1.5	1	26	0	200	**FA**
(Health Valley):								
Granola O, Apple/Cin.	1 Cup	160	0	4	35	4	13	
Granola, Date &								
Almond	1 Cup	270	0	8	68	9	38	
(Healthy Choice) Raisin/								
Almonds	1 Cup	160	1.6	3	36	3	192	
(Kellogg's):								
Apple Cinnamon								
Squares	1 Cup	240	1.3	5	59	7	20	**F**
Apple Jacks	1 Cup	110	0	2	27	1	135	**FA**
Apple Raisin Crisp	1 Cup	180	0	3	46	4	340	**F**
Cinnamon Mini Buns ..	1 Cup	160	0.7	1	36	1	280	**FA**
Double Dip Crunch	1 Cup	147	0	3	36	0	213	**FA**
Froot Loops	1 Cup	120	1	1	26	1	150	**FA**
Granola-LF	1 Cup	420	6	10	86	6	240	**FA**
Granola W/Raisins,								
LF	1 Cup	315	4.5	8	65	5	202	**FA**
Just Right, Fruit and								
Nuts............................	1 Cup	210	1.5	4	46	3	260	**FA**
Müeslix Golden								
Crunch	1 Cup	280	6.7	8	53	8	373	**FA**
Müeslix Crispy Blend..	1 Cup	300	4.5	6	63	6	285	**FA**
Nut & Honey Crunch								
Oh's............................	1 Cup	160	3.3	4	31	3	267	**FA**
Nutri-Grain Nuggets....	1 Cup	360	2	14	86	14	700	**FA**
Product 19	1 Cup	110	0	3	25	1	280	**FA**
(Nature Valley) Granola .	1 Cup	503	19.6	12	76	4	232	**FA**
(Post):								
Alpha Bits	1 Cup	130	1	3	27	1	210	**FA**
Fruit & Fibre,								
Date/Raisin/Walnut	1 Cup	210	3	4	46	6	260	**FA**
Grape Nuts	1 Cup	400	2	12	94	10	700	**FA**
(Quaker):								
Life	1 Cup	172	2.5	8	30	4	237	**F**
100% Natural, LF,								
Raisin	1 Cup	380	6	8	80	6	190	
Oat								
(General Mills):								
Apple Cinnamon								
Cheerios..................	1 Cup	160	2.7	3	33	1	213	**FA**

	Serv.	K-Cal.	Fat	Prot.	Carb.	Fib.	Sod.	FAC
Cheerios......................	1 Cup	110	2	3	23	3	280	FA
Lucky Charms.............	1 Cup	120	1	2	25	1	210	FAC
Oatmeal Crisp, Almond	1 Cup	220	5	6	42	4	250	F
(Kellogg's) Nut & Honey Crunch	1 Cup	176	3.2	3	36	1	296	FA
(Nature Valley) Toasted Oats & Honey.............	1 Cup	333	13.3	8	48	4	120	A
(Post) Honey Bunches of Oats	1 Cup	160	2	3	33	1	253	FA
(Quaker):								
100% Natural, Oat/ Honey	1 Cup	440	16	10	64	6	50	
Cinnamon Oat Life	1 Cup	190	2	5	39	4	220	
Cinnamon Oat Squares...................	1 Cup	230	2.5	7	48	5	260	F
Quaker Oat Squares ..	1 Cup	220	3	7	44	4	260	F
Toasted Oatmeal, Original	1 Cup	160	1.3	4	33	3	280	
Rice								
(Barbara's Bakery) Brown Rice Crisps......	1 Cup	120	1	2	25	1	125	
(Health Valley):								
Crisp Brown Rice	1 Cup	110	0	1	30	1	0	
Organic Crisp Brown Rice	1 Oz	90	1	2	21	2	3	
(Kellogg's):								
Apple Cinnamon Rice Krispies....................	1 Cup	147	0	3	36	1	293	FA
Cocoa Krispies	1 Cup	160	0.7	3	36	0	253	FA
Kenmei Rice Bran	1 Cup	147	1.3	3	33	1	333	FA
Rice Krispies..............	1 Cup	88	0	2	21	1	256	FA
Rice Krispies Treats ...	1 Cup	160	2	1	33	0	227	FA
Special K	1 Cup	110	0	6	21	1	250	FA
(Quaker) Puffed Rice, Plain	1 Cup	50	0	1	12	0	0	
(Ralston Purina) Rice Chex.............................	1 Cup	120	0	2	27	0	230	F
Wheat								
(General Mills):								
Crispy Wheats N Raisins......................	1 Cup	190	1	4	44	4	270	FA
Total Raisin Bran........	1 Cup	180	1	4	43	5	240	FAC
Wheaties.....................	1 Cup	110	1	3	24	3	220	FA
(Health Valley) Puffed Wheat, LT	1 Cup	100	0	4	22	3	0	
(Kellogg's):								
Blueberry Squares......	1 Cup	240	1.3	5	59	7	20	F

	Serv.	K-Cal.	Fat	Prot.	Carb.	Flb.	Sod.	FAC
(Cereal, Ready-to-Serve cont.)								
Frosted Mini Wheat,								
Bite Size..................	1 Cup	190	1	5	45	6	0	F
Raisin Squares	1 Cup	240	1.3	5	59	7	0	F
Smacks	1 Cup	147	0.7	3	35	1	100	FA
Strawberry Squares....	1 Cup	180	1	4	44	5	10	F
(Nabisco):								
Frosted Wheat Bites...	1 Cup	190	1	4	44	5	10	F
Fruit Wheats,								
Strawberry	1 Cup	227	0.7	5	55	5	20	FA
Shredded Wheat,								
Spoon Size..............	1 Cup	170	0.5	5	41	5	0	F
(Post) *Fruit & Fibre,*								
Peach/Raisin/Almond..	1 Cup	210	3	4	46	6	270	FA

Cereal, Hot (Also See Grits)
(All values for dry cereal)
Barley
(Arrowhead Mills):

	Serv.	K-Cal.	Fat	Prot.	Carb.	Flb.	Sod.	FAC
....	⅓ Cup	140	1	5	35	6	0	
Banana Nut..................	⅓ Cup	170	2.5	4	39	6	240	
Brown Rice								
(Arrowhead Mills) *Rise &*								
Shine...........................	¼ Cup	150	1	3	32	2	0	
(Lundberg):								
Cinnamon/								
Raisin	⅓ Cup	190	1.5	3	42	4	0	
Organic	⅓ Cup	190	2	4	43	3	0	
Sweet Almond	⅓ Cup	200	3.5	3	40	4	0	
(Nabisco) *Cream of Rice*	¼ Cup	170	0	3	38	1	0	
Bulgar								
(Arrowhead Mills)	¼ Cup	150	0.5	3	30	1	0	
(Krusteaz) *Ala*	¼ Cup	150	0.5	4	32	8	5	
Farina								
Enriched	¼ Cup	160	0.3	3	26	1	1	
(Bob's Red Mill) WW	¼ Cup	160	1	5	33	2	1	
Multigrain								
(Bob's Red Mill) 5-Grain	⅓ Cup	140	1	5	29	1	0	
(Fantastic) Maple/Rai-								
sin/3 Grain	¼ Cup	180	1	5	42	5	240	
Peachberry Wheat &								
Oat............................	¼ Cup	190	1.5	5	42	5	260	
Oat Bran, Instant								
(Arrowhead Mills)	⅓ Cup	150	2.5	8	23	7	0	A
(Nabisco) *Honey*	1 Pkt	110	2	3	26	5	160	A
Regular	1 Pkt	80	2	4	20	5	0	A
Oatmeal, Instant								
(Arrowhead Mllls):								
....	1 Pkt	110	2	4	19	2	0	FA

	Serv.	K-Cal.	Fat	Prot.	Carb.	Fib.	Sod.	FAC
Cinnamon/Raisin								
Almond	1 Pkt	130	2	5	24	2	0	**FA**
Maple/Apple Spice	1 Pkt	130	2	4	25	2	40	**FA**
(Fantastic):								
Apple/Cinnamon	⅓ Cup	170	2	6	37	4	240	**FA**
Cranberry/Orange	⅓ Cup	180	2	6	38	4	210	**FA**
(Mother's)	1 Cup	300	6	10	54	8	0	**FA**
(Quaker):								
Apple/Raisin/								
Walnut	1 Pkt	140	2.5	3	27	3	160	**FA**
Blueberry/Cream	1 Pkt	130	2.5	3	27	2	140	**FA**
Cinnamon Graham	1 Pkt	150	2.5	4	30	3	170	**FA**
Cinnamon/Spice	1 Pkt	170	2	4	36	3	290	**FA**
Cinnamon Toast	1 Pkt	130	2	3	27	2	160	**FA**
Honey Nut	1 Pkt	130	3	3	25	2	210	**FA**
Raspberry	1 Pkt	150	3	4	29	3	170	**FA**
Oat								
Maypo	½ Cup	190	2	6	36	3	0	**A**
(Quaker) Old-Fashioned	½ Cup	150	3	6	27	4	0	**FA**
Quick	½ Cup	150	3	6	27	4	0	**FA**
Wheat								
(Arrowhead Mills):								
Bear Mush	¼ Cup	160	1	5	33	2	0	
Cracked	¼ Cup	140	0.5	5	29	6	0	
(Fantastic) *Wheat N'*								
Berries	¼ Cup	170	1	5	40	5	230	
(Krusteaz) *Zoom*	⅓ Cup	120	0.5	6	23	6	0	
Malt-O-Meal	3 Tbsp	120	0	4	26	1	0	
(Nabisco) *Cream of*								
Wheat	1 Tbsp	120	0	3	25	1	0	
(Ralston)	½ Cup	130	1	6	27	6	0	
Wheatena	⅓ Cup	150	0	5	32	5	0	

Chard—Swiss Chard

Raw	1 Cup	7	0.1	1	1	1	77	**A**
Boiled	1 Cup	35	0.1	3	7	4	313	**FA**

Chayote

Raw	1 Cup	33	0.4	1	7	NV	6	

Cheese

American
(Healthy Choice)								
White, Singles	1 Slice	30	0	5	2	1	290	
(Kraft):								
(1 Oz)	1 Slice	110	9	5	1	0	460	
LT (1 Oz)	1 Slice	70	4	6	2	0	420	**C**
(Light N Lively) LF (1 Oz)	1 Slice	67	3.3	7	3	0	373	**C**

	Serv.	K-Cal.	Fat	Prot.	Carb.	Fib.	Sod.	FAC
(Cheese cont.)								
(Nucoa) *Smart Beat,*								
FF..........................	1 Slice	25	0	4	3	0	180	
(Wt Watchers) LS	1 Slice	15	0	3	1	0	75	
Blue								
(1 cup crumbled weighs approximately 4 Oz)								
(Denmark's Finest).........	1 Oz	110	9	6	0	0	330	
(Kraft)............................	1 Oz	100	9.1	6	1	0	331	
(Sargento) Crumbled......	4 Oz	400	32	24	4	0	1,520	AC
(Stella)...........................	1 Oz	100	8	6	1	0	380	
Brie								
(Pere).............................	1 Oz	90	8	5	0	0	170	
(Rouge Et Noir)..............	1 Oz	90	7	6	0	0	210	
(Sargento)......................	1 Oz	95	7.4	6	0	0	178	
Camembert								
(Rouge Et Noir)..............	1 Oz	90	7	6	0	0	210	
(Sargento)......................	1 Oz	85	6.9	6	0	0	239	
Colby								
(Lorraine Lites) LF	1 Oz	90	6	8	1	0	140	C
(Pauly) LS, LF.................	1 Oz	70	3	10	1	0	50	C
(Sargento)......................	1 Cup	440	36	24	2	0	760	AC
Cheddar								
(1 cup weighs approximately 4 oz)								
(Cabot) Vermont............	1 Oz	110	9	7	1	0	180	
(Dorman's) LS, LF	1 Oz	80	5	8	1	0	140	C
(Kraft):								
Chunk.........................	1 Oz	110	9	7	1	0	180	C
Mild, LF.....................	1 Oz	80	5	9	0	0	220	C
Sharp, LF...................	1 Oz	80	5	9	1	0	220	C
(Light N Lively)..............	1 Oz	70	4	6	2	0	380	C
(Pauly) LS, LF.................	1 Oz	70	3	10	1	0	50	C
(Sargento):								
(1 Oz).........................	1 Slice	110	9	6	1	0	160	C
Mootown, LT..............	1 Oz	60	4	7	1	0	170	C
New York...................	1 Oz	114	9.4	7	0	0	176	C
Shredded	1 Cup	440	36	24	4	0	640	AC
Shredded, LT..............	1 Cup	280	18	32	2	0	1,800	AC
(Wt Watchers)	2 Slice	30	0	5	3	0	320	
Cottage								
(1 cup weighs approximately 8 Oz)								
(Crowley):								
1% Milkfat....................	1 Cup	180	2	28	8	0	780	
4% Milkfat....................	1 Cup	240	10	28	8	0	780	
(R.W. Knudsen):								
FF..............................	1 Cup	160	0	30	8	0	740	
2% Milkfat..................	1 Cup	200	5	28	10	0	800	
4% Milkfat..................	1 Cup	240	10	28	8	0	800	
(Lucerne) FF	1 Cup	140	0	28	8	0	840	
(Nancy's) LF...................	1 Cup	160	1	28	6	0	920	

	Serv.	K-Cal.	Fat	Prot.	Carb.	Flb.	Sod.	FAC
(Wt Watchers):								
1% Milkfat..................	1 Cup	180	2	28	8	0	920	
2% Milkfat..................	1 Cup	200	4	28	8	0	920	
Cream								
(2 tbsp weigh approximately 1 Oz)								
(Healthy Choice)	1 Tbsp	13	0	2	1	0	100	
(Horizon) Organic...........	1 Tbsp	50	5	1	1	0	50	
(Kraft):								
Philadelphia	1 Tbsp	50	5	1	1	0	45	
Philadelphia, FF..........	1 Tbsp	13	0	2	1	0	85	
Philadelphia, LT..........	1 Tbsp	35	2.5	2	1	0	75	
Philadelphia, Smoked								
Salmon	1 Tbsp	50	4.5	1	1	0	100	
Philadelphia, Soft........	1 Tbsp	50	5	1	1	0	50	
Philadelphia,								
Whipped..................	1 Tbsp	37	3.7	1	0	0	32	
Philadelphia, W/								
Chives/Onion...........	1 Tbsp	55	5	1	1	0	55	
Edam								
(May Bud)......................	1 Oz	100	8	6	1	0	260	C
(Sargento)......................	1 Oz	101	7.9	7	0	0	274	C
Farmer								
(Healthy Choice) FF.......	1 Cup	180	0	36	8	0	800	C
(Queso Fresco)	1 Cup	357	20.5	30	13	0	323	C
(Sargento)......................	1 Oz	102	8	7	1	0	129	C
Feta								
(Alpine Lace) LF	1 Oz	50	3	5	1	0	370	
(Atheno):								
....	1 Oz	80	6	5	0	0	320	
Brine Pack	1 Oz	80	6	5	0	0	320	
Oil Pack	1 Oz	170	17	3	0	0	135	
(Sargento)......................	1 Oz	80	6	4	1	0	320	
Fontina								
(Denmark's Finest).........	1 Oz	90	7	7	0	0	160	C
(Sargento)......................	1 Oz	110	8.6	7	0	0	227	
Gjetost								
(Sargento)......................	1 Oz	132	8.4	3	12	0	170	
Goat								
Hard..............................	1 Oz	128	10.1	9	1	0	98	C
Semi-soft	1 Oz	103	8.5	6	1	0	146	
Soft	1 Oz	76	6.0	5	0	0	104	
Chaurie, Spreadable	1 Oz	50	4	3	1	0	120	
Couturier, Fresh	1 Oz	70	6	5	0	0	20	
Gorgonzola								
(Stella)	1 Oz	80	9	6	0	0	390	
Gouda								
(Holland)	1 Oz	110	8	7	0	0	250	C
(May Bud)......................	1 Oz	100	8	7	0	1	210	C
(Sargento)......................	1 Oz	101	7.8	7	1	0	232	C

	Serv.	K-Cal.	Fat	Prot.	Carb.	Fib.	Sod.	FAC
(Cheese cont.)								
Havarti								
(Denmark's Finest).........	1 Oz	120	10	5	0	0	150	C
(Sargento).....................	1 Oz	118	10.6	5	0	0	200	C
Lappi								
(Finlandia).....................	1 Oz	100	8	7	0	0	160	C
Limburger								
(Honey Creek)...............	1 Oz	90	8	6	0	0	240	
(Sargento).....................	1 Oz	93	7.7	6	0	0	227	
Mexican								
(Healthy Choice) FF.......	1 Cup	180	0	36	8	0	800	AC
Queso Anejo	1 Oz	104	8.4	6	1	0	323	
Queso Asadero	1 Cup	402	32	26	3	0	722	AC
(Ranchero) Fresco	1 Oz	80	6	6	0	0	220	
(Sargento) Blanco	1 Oz	104	8.5	7	0	0	178	
(Sargento) Blend............	1 Cup	440	36	24	2	0	800	AC
Monterey Jack								
(Dormans)								
LS.................................	1 Oz	80	5	8	1	0	140	C
(Kraft) Jalapeño..............	1 Oz	110	9	7	1	0	190	C
LF.................................	1 Oz	80	5	9	0	0	220	AC
(Sargento) Shredded......	1 Cup	400	36	24	0	0	760	C
Sliced	1 Slice	100	9	6	0	0	190	C
Mozzarella								
(1 cup shredded weighs approximately 4 Oz)								
(Dormans) LS.................	1 Oz	80	4	9	1	0	140	C
(Healthy Choice):								
FF.................................	1 Oz	45	0	10	1	1	200	C
Shredded, FF..............	1 Cup	180	0	36	8	0	800	AC
String, FF....................	1 Oz	45	0	9	1	0	200	C
(Kraft) Shredded, RF	1 Cup	320	20	36	2	0	840	AC
(Polly-O) LT...................	1 Oz	60	2.5	7	0	0	230	
(Polly-O) Whole Milk	1 Oz	80	6	6	0	0	220	
(Precious):								
FF.................................	1 Oz	30	0	7	1	0	290	
LF.................................	1 Oz	70	3	8	1	0	180	
Part Skim	1 Oz	80	6	8	1	0	150	
(Sargento) Shredded......	1 Cup	320	24	28	4	0	600	AC
Shredded, LT..............	1 Cup	280	12	32	2	0	560	AC
Muenster								
(Dormans) LS.................	1 Oz	80	5	8	0	0	140	C
(Finlandia)	1 Oz	110	9	7	0	0	180	C
LT.................................	1 Oz	80	4	8	0	0	180	
(Sargento) Sliced	1 Slice	100	9	6	1	0	200	AC
Neufchatel								
(2 tbsp weigh approximately 1 Oz)								
Organic (Horizon)...........	1 Oz	70	6	3	0	0	120	
Philadelphia (Kraft).........	1 Oz	70	6	3	1	0	120	

	Serv.	K-Cal.	Fat	Prot.	Carb.	Fib.	Sod.	FAC
Parmesan								
(1 cup weighs approximately 4 Oz)								
(Kraft) Cube....................	1 Tbsp	20	1	2	0	0	55	
Grated.........................	2 Tsp	20	1.5	2	0	0	85	
(Sargento):.....................	1 Oz	111	7.3	10	1	0	454	C
Shredded	1 Cup	440	28	36	4	0	1,200	AC
W/Romano..................	1 Cup	440	28	36	4	0	1,360	AC
(Stella)	1 Oz	100	7	9	0	0	390	C
(Wt Watchers) FF	1 Tbsp	20	0	2	2	0	60	
Provolone								
(Dormans) LS.................	1 Oz	80	4	9	1	0	140	C
(Kraft) Sliced	1 Slice	150	11	11	0	0	370	C
(Sargento) Sliced	1 Slice	100	8	7	0	0	190	C
(Stella)	1 Oz	100	8	7	0	0	290	C
Ricotta								
(1 cup weighs approximately 9 Oz)								
(Frigo) FF	1 Cup	190	1.6	34	10	0	488	AC
(Frigo) LF	1 Cup	257	7.4	37	11	0	390	C
(Gardenia) LF	1 Cup	258	11.2	31	9	0	634	C
(Precious):								
FF.............................	1 Cup	240	0	40	20	0	240	C
LF.............................	1 Cup	280	12	24	12	0	180	C
Part Skim...................	1 Cup	400	24	32	8	0	320	C
(Sargento):								
LT.............................	1 Cup	240	10	20	12	0	220	C
Part Skim...................	1 Cup	320	20	28	8	0	300	AC
Old-Fashioned	1 Cup	360	24	28	12	0	300	AC
Romano								
(Sargento)......................	1 Oz	110	7.6	9	1	0	340	C
(Stella)	1 Oz	100	8	8	1	0	390	C
Roquefort								
(Societe)	1 Oz	110	9	5	0	0	460	C
String								
(Horizon) Organic,								
Mozzarella..................	1 Oz	80	5	7	0	0	170	C
(Kraft) Part Skim,								
Mozzarella..................	1 Item	80	6	7	1	0	240	
(Precious) Mozzarella	1 Oz	80	5	8	1	0	180	C
(Sargento):								
Mootown, LT..............	1 Piece	60	3	7	1	0	200	C
Mootown Snack..........	1 Piece	70	5	6	1	0	170	C
Smoked......................	1 Oz	79	4.9	8	1	0	150	C
Swiss								
(County Line) LS, RF.....	1 Oz	80	4	10	1	0	50	C
(Deli Light) LS...............	1 Oz	100	8	8	0	0	8	C
(Dormans) LS, LF..........	1 Oz	90	5	10	0	0	60	C
(Kraft) LS......................	1 Oz	110	8	8	1	0	10	C
(Kraft) Natural...............	1 Oz	90	5	10	1	0	70	C
(Light N Lively)...............	1 Oz	70	3	6	2	0	350	C

	Serv.	K-Cal.	Fat	Prot.	Carb.	Fib.	Sod.	FAC
(Cheese cont.)								
(Pauly) LS, RF	1 Oz	97	7	9	1	0	32	C
(Sargento):								
Jarlsberg	1 Slice	120	9	9	1	0	160	AC
Shredded	1 Cup	440	32	32	0	0	160	C
Sliced	1 Slice	80	6	6	0	0	30	C
Sliced, LT....................	1 Slice	80	4	9	1	0	50	C
(Tine) LT.....................	1 Oz	70	35	9	0	0	130	C
(Wt Watchers) FF	1 Slice	15	0	3	1	0	140	

Cheese Alternative, Rice
	Serv.	K-Cal.	Fat	Prot.	Carb.	Fib.	Sod.	FAC
(Soyco) Mozzarella	1 Oz	40	2	4	1	0	240	CA
Parmesan....................	2 Tsp	15	0.5	2	1	0	80	

Cheese, Alternative, Soy
Cheddar
	Serv.	K-Cal.	Fat	Prot.	Carb.	Fib.	Sod.	FAC
(Rella)	1 Oz	60	3	5	2	0	290	CA
(Sargento) Shredded......	1 Cup	360	28	20	8	0	1,680	C
(Soya Kaas) FF..............	1 Oz	40	0	7	2	0	250	
Cream Cheese								
(Rella) Vegan	1 Tbsp	40	3	0	3	0	42	
(Soya Kaas)	1 Tbsp	100	9	3	1	0	110	
(Tofutti)	1 Tbsp	40	4	1	1	NV	68	
Monterey Jack								
(Soya Kaas)	1 Oz	70	5	6	1	0	250	
Mozzarella								
(Nutofu) FF.....................	1 Oz	40	0	7	2	0	220	
(Rella)	1 Oz	60	3	5	2	0	290	CA
(Sargento) Shredded......	1 Cup	320	24	24	2	0	1,280	C
(Savoldi)	1 Oz	80	7	4	1	0	330	
Parmesan								
(Soyco)	1 Tsp	8	0.3	1	0	0	40	

Cheese Food
	Serv.	K-Cal.	Fat	Prot.	Carb.	Fib.	Sod.	FAC
(Cracker Barrel):								
Sharp Cheddar	1 Tbsp	50	4	3	2	0	145	
Sharp Cheddar, RF	1 Oz	80	5	9	1	0	220	C
(Kraft):								
American, Sliced........	1 Oz	92	6.7	5	3	0	383	
Garlic............................	1 Oz	90	7	5	2	0	370	
Jalapeño	1 Oz	90	7	5	2	0	370	
Jalapeño, Singles	1 Oz	93	6.7	5	3	0	440	
Monterey, Singles.......	1 Oz	93	6.7	5	3	0	387	
Pimento, Singles.........	1 Oz	90	6.8	6	2	0	390	
Sharp, Singles	1 Oz	93	8	5	1	0	400	
Swiss, Singles	1 Oz	93	6.7	5	1	0	427	C
(Nucoa) *Smart Beat*,								
Nondairy, FF...............	1 Slice	25	0	4	3	0	220	

	Serv.	K-Cal.	Fat	Prot.	Carb.	Flb.	Sod.	FAC
(Sargento) Swiss Almond Nut Log.............	1 Oz	94	7.4	6	2	0	349	C
(Velveeta):								
Mexican, Shredded.....	1 Cup	520	36	32	12	0	2,160	AC
Shredded	1 Cup	520	36	32	12	0	2,000	AC

Cheese Snack

	Serv.	K-Cal.	Fat	Prot.	Carb.	Flb.	Sod.	FAC
(Barbara's):								
Puffs.............................	1 Cup	200	13.3	3	21	0	173	
Puffs, Bakes	1 Cup	107	7.3	1	9	0	127	
Puffs, Jalapeño...........	1 Cup	200	12	3	20	0	333	
(Bearitos) Puffs, Original	1 Oz	160	10	2	14	NV	260	
(Frito-Lay):								
Chee-tos Chip, LT	1 Oz	120	6	2	16	1	270	
Chee-tos Curls..........	1 Oz	150	9	2	16	1	280	
(General Mills) *Chex Mix*, Traditional	1 Oz	117	3.2	3	20	1	252	F
(Health Valley):								
Puffs, LT	1 Oz	160	8	4	16	0	140	
Puffs, Original, FF	1 Cup	73	0	2	15	1	173	
Puffs, W/Green Onion, FF.............................	1 Cup	73	0	2	15	1	173	
(Ultra Slim-Fast) Curl-Lite	1 Oz	110	3	2	20	3	360	
(Wt Watchers) Curls	1 Oz	140	5.0	2	20	0	170	

Cheese, Spreads

(2 tbsp weigh approximately 1 Oz)

	Serv.	K-Cal.	Fat	Prot.	Carb.	Flb.	Sod.	FAC
(Alouette) Garlic Herb	2 Tbsp	50	4	2	1	0	120	
Vegetable....................	1 Oz	60	4.5	3	1	0	120	
(Cheez Whiz):								
....	1 Tbsp	45	3.5	3	1	0	280	
Hot Salsa....................	1 Tbsp	45	3.5	3	1	0	265	
Jalapeño	1 Tbsp	45	4	3	1	0	265	
(Kraft):								
American.....................	1 Oz	80	6	4	2	0	470	
Bacon..........................	1 Oz	80	7	5	1	0	560	
Jalapeño Loaf.............	1 Oz	80	6	5	2	0	470	
(Mohawk Valley) Limburger....................	1 Tbsp	40	3.5	2	0	0	250	
(Nabisco):								
American, *Easy Cheese*.....................	1 Tbsp	50	3.5	3	1	0	200	
Cheddar & Bacon.......	1 Tbsp	50	3.5	3	2	0	205	
Cheddar, *Easy Cheese*	1 Tbsp	50	3.5	3	2	0	205	
Nacho, *Easy Cheese* .	1 Tbsp	50	3.5	3	2	0	195	
Sharp Cheddar, *Easy Cheese*........................	1 Tbsp	50	3.5	3	2	0	220	

	Serv.	K-Cal.	Fat	Prot.	Carb.	Flb.	Sod.	FAC
(Cheese cont.)								
(Rondele):								
French Onion	1 Oz	95	9	2	2	0	205	
Garden Veg	2 Tbsp	90	9	2	1	0	180	
(Squeez-A-Snak):								
Bacon	1 Oz	80	7	5	1	0	500	
Garlic	1 Oz	80	7	5	1	0	430	
Hickory Smoke	1 Oz	80	7	5	1	0	440	
Jalapeño	1 Oz	80	6	5	1	0	510	
Sharp	1 Tbsp	45	4	3	0	0	220	
(Velveeta) Hot Mexican	1 Oz	80	6	5	2	0	520	

Cherimoya
Raw	1 Item	514	2.2	7	131	13	NV	A
Raw	6 Oz	160	.7	2	41	4	NV	A

Cherry
Fresh
Sweet (5 Oz)	1 Cup	90	1	1	19	3	0	A
Sweet	1 Item	5	0.1	0	1	0	1	
Sour	1 Cup	78	0.5	2	19	2	25	A

Canned, Sweet-Packed W/
Extra Heavy Syrup	1 Cup	266	0.4	2	69	4	8	
Heavy Syrup	1 Cup	213	0.4	2	55	4	8	
Juice	1 Cup	135	0.1	2	35	4	8	
Light Syrup	1 Cup	169	0.4	2	44	2	8	
Water	1 Cup	114	0.3	2	29	4	2	

Canned, Sour-Packed W/
Extra Heavy Syrup	1 Cup	298	0.2	2	76	2	18	
Heavy Syrup	1 Cup	233	0.3	2	60	3	18	
Light Syrup	1 Cup	189	0.3	2	49	2	18	
Water	1 Cup	88	0.2	2	22	3	17	

Frozen
Sweet, Sweetened	1 Cup	231	0.3	3	58	5	3	
Sour, Unsweetened	1 Cup	71	0.7	1	17	2	2	

Maraschino
W/Stems (S & W)	1 Item	10	0	0	3	0	0	

Cherry Juice
Black Cherry (Heinke's)	1 Cup	180	0	2	43	NV	40	
Black Cherry (R.W. Knudsen)	1 Cup	180	0	2	43	NV	40	
Cider (R.W. Knudsen)	1 Cup	130	0	0	33	NV	35	
Juicy Juice (Libby's)	1 Cup	130	0	1	32	0	10	
Nectar (Santa Cruz Farms)	1 Cup	110	0	0	26	NV	20	

Chervil
Dried (McCormick)	1 Tsp	2	0	0	0	0	1	

	Serv.	K-Cal.	Fat	Prot.	Carb.	Fib.	Sod.	FAC
Chestnut, Chinese								
Raw	1 Oz	64	0.3	1	14	NV	1	
Dried	1 Oz	103	0.5	2	23	NV	1	A
Dried	2 Oz	206	1.0	4	45	NV	3	FA
Chestnut, European—Italian—Sweet								
Raw, Shelled, Peeled	1 Oz	56	0.4	0.5	13	0	1	
Dried, Shelled, Peeled ...	1 Oz	105	1.1	1	22	1	11	
Roasted, Shelled	1 Oz	70	0.6	0.9	15	3	1	
Chestnut Puree								
(Faugier)	2 Tbsp	30	0	0	6	1	0	
Chestnut Spread								
(Faugier)	2 Tbsp	80	0	0	20	0	0	
Chicken								
Back								
Meat Only, Roasted	4 Oz	271	14.9	32	0	0	109	
Meat Only, Stewed	4 Oz	238	12.7	29	0	0	24	
Meat/Skin, Roasted	4 Oz	340	23.8	29	0	0	96	
Meat/Skin, Stewed	4 Oz	295	20.7	23	0	0	73	
Breast								
Meat Only, Roasted	4 Oz	186	4.0	35	0	0	17	
Meat Only, Stewed	4 Oz	172	3.5	33	0	0	15	
Meat/Skin, Batter-fried ...	4 Oz	298	15.2	29	10	0	23	
Meat/Skin, Roasted	4 Oz	222	8.8	34	0	0	80	
Dark Meat								
Meat Only, Roasted	4 Oz	232	11.0	31	0	0	105	
Meat Only, Stewed	4 Oz	218	10.2	29	0	0	84	
Meat/Skin, Roasted	4 Oz	287	17.9	30	0	0	99	
Meat/Skin, Stewed	4 Oz	266	16.7	27	0	0	80	
Drumstick								
Meat Only, Fried	4 Oz	221	9.2	32	0	0	109	
Meat Only, Roasted/ Broiled	4 Oz	195	6.4	32	0	0	14	
Meat Only, Stewed	4 Oz	192	6.5	31	0	0	91	
Meat/Skin, Batter-fried ...	4 Oz	303	17.8	25	9	0	305	
Meat/Skin, Roasted/ Broiled	4 Oz	244	12.6	31	0	0	102	
Meat/Skin, Stewed	4 Oz	232	12.1	29	0	0	87	
Leg								
Meat Only, Broiled	4 Oz	220	9.7	31	0	0	14	
Meat Only, Fried	4 Oz	235	10.5	32	1	0	108	
Meat Only, Stewed	4 Oz	209	9.1	30	0	0	88	
Meat/Skin, Roasted	4 Oz	268	15.5	30	0	0	100	
Meat/Skin, Stewed	4 Oz	247	14.5	27	0	0	12	

	Serv.	K-Cal.	Fat	Prot.	Carb.	Fib.	Sod.	FAC
(Chicken cont.)								
Light Meat								
Meat Only, Fried	4 Oz	218	6.3	37	1	0	92	
Meat Only, Roasted	4 Oz	196	5.1	35	0	0	87	
Meat Only, Stewed	4 Oz	181	4.5	33	0	0	74	
Meat/Skin, Batter-fried	4 Oz	313	17.4	27	11	0	324	
Meat/Skin, Roasted	4 Oz	251	12.3	33	0	0	85	
Meat/Skin, Stewed	4 Oz	229	11.4	30	0	0	72	
Liver								
Simmered	4 Oz	178	6.2	28	1	0	16	FA
Thigh								
Meat Only, Roasted	4 Oz	238	12.3	29	0	0	14	
Meat Only, Stewed	4 Oz	224	11.3	29	0	0	13	
Meat/Skin, Batter-fried	4 Oz	309	18.5	24	10	0	20	
Meat/Skin, Roasted/ Broiled	4 Oz	275	17.3	28	0	0	13	
Meat/Skin, Stewed	4 Oz	284	18	28	0	0	87	
Wing								
Meat Only, Fried	4 Oz	240	10.4	34	0	0	103	
Meat Only, Roasted	4 Oz	230	9.3	35	0	0	104	
Meat Only, Stewed	4 Oz	204	8.1	31	0	0	15	
Meat/Skin, Batter-fried	4 Oz	369	24.8	23	12	0	23	
Meat/Skin, Roasted	4 Oz	329	22.1	31	0	0	93	
Meat/Skin, Stewed	4 Oz	283	22.5	26	0	0	76	
Chicken, Alternative								
Canned								
(Loma Linda) *Chik'n*								
Fried W/Gravy	2.6 Oz	193	15.4	11	3	2	407	
(Worthington):								
Diced Chik (8 Oz)	1 Cup	226	14	22	3	3	942	
Fried Chik	1.6 Oz	58	4	5	1	1	214	
Sliced (1 Oz)	1 Slice	45	4	2	1	NV	165	
Frozen								
(Loma Linda) *Chik*								
Nuggets	0.5 Oz	49	3.2	2	3	1	142	
Fried Chik'n	2 Oz	180	15	11	<1	<1	500	
(Morningstar) *Chik*								
Patties	2.5 Oz	177	9.8	7	15	2	536	
(Worthington):								
Chicken, Meatless	3.2 Oz	180	13	11	4	4	610	
Chicken, Meatless, Diced	1 Cup	226	14	20	4	4	942	
Crispychik Patties	2.5 Oz	175	9.4	8	15	4	596	
Shikstiks	1.7 Oz	111	7.3	9	3	2	355	
Vegetarian Chicken Pie	8 Oz	450	27	9	44	8	1080	

	Serv.	K-Cal.	Fat	Prot.	Carb.	Fib.	Sod.	FAC
Chicken, Canned								
Breast (Hormel)	2 Oz	60	1.5	12	0	0	200	
Chunk (Hormel)	2 Oz	70	3	12	0	0	200	
Chunk in Water (Valley Fresh)	2 Oz	70	1	15	0	0	130	
Spread (Underwood)	¼ Cup	120	8	9	2	9	390	
Stew (Dinty Moore)	1 Cup	220	11	12	16	2	980	
White Premium (Swanson)	2.5 Oz	80	2	15	1	0	240	
Chicken Entree and Dinner, Frozen								
A La King								
(Le Menu) *Lightstyle*	8.24 Oz	240	5	19	29	NV	670	
(Stouffer's)	9.5 Oz	320	10	15	43	3	750	
A L'Orange								
(Healthy Choice)	9 Oz	260	2	23	38	NV	340	
(Smart Ones)	8 Oz	200	1	12	35	2	320	
(Stouffer's) *Lean Cuisine*	9 Oz	260	2.5	19	40	1	260	
Barbecue								
(Banquet)	9 Oz	320	12	18	36	3	800	
(Healthy Choice):								
Mesquite	10.5 Oz	320	2	19	55	6	290	A
Smokey	12.75 Oz	380	5	25	57	7	450	A
(Light and Elegant)	8 Oz	300	6	26	35	3	900	
(Stouffer's) *Lean Cuisine:*								
Rice Pilaf	8.75 Oz	260	6	20	32	NV	500	A
W/Honey	8.5 Oz	250	4.5	18	35	6	560	
(Tysons) *Healthy Portions*	10.8 Oz	258	9.8	18	49	6	588	
(Wt Watchers)	9 Oz	230	2.5	20	33	4	440	A
Cacciatore								
(Healthy Choice)	12.5 Oz	260	3	22	36	6	510	A
(Light Balance)	8.25 Oz	200	1	12	37	3	730	A
(Stouffer's) Dinner	11.25 Oz	310	11	25	29	3	1,135	A
(Stouffer's) *Lean Cuisine,* W/Vegetables	10.75 Oz	280	7	22	31	NV	570	
(Swanson) *Home-style*	1 Oz	24	0.7	1	3	0	94	
Chow Mein								
(Banquet)	9 Oz	210	7	9	28	3	850	
(Healthy Choice)	9 Oz	240	5	20	29	NV	530	
(Le Menu) LT	10 Oz	260	4	18	37	1	830	A
(Stouffer's)	8 Oz	130	4	13	11	1	1,080	A
(Stouffer's) *Lean Cuisine,* W/Rice	9 Oz	210	5	13	28	2	510	
(Wt Watchers)	9 Oz	200	2	12	34	3	490	A
Cordon Bleu								
(Le Menu) *Lightstyle* Dinner	11 Oz	460	20	23	47	NV	850	A
(Wt Watchers)	9 Oz	230	4.5	15	31	2	650	A

	Serv.		K-Cal.	Fat	Prot.	Carb.	Fib.	Sod.	FAC
(Chicken Entree and Dinner, Frozen cont.)									
Dijon									
(Healthy Choice)	11	Oz	280	4	21	41	9	410	
(Le Menu) Light Style	8	Oz	240	7	22	21	NV	500	A
Enchilada									
(Don Miguel)..................	12	Oz	410	8	17	67	10	1,220	
(Healthy Choice) Suiza..	10	Oz	270	4	14	43	5	440	
(Healthy Choice)									
Suprema	13.4	Oz	390	9	17	60	8	390	AC
(Stouffer's) W/Rice	10	Oz	370	14	16	45	3	970	C
Fettucini									
(Budget Gourmet)	10	Oz	380	19	20	33	3	810	
(Healthy Choice) Alfredo	8.5	Oz	260	4.5	22	35	3	410	
(Stouffer's) Lean Cuisine	9	Oz	270	6	22	33	2	580	
(Ultra Slim-Fast)	12	Oz	400	10	31	46	6	780	A
(Wt Watchers)	10	Oz	290	7	19	39	4	590	
Fiesta									
(Light Balance)...............	8.25	Oz	210	3	10	37	NV	640	
(Stouffer's) Lean Cuisine,									
W/Rice/Veg................	8.5	Oz	260	5	19	35	3	550	
(Wt Watchers)	8.5	Oz	220	2	12	38	5	480	
Français									
(Tyson)	9	Oz	258	9.9	19	23	6	794	A
(Wt Watchers)	8.5	Oz	150	1	14	21	4	390	
Fried									
(Banquet)........................	9	Oz	470	27	21	35	6	980	
(Banquet) White Meat....	8.75	Oz	470	28	22	33	6	1,100	
(Stouffer's) Homestyle,									
W/Potato	7	Oz	330	16	18	29	3	780	C
(Swanson):									
Dinner, Dark	10	Oz	550	28	24	50	4	1,530	
Dinner, White.............	10.5	Oz	560	26	27	54	5	1,710	
Hungry Man, Dinner,									
Dark........................	13.75	Oz	810	41	34	76	9	1,710	
Hungry Man, Dinner,									
White	14.5	Oz	810	40	35	77	7	2.060	
M. Potatoes, Entree ...	7	Oz	400	21	19	34	2	1,120	
Garlic									
(Banquet)........................	9	Oz	220	7	10	29	4	1,040	
(Healthy Choice) Hearty									
Handful......................	6	Oz	330	5	20	53	6	600	A
(Healthy Choice) Milano	9.5	Oz	240	4	18	34	3	510	A
Glazed									
(Budget Light).................	9	Oz	300	2	15	56	1	920	
(Healthy Choice)									
Southwestern	12.5	Oz	300	3	20	48	6	430	A
(Le Menu) Lightstyle									
Dinner, Breast.............	10	Oz	230	3	25	25	NV	480	
(Light and Elegant)	8	Oz	230	4	24	25	NV	655	

	Serv.	K-Cal.	Fat	Prot.	Carb.	Fib.	Sod.	FAC
(Stouffer's) *Lean Cuisine,*								
W/Rice/Veg	8.5 Oz	240	6	22	24	2	460	
(Wt Watchers)	9.25 Oz	240	6	18	29	4	550	
Grilled								
(Tyson) W/Corn & Beans	9 Oz	234	3.9	19	30	7	589	
(Wt Watchers)	8 Oz	130	1	12	20	3	460	
(Wt Watchers) Suiza	8.5 Oz	240	6	22	25	3	590	
Herb								
(Le Menu) *Lightstyle*	10 Oz	240	7	27	18	NV	400	A
(Light and Healthy)								
Breast	11 Oz	240	7	23	28	6	430	
(Stouffer's) *Lean Cuisine,*								
Cafe Classic	8 Oz	210	5	17	25	4	430	A
Honey Mustard								
(Healthy Choice)	9.5 Oz	260	2	21	40	4	550	A
(Stouffer's) *Lean Cuisine*	7.5 Oz	270	5	16	39	3	580	A
(Wt Watchers)	8.5 Oz	200	2	13	33	36	340	
Imperial								
(Healthy Choice)	9 Oz	230	4	17	31	3	470	
(Wt Watchers)	8.5 Oz	200	3	18	25	4	420	
Italian								
(Right Course)	9.5 Oz	280	8	24	29	NV	560	A
(Stouffer's) *Lean Cuisine*	9 Oz	270	6	22	31	3	560	
(Tyson) *Healthy Portion*	11.5 Oz	328	6.7	24	43	5	664	A
(Tyson) Pasta & Vegs	9 Oz	193	3.7	21	19	3	436	
Mandarin								
(Budget Gourmet Light)	10 Oz	250	5	16	37	4	850	
(Healthy Choice)	10 Oz	280	2.5	20	44	4	520	A
(Stouffer's) *Lean Cuisine,*								
Lunch Express	9.75 Oz	270	6	12	41	2	520	
Marsala								
(Healthy Choice) W/								
Vegetables	11.5	220	1	22	32	3	440	
(Stouffer's) *Lean Cuisine*	8 Oz	180	4	22	13	5	470	A
(Wt Watchers)	9 Oz	150	2	10	22	6	500	
Mesquite								
(Tyson) W/Corn/Peas/								
Potato	9 Oz	308	7.1	23	38	6	593	
(Ultra Slim-Fast) W/Rice	12 Oz	360	1	29	61	0	170	A
Nuggets								
(Banquet)	6.75 Oz	410	21	18	38	4	650	
(Swanson) Dinner	9.5 Oz	440	19	18	48	4	980	
Oriental								
(Banquet)	9 Oz	260	9	12	34	4	610	
(Healthy Choice)	11.25 Oz	200	1	19	32	NV	440	A
(Healthy Choice) W/								
Peanut Sauce	9.5 Oz	280	5	29	31	NV	400	
(Stouffer's) *Lean Cuisine*	9.5 Oz	230	6	22	23	2	790	A

	Serv.		K-Cal.	Fat	Prot.	Carb.	Fib.	Sod.	FAC
(Chicken Entree and Dinner, Frozen cont.)									
(Stouffer's) *Lean Cuisine,* Vermicelli W/Vegs	9	Oz	260	6	21	30	3	530	
Parmigiana									
(Banquet)........................	9.5	Oz	290	15	14	27	3	900	
(Healthy Choice)	11.5	Oz	300	4	20	47	5	490	A
(Le Menu) Dinner...........	11.75	Oz	410	20	26	31	NV	1,030	
(Light and Elegant)	8	Oz	260	6	28	23	2	685	A
(Light and Healthy)	11	Oz	260	8	22	29	5	420	
(Stouffer's) *Homestyle*....	11	Oz	320	10	27	30	4	890	
(Stouffer's) *Lean uisine*..........................	11	Oz	240	7	20	25	4	580	AC
(Wt Watchers)	10	Oz	310	7	21	39	4	500	
Sesame									
(Healthy Choice)	9.75	Oz	240	3	16	38	3	600	
(Healthy Choice) Shanghai....................	12	Oz	310	5	24	42	5	460	
(Right Course)................	10	Oz	320	9	25	34	NV	590	
Southern-Fried									
(Banquet)........................	8.75	Oz	520	31	26	32	4	1,410	
(Wt Watchers)	8	Oz	280	11	19	25	1	590	
Sweet and Sour									
(Budget Gourmet)	10	Oz	330	5	18	55	4	700	A
(Healthy Choice)	10	Oz	310	5	23	42	5	250	
(Le Menu) Dinner...........	11.25	Oz	400	18	19	41	NV	1,020	A
Lightstyle Dinner..........	10	Oz	250	7	18	29	NV	530	A
(Stouffer's) *Lean Cuisine,* W/Vegetables...............	10.5	Oz	260	2.5	17	43	3	440	A
(Ultra Slim-Fast)	12	Oz	330	2	20	57	2	160	
Tenders									
(Right Course) Barbecue	8.75	Oz	270	6	20	35	NV	590	A
(Right Course) W/ Peanut....................	9.25	Oz	330	10	27	32	NV	570	
(Stouffer's) *Homestyle*....	6.5	Oz	380	18	21	33	4	1,060	C
(Tyson) Glazed W/ Pilaf & Veg	9	Oz	236	5.8	16	30	2	450	A
Teriyaki									
(Banquet)........................	9	Oz	230	6	11	32	3	1,110	
(Healthy Choice)	12.25	Oz	270	2	21	42	5	420	
(Healthy Choice) W/ Pasta...........................	12.5	Oz	350	3	24	58	NV	370	

Chicken Entree, Canned

	Serv.		K-Cal.	Fat	Prot.	Carb.	Fib.	Sod.	FAC
(La Choy) Chicken Chow Mein	1	Cup	80	3.5	8	6	3	1,352	
(Libby's) Chicken Vienna Sausage......................	1	Item	33	2.7	2	0	0	150	

	Serv.	K-Cal.	Fat	Prot.	Carb.	Fib.	Sod.	FAC
(Swanson) Chicken A La King	1 Cup	320	22	15	17	0	1,080	
(Swanson) Chicken & Dumplings	1 Cup	260	13	13	22	0	1,120	

Chicken Entree, Packaged
(Prepared as indicated on package)
(Betty Crocker) *Chicken Helper.*

	Serv.	K-Cal.	Fat	Prot.	Carb.	Fib.	Sod.	FAC
Cheesy Broccoli	7 Oz	310	9	24	34	NV	790	
Creamy Chicken	8.2 Oz	330	13	26	29	NV	820	
Creamy Mushroom	8 Oz	320	11	25	31	NV	810	
Fettucini Alfredo	7.5 Oz	320	12	26	27	NV	780	
Stir-Fried Mix	7 Oz	370	14	25	36	NV	950	

Chicken Entree, Refrigerated
(Chicken By George):

	Serv.	K-Cal.	Fat	Prot.	Carb.	Fib.	Sod.	FAC
Lemon Herb	4 Oz	120	3	20	3	0	800	
Mustard Dill	4 Oz	140	5	20	2	0	650	
Roasted	4 Oz	110	3	20	1	0	500	

Chicken, Fast Food

	Serv.	K-Cal.	Fat	Prot.	Carb.	Fib.	Sod.	FAC
(Arby's) *Cordon Bleu*	8.5 Oz	623	33	38	46	5	1,594	
(Burger King) *Tenders*	0.5 Oz	38	2	3	2	0	88	
(Carl's Jr) *Stars*	0.5 Oz	38	2.3	2	2	0	75	
(Jack In The Box):								
Fajita Pita	6.7 Oz	290	8	24	29	3	700	C
Strips	4 Oz	290	13	25	18	0	700	
Taquitos	4.7 Oz	350	15	19	34	4	570	
Teriyaki Bowl	15.5 Oz	580	1.5	28	115	6	1,220	A
(KFC):								
Breast, *Original*	3.7 Oz	260	14	25	8	NV	609	
Breast/Wing W/Skin	6.2 Oz	335	18.7	40	1	0	1,104	
Breast, *Extra Tasty Crispy*	6 Oz	470	28	31	25	1	930	
Drumstick, *Original*	2 Oz	130	7	13	4	0	210	
Nuggets	0.5 Oz	47	3	3	3	NV	144	
Thigh, *Extra Tasty Crispy*	4.2 Oz	370	25	19	18	2	540	
Thigh, *Original*	3.2 Oz	260	17	19	9	1	570	
Wing, *Hot & Spicy*	2 Oz	210	15	10	9	1	340	
Wing, *Original*	2 Oz	150	8	11	7	0	380	
(McDonald's) *Fajita*	3 Oz	190	8	11	20	NV	310	
(McDonald's) *Nuggets*	2.5 Oz	200	12	12	10	0	350	
(Wendy's) *Nuggets*	3.2 Oz	280	20	14	12	0	600	

Chicken Fat

	Serv.	K-Cal.	Fat	Prot.	Carb.	Fib.	Sod.	FAC
(Empire)	1 Tbsp	120	13	0	0	0	0	

	Serv.	K-Cal.	Fat	Prot.	Carb.	Fib.	Sod.	FAC
Chicken, Luncheon Meat								
Breast								
(Healthy Choice) FF.......	1 Slice	8	0	2	0	0	78	
(Hillshire Farm) Smoked	1 Slice	10	0.1	2	1	0	95	
(Oscar Mayer) FF	1 Slice	11	0	2	0	0	162	
W/Honey, Thin............	1 Slice	15	0.4	3	1	0	185	
(Louis Rich):								
Deluxe..........................	1 Slice	30	0.5	5	1	0	330	
Thin.............................	1 Slice	15	0.4	2	0	0	155	
W/Honey, *Carving Bird*.	1 Slice	23	0.3	5	1	0	265	
Roll								
(Tyson) White.................	1 Slice	31	1.9	3	0	0	148	
Smoked								
(Healthy Choice)	1 Slice	35	1	6	0	0	210	
(Mr. Turkey) Deli Cut,								
FF.................................	1 Slice	9	0	2	1	0	119	
(Tyson) FF......................	1 Slice	17	0.1	4	0	0	218	
Chicken, Luncheon Meat, Alternative								
(White Wave)	2 Slices	80	0	12	8	0	260	
(Worthington) Chicken ...	2 Slices	80	4.5	9	1	1	370	
Chic-Ketts	1 Oz	60	3.3	7	1	1	195	
Chicken Potpie, Frozen								
(Banquet)......................	7 Oz	350	18	10	36	3	950	A
(Marie Callender's).........	10 Oz	680	44	1	54	3	920	
(Sheltons) White Flour ...	10 Oz	230	10	15	18	1	370	A
(Sheltons) Whole Wheat	10 Oz	230	10	16	18	3	370	A
(Stouffer's)	10 Oz	560	36	20	40	4	1,050	A
(Stouffer's) *Lean Cuisine*	9.5 Oz	320	10	18	39	3	0	A
(Swanson)	8 Oz	470	21	14	56	7	950	
(Swanson) *Hungry Man*.	14 Oz	650	35	19	64	3	1,470	A
Chicken Sauce								
(Lipton) *Chicken Tonight:*								
Country French............	1 Cup	260	22	1	12	2	1,720	
Creamy Mushrooms ...	1 Cup	220	18	1	10	2	1,500	
Creamy Primavera......	1 Cup	180	12	1	14	4	1,500	
Herbed with Wine.......	1 Cup	160	12	1	12	2	1,340	
Chickpea (See Bean, Garbanzo)								
Chickpea Flour (See Garbanzo Flour)								
Chicory								
Greens, Raw, Chopped .	1 Cup	41	0.5	3	8	7	81	FA
Witloof, Raw..................	1 Cup	15	0.1	1	4	3	2	
Witloof, Raw..................	4 Oz	19	0.1	1	5	4	2	F

	Serv.	K-Cal.	Fat	Prot.	Carb.	Fib.	Sod.	FAC
Chicory Roots								
Raw	1 Cup	66	0.2	1	16	NV	45	
Raw	1 Tbsp	8	0	0	2	NV	6	
Chili, Canned								
(Bearitos) LF	1 Cup	150	1	9	20	5	550	A
(Campbell's) Zesty								
Sauce	1 Cup	260	6	12	42	12	980	
(Chef Boyardee) W/Beef	1 Cup	310	18	12	25	7	1,040	A
(Eden) Organic FF	1 Cup	260	0	18	42	14	500	A
(Gebhardt):								
	1 Cup	268	2.0	14	61	14	1,260	
Spicy	1 Cup	200	3.1	14	39	15	1,308	
(Hormel):								
No Beans	1 Cup	410	30	19	16	3	950	A
W/Beans, Chunky	1 Cup	330	16	17	30	8	1,040	
W/Turkey, Beans	1 Cup	200	3	18	25	5	1210	A
(Hunts):								
	1 Cup	174	1.9	12	34	11	1,194	
Open Range	1 Cup	281	16	17	25	10	1,291	
(Just Rite)	1 Cup	379	26.5	18	31	13	1,233	
(Luck's)	1 Cup	240	2	12	40	12	620	
(S & W):								
	1 Cup	220	2	14	46	12	1,160	
Homestyle	1 Cup	160	0	14	38	12	1,260	A
Hot Chipotle	1 Cup	180	0	14	42	12	1,140	
Sun Vista	1 Cup	220	2	14	48	14	720	
(Sheltons):								
W/Chicken	1 Cup	210	3	21	26	7	970	
W/Turkey	1 Cup	210	4	19	26	4	990	A
(Wolf):								
Turkey W/Beans	1 Cup	198	1.5	18	28	7	746	A
W/Beans	1 Cup	330	18	19	30	9	1,050	A
Vegetarian								
(Bearitos) LF	1 Cup	190	1	10	36	6	550	A
(Bearitos) Spicy, LF	1 Cup	190	1	10	36	5	550	A
(Health Valley):								
Black Bean FF	1 Cup	160	0	14	30	14	320	
Black Bean, Vegetar-								
ian FF	1 Cup	160	0	14	30	14	320	
3 Bean FF	1 Cup	160	0	14	30	14	320	
(Hormel) FF	1 Cup	200	0	12	38	9	830	A
(Natural Touch)	1 Cup	268	12.3	18	22	11	1,329	
(Worthington)	1 Cup	294	15	19	21	9	1,134	
Chili, Frozen								
(Stouffer's) Con Carne								
W/Beans	8.7 Oz	270	10	15	29	8	1,130	

	Serv.	K-Cal.	Fat	Prot.	Carb.	Fib.	Sod.	FAC
(Chili, Frozen cont.)								
(Stouffer's) *Lean Cuisine*, Three Bean W/ Rice	9 Oz	210	6	8	32	7	460	A
(Swanson) Con Carne, *Homestyle*	8.25 Oz	270	10	20	26	0	740	

Chili Peppers (See Pepper, Chile)

Chili Powder
Dried	1 Oz	69	1.3	4	11	7	7	
(Gebhardt)	1 Tsp	3	0.2	0	1	0	1	
Quick Seasoning	1 Tbsp	14	0.3	0	3	0	204	
(Old El Paso) Seasoning Mix	1 Tbsp	25	0.5	0	4	1	770	

Chili Sauce
(Del Monte)	1 Tbsp	20	0	0	5	0	480	
Hot Dog (Hunt's)	1 Tbsp	15	0.8	1	2	1	64	
Hot Dog (Gebhardt)	1 Tbsp	14	0.8	1	2	0.5	66	
Hot Dog (Wolf)	1 Tbsp	15	1	1	2	0	90	
(Hunt's)	1 Tbsp	17	0.1	0	4	0	196	
Steakhouse (S & W)	1 Tbsp	15	0	0	4	0	180	

Chimichanga
(Don Miguel):								
Bean/Cheese	7 Oz	460	17	17	59	8	1,040	AC
Chicken	7 Oz	390	12	17	54	5	910	A
Chicken/Cheese	7 Oz	450	18	18	52	3	950	A
(Old El Paso):								
Beef	4.5 Oz	360	20	9	37	3	470	
Chicken	4.5 Oz	340	16	11	39	2	540	

Chinese Apple (See Pomegranate)

Chinese Date (See Jujube)

Chinese Gooseberry (See Kiwifruit)

Chinese Grapefruit (See Pomelo)

Chinese Kale (See Broccoli, Chinese)

Chinese Okra (See Looffah)

Chinese Parsley (See Coriander, Leaf)

Chinese Radish (See Daikon)

	Serv.	K-Cal.	Fat	Prot.	Carb.	Fib.	Sod.	FAC

Chinese Star Fruit (See Carambola)

Chinese White Cabbage (See Bok Choy)

Chinese Yam (See Jicama)

Chips (See individual listings)

Chives

Raw	1 Tsp	0	0	0	0	0	1	
Raw	1 Cup	14	0.3	2	2	1	1	**FA**
Dried (McCormick)	1 Tsp	1	0	0	0	0	0	
Freeze-dried (McCormick)	1 Tsp	1	0	0	0	0	0	

Chocolate, Baking
Bar

(Baker's):								
Semisweet	1 Oz	130	9	2	17	2	0	
Sweet, German's	1 Oz	120	9	2	16	1	0	
Unsweetened	1 Oz	140	14	3	9	4	0	
White	1 Oz	160	9	2	17	0	25	
(Barra) Mexican	1 Oz	110	3	1	18	0	0	
(Hershey's) Unsweetened, Premium	1 Oz	180	14	4	8	4	3	
(Nestlé) Semisweet	1 Oz	160	9	2	16	NV	0	

Chips

(Baker's):								
Milk Chocolate	1 Oz	140	8	2	18	NV	25	
Milk Chocolate, Real	1 Tbsp	80	4.6	1	10	NV	14	
Semisweet, Real	1 Chip	2	0.1	0	0	0	0	
(Hersheys):								
Milk Chocolate	1 Tbsp	79	4.2	1	9	0	16	
RF	1 Tbsp	60	3.5	1	10	0	0	
Semisweet	1 Tbsp	80	4	0	10	NV	0	
Sweet, German	1 Tbsp	67	4	1	9	1	0	
Tofu Chocolate	1 Tbsp	54	4	1	5	NV	13	

Chocolate Milk (See Milk, Chocolate)

Chocolate Syrup and Toppings

(Baskin Robbins):								
Hot Fudge	1 Tbsp	50	1.5	1	9	0	23	
Hot Fudge, FF	1 Tbsp	45	0	1	10	0.5	48	

	Serv.	K-Cal.	Fat	Prot.	Carb.	Flb.	Sod.	FAC
(Chocolate Syrup and Toppings cont.)								
(Hershey's):								
	1 Tbsp	51	0.2	0	12	1	10	
Hot Fudge	1 Tbsp	65	2.3	1	10	0	77	
Hot Fudge, FF	1 Tbsp	50	0	1	11	0	67	
LT-FF	1 Tbsp	25	0	0	6	NV	17	
W/Mint FF	1 Tbsp	50	0	0	13	NV	15	
(Kraft):								
Fudge	1 Tbsp	70	2	1	12	0	50	
FF (Kraft)	1 Tbsp	55	0	1	13	1	15	
(Nestlé) *Quik*	1 Tbsp	50	0.3	1	12	0	15	
(Mrs. Richardson's)								
Fudge	1 Tbsp	65	3	1	10	NV	27	
(Smucker's):								
	1 Tbsp	65	1	1	13	NV	17	
Fudge	1 Tbsp	80	7.5	1	8	NV	25	

Chow Mein

	Serv.	K-Cal.	Fat	Prot.	Carb.	Flb.	Sod.	FAC
(Chun King):								
Beef	1 Cup	79	1	8	11	3	720	
Chicken	1 Cup	98	3	8	11	3	1,123	
Pork	1 Cup	78	2.2	7	9	2	1,183	
(Fantastic):								
Mandarin, Prepared	1 Cup	272	2.4	10	53	5	1,152	A
W/Tofu, Prepared	1 Cup	330	5	22	51	5	1,130	A

Chow Mein Noodles (See Noodle, Chinese)

Chub—Cisco

	Serv.	K-Cal.	Fat	Prot.	Carb.	Flb.	Sod.	FAC
Raw	3 Oz	85	1.5	5	0	0	48	
Smoked	3 Oz	150	10	14	0	0	405	

Chutney

	Serv.	K-Cal.	Fat	Prot.	Carb.	Flb.	Sod.	FAC
(Crosse & Blackwell):								
Apple Curry	1 Tbsp	25	0.9	0	7	0	20	
Major Grey	1 Tbsp	60	0	0	14	0	170	
(Sharwoods):								
Hot, Bengal	1 Tbsp	45	0	0	11	0	252	
Mango & Ginger	1 Tbsp	47	0	0	12	0	233	

Cilantro (Also See Coriander, leaf)

	Serv.	K-Cal.	Fat	Prot.	Carb.	Flb.	Sod.	FAC
Fresh	¼ Cup	1	0	0	0	0	1	
Fresh	1 Oz	6	.2	1	1	0	8	
Dried (McCormick)	1 Tsp	2	0	0	0	0	4	

Cinnamon

	Serv.	K-Cal.	Fat	Prot.	Carb.	Flb.	Sod.	FAC
Ground (McCormick)	1 Tsp	7	0	0	2	1	0	

	Serv.	K-Cal.	Fat	Prot.	Carb.	Flb.	Sod.	FAC
Citron								
Candied (S & W)	1 Piece	2	0	0	1	0	1	
Clam								
Fresh								
Raw	3 Oz	63	0.8	11	2	0	48	A
Breaded, Fried	3 Oz	172	9.5	12	9	0	309	A
Broiled	3 Oz	126	1.7	22	4	0	95	A
Canned								
Baby, Whole (S & W)	1 Cup	200	6	32	8	0	1,040	
Chopped (Progresso).....	1 Cup	140	2	24	4	0	280	
Chopped (S & W)	1 Cup	80	0	16	4	0	1,440	
Minced (Gorton's)...........	1 Cup	80	0	16	4	0	1,440	
Minced (Progresso)........	1 Cup	100	0	16	8	0	1,000	
Frozen								
(Gorton's) Crunchy,								
Fried............................	3 Oz	260	17	9	17	0	300	
(Mrs. Paul's)	2.5 Oz	200	9	10	21	0	450	
Clam Juice								
....	1 Tbsp	0	0	0	0	0	46	

Clam Sauce (See Pasta Sauce, Clam)

Clarified Butter (See Butter, Clarified)

	Serv.	K-Cal.	Fat	Prot.	Carb.	Flb.	Sod.	FAC
Cloves								
Ground............................	1 Tsp	7	0.4	0	1	1	5	
Whole	1 Tsp	5	0.3	0	1	0	4	

Club Soda (See Soft Drink, Unflavored)

Coating Mix (See Seasoning and Coating Mix)

	Serv.	K-Cal.	Fat	Prot.	Carb.	Flb.	Sod.	FAC
Cobbler								
(Marie Callender's):								
Apple.............................	4.2 Oz	350	18	2	45	2	170	A
Blueberry......................	4.2 Oz	340	18	3	42	2	220	
Cherry	4.2 Oz	390	19	3	50	0	100	
Peach...........................	4.2 Oz	370	18	3	47	0	170	
(Mrs. Smith's):								
Blackberry	⅛ Item	250	9	3	38	3	250	
Peach...........................	⅛ Item	240	9	3	38	3	250	

Cocktail (See Alcoholic Beverage, Mixed Drink)

	Serv.	K-Cal.	Fat	Prot.	Carb.	Flb.	Sod.	FAC
Cocktail Sauce								
(Crosse & Blackwell)......	¼ Cup	110	0	1	25	0	790	
(Del Monte)	¼ Cup	100	0	1	24	0	910	
(Heinz)	¼ Cup	60	0	1	14	0	680	

	Serv.	K-Cal.	Fat	Prot.	Carb.	Fib.	Sod.	FAC
Cocoa Butter Oil								
....	1 Tbsp	120	13.6	0	0	0	0	
Cocoa, Mix								
(Land O Lakes)	1.2 Oz	160	5	4	24	0	135	
(Swiss Miss):								
FF............................	0.5 Oz	52	0.3	4	9	1	185	
Hot, LT......................	0.7 Oz	76	0.6	2	18	2	177	
Milk Chocolate	1 Oz	118	2.7	1	22	1	118	
NSA............................	0.5 Oz	54	1	2	10	1	165	
(Wt Watchers) FF	0.7 Oz	70	0	6	10	1	160	C
Cocoa, Unsweetened								
(Droste)...........................	1 Tbsp	15	1	1	2	1	35	
(Ghirardelli).....................	1 Tbsp	20	1.5	1	3	2	0	
(Hershey's)	1 Tbsp	20	0.5	1	3	1	0	
(Hershey's) *European*	1 Tbsp	20	0.5	1	3	0	0	
Coconut								
Raw								
Shredded........................	1 Cup	283	26.8	3	12	7	16	
Shredded........................	1 Oz	101	9.8	2	1	1	1	
Dried, Sweetened								
(Baker's):								
Flakes	½ Cup	280	18	4	28	4	180	
Flakes, Toasted	½ Cup	350	25.5	4	26	NV	128	
Shredded, Premium....	½ Cup	240	16	0	24	4	140	
Coconut Cream								
Raw, From Grated Meat	1 Cup	792	83.2	9	16	5	10	
Canned, Sweetened.......	2 Tbsp	120	5	0	20	NV	10	
Coconut Milk								
Raw	1 Cup	552	57.2	6	13	5	36	
(Taste of Thai)	1 Cup	440	44	4	8	0	60	
LT	1 Cup	140	12	0	8	0	60	
Coconut Oil								
(Hain).............................	1 Tbsp	120	14	0	0	0	0	
Cod								
Atlantic								
Raw	3 Oz	70	0.6	15	0	0	46	
Broiled	3 Oz	90	0.7	20	0	0	67	
Dry, Salted	3 Oz	246	2	53	0	0	5,973	
Smoked	3 Oz	72	0.8	15	0	0	718	
Pacific								
Raw	3 Oz	69	0.5	15	0	0	61	
Broiled	3 Oz	90	0.7	20	0	0	78	

	Serv.	K-Cal.	Fat	Prot.	Carb.	Flb.	Sod.	FAC
Frozen, Prepared								
Breaded, LT (Mrs.								
Paul's)........................	1 Item	240	50	22	11	0	430	
Cod Liver Oil								
(Hain)...............................	1 Tbsp	120	14	0	0	0	0	**A**
Coffee								
Brewed	1 Cup	5	0	0	1	0	3	
Brewed, Decaffeinated...	1 Cup	5	0	0	1	0	5	
Cappuccino.....................	1 Cup	88	4	4	7	0	64	
Cappuccino,								
Decaffeinated..............	1 Cup	88	4	4	7	0	64	
Decaffeinated								
(Sanka)	1 Cup	3	0	0	1	0	0	
Espresso......................	1 Cup	5	0	0	1	0	5	
Espresso, Decaffeinated	1 Cup	5	0	0	1	0	5	
Instant, Prepared.......	1 Cup	5	0	0	1	0	7	
Regular, Instant Powder	1 Tsp	4	0	0	1	0	1	
Coffee Alternative, Mix								
(Inka)	1 Tsp	0	0	0	1	0	3	
(Kafree Roma)...............	1 Tsp	8	0	0	2	NV	3	
(Pero).............................	1 Tsp	1	0	0	1	0	0	
(Postum)	1 Tsp	10	0	0	3	0	0	

Cola (See Soft Drink, Cola)

Cold Cuts (See individual listings)

Cole (See Kale)

Coleslaw Dressing (See Salad Dressing, Bottled, Cole Slaw)

	Serv.	K-Cal.	Fat	Prot.	Carb.	Flb.	Sod.	FAC
Collard								
Raw, Chopped	1 Cup	12	0	1	1	1	4	
Boiled................................	1 Cup	35	0.2	2	8	4	21	**FAC**

Condiments (See individual listings)

	Serv.	K-Cal.	Fat	Prot.	Carb.	Flb.	Sod.	FAC
Cookie								
Almond (Also See Cookie, Biscotti)								
(Stella D'Oro) Chinese								
Dessert........................	1 Item	169	8.9	2	20	NV	NV	
(Sunshine) *Crescents*.....	1 Item	38	1.5	1	6	0	26	
(Westbrae) W/Honey......	1 Item	110	4	1	17	1	135	
Animal Cracker								
(Barbara's Bakery)	1 Item	16	0.6	0	3	0	13	

	Serv.	K-Cal.	Fat	Prot.	Carb.	Fib.	Sod.	FAC
(Cookie cont.)								
(Mother's) *Zoo Pals*	1 Item	28	1.5	2	4	NV	10	
(Nabisco) *Barnum's*								
Animals	1 Item	12	0.3	0	2	0	13	
(Sunshine)	1 Item	10	0.3	0	1	0	7	
Apple								
(Auburn Farms) *Jam-*								
mer, Organic, FF	1 Item	40	0	1	10	1	33	
(Bakery Wagon) Cobbler								
FF.................................	1 Item	70	0	1	16	0	50	
Oatmeal	1 Item	90	3	1	14	1	65	
(Health Valley) Jumbo,								
W/Raisin, FF...............	1 Item	80	0	2	19	3	35	
W/Spice, FF................	1 Item	33	0	1	8	1	17	
(Nabisco) *Newton*, FF....	1 Item	50	0	1	12	1	30	
(Sunshine) *Golcoon*								
Fruit, LF	1 Item	70	1	1	15	1	60	
(Wt Watchers) Bar W/								
Raisin..........................	1 Item	70	2	1	14	2	60	
(Westbrae) Dutch	1 Item	110	4	1	17	0	140	
Apricot								
(Health Valley)								
Delights, FF	1 Item	33	0	1	8	1	17	
Tart (Healthy Choice).....	1 Item	55	0.7	1	11	0	25	
(Pepperidge Farm)								
W/Raspberry...............	1 Item	47	2	1	7	0	37	
Arrowroot								
(Nabisco) Biscuit	1 Item	20	0.5	0	3	1	15	
Biscotti								
(Allegria)								
Amaretto	1 Item	90	2	2	16	1	70	
Chocolate....................	1 Item	180	8	3	24	1	60	
(La Tempesta)								
Chocolate....................	1 Item	150	6	4	24	3	80	
(Musso's)......................	1 Item	110	5	3	16	1	30	
(Sapori) Almond	1 Item	147	5	3	22	2	37	
(Semifreddi's) Almond....	1 Item	147	8	4	16	2	20	
(Slendido) Hazelnut								
Chocolate Chip	1 Item	150	10	3	12	2	50	
W/Almond/Orange	1 Item	100	3.5	3	15	2	25	
Butter								
(Cookietree) Sugar.........	1 Item	120	4.5	2	18	0	120	
(Delicious) Frosted	1 Item	88	5	1	11	0	44	
(Keebler) *Buttercup*........	1 Item	23	0.8	0	4	0	38	
(Lu) *Petite Beurre*	1 Item	40	1	1	7	NV	45	
(Pepperidge Farm)								
Chessman...................	1 Item	40	1.7	1	6	0	27	
(Sunshine)	1 Item	28	1.2	0	4	0	27	

	Serv.	K-Cal.	Fat	Prot.	Carb.	Fib.	Sod.	FAC
Caramel								
(Barbara's) Mini-								
Caramel Apple, FF	1 Item	18	0	0	4	0	21	
(Little Debbie) Bar..........	1 Item	160	8	1	22	0	85	
(Pepperidge Farm)								
Pecan.........................	1 Item	130	7	2	16	1	55	
Cherry								
(Auburn Farms) Choco-								
late FF	1 Item	40	0	1	10	1	40	
(Pepperidge Farm)								
Cobbler	1 Item	70	2.5	1	11	0	45	
Chocolate								
(Auburn Farms):								
Jammer, Chewey........	1 Item	40	0.3	1	10	1	33	
Mint, FF	1 Item	45	0	1	10	1	48	
(Barbara's):								
Double Chocolate								
Fudge	1 Item	60	2.5	1	9	1	40	
Mini Double								
Chocolate, FF	1 Item	17	0	0	4	0	23	
(Cookietree):								
Chunk..........................	1 Item	120	5	2	18	0	115	
Fudge, FF	1 Item	120	0	2	27	1	180	
Macaroon	1 Item	130	6	2	17	1	85	
(Health Valley):								
Caramel Centers,								
FF............................	1 Item	35	0	1	9	2	10	
Fudge Centers, FF	1 Item	35	0	1	9	2	10	
Mint Fudge Centers,								
FF............................	1 Item	35	0	1	9	2	10	
(Hydrox)								
....	1 Item	50	2.3	1	7	0	42	
LF..............................	1 Item	47	1.3	0	8	0	47	
(Keebler) *Elfin Coolights*,								
Fudge........................	1 Item	55	1.3	1	10	0	50	
(Nabisco):								
Covered Ritz...............	1 Item	50	3	1	6	0	32	
Famous Wafers	1 Item	28	0.8	0	5	0	46	
Mallomars	1 Item	60	2.5	1	9	1	18	
Marshmallow								
Pinwheel....................	1 Item	130	5	1	21	1	35	
Oreo.............................	1 Item	53	2.3	1	8	0	73	
Sandwich, LF..............	1 Item	50	1.3	1	10	1	95	
Snackwell's, Choco-								
late Sandwich..........	1 Item	55	1.2	1	10	1	110	
Snackwell's, Devil								
Foods, FF................	1 Item	50	0	1	12	0	30	
Snaps..........................	1 Item	20	0.7	0	3	0	26	

	Serv.	K-Cal.	Fat	Prot.	Carb.	Flb.	Sod.	FAC
(*Cookie cont.*)								
(Pepperidge Farm):								
Beacon Hill, Walnut....	1 Item	130	7	2	16	1	100	
Chunk..........................	1 Item	130	6	1	16	2	35	
Macadamia	1 Item	130	6	1	16	1	55	
Milano	1 Item	60	3.3	1	7	0	27	
(Sunshine) *Vienna*								
Fingers	1 Item	65	1.8	1	11	0	63	
(Ultra Slim-Fast) Sand-								
wich Creme.................	1 Item	43	1	0	8	0	43	
(Wt Watchers)								
Sandwich	1 Item	70	1.8	1	12	1	80	
Chocolate Chip								
(Barbara's):								
....	1 Item	80	4	1	10	1	60	
Snackimals.................	1 Item	15	0.6	0	2	0	11	
(Chip-A-Roos) Mini........	1 Item	32	1.6	0	4	0	28	
(Cookietree):								
Dark Chunk...............	1 Item	120	5	2	18	0	110	
W/Pecan	1 Item	130	5	2	18	0	95	
(Dunkaroos) W/Vanilla								
Frosting	1 Item	120	4.5	1	21	1	65	
(Grandma's) Big	1 Item	190	9	2	25	1	130	
(Health Valley) FF..........	1 Item	33	0	1	8	1	7	
(Keebler):								
Bite Size	1 Item	20	1.1	0	3	0	14	
Cooluxe.....................	1 Item	80	4.5	1	9	0	60	
RF	1 Item	70	3	1	11	0	70	
Old-Fashioned.............	1 Item	80	4	1	10	0	60	
Soft Batch...................	1 Item	80	3.5	1	10	1	70	
(Mother's)	1 Item	80	4	1	10	0	52	
(Nabisco):								
Chips Ahoy	1 Item	53	2.7	1	7	0	35	
Chips Ahoy, Chewy	1 Item	57	2.7	0	8	0	42	
Chips Ahoy, Pecan								
Chunk	1 Item	100	6	1	10	NV	65	
Chips Ahoy, RF	1 Item	50	2	1	8	0	50	
Chips Ahoy, White								
Fudge Chunk...........	1 Item	90	5	1	10	NV	75	
Snackwell's, LF...........	1 Item	10	0.3	0	2	0	13	
Snaps..........................	1 Item	21	0.7	0	3	0	16	
(Pepperidge Farm):								
....	1 Item	47	2.3	1	6	0	22	
Chesapeake.................	1 Item	140	8	2	15	1	100	
Nantucket....................	1 Item	130	7	1	16	1	75	
(Pillsbury)......................	1 Item	130	6	1	17	1	85	
(Sunshine) Oatmeal	1 Item	57	2.7	1	8	1	43	
(Wt Watchers)	1 Item	70	2.5	1	11	1	45	

	Serv.	K-Cal.	Fat	Prot.	Carb.	Fib.	Sod.	FAC
(Westbrae):								
....	1 Item	110	4	1	18	1	125	
W/Pecan	1 Item	110	5	1	18	1	110	
Cranberry								
(Nabisco) *Newton*, FF....	1 Item	50	0	1	12	1	48	
(Sunshine) Golcoon, LF.	1 Item	70	1	1	15	1	60	
Date								
(Bakery Wagon)								
Oatmeal	1 Item	90	2.5	1	17	1	90	
(Health Valley) Delight,								
FF................................	1 Item	33	0	1	8	1	17	
(Pepperidge Farm)								
W/Pecan	1 Item	55	2.5	1	8	NV	20	
Fig								
(Bakery Wagon):								
FF................................	1 Item	70	0	1	16	1	65	
WW, FF	1 Item	70	0	1	17	1	60	
(Keebler) Bar..................	1 Item	60	2	2	11	NV	70	
(Nabisco):								
Newton........................	1 Item	55	1.3	1	10	1	60	
Newton, FF	1 Item	50	0	1	11	1	58	
(Sunshine):								
Bar	1 Item	55	1.3	1	10	1	30	
Golcoon, FF	1 Item	60	0	1	13	1	50	
(Ultra Slim-Fast)	1 Item	60	0.5	0	14	1	70	
(Wt Watchers) FF...........	1 Item	70	0	1	16	0	50	
Fortune								
(La Choy)	1 Item	28	0.1	0	7	0	1	
Fudge								
(Cookietree) Double	1 Item	120	5	2	18	1	70	
(Keebler):								
Double.........................	1 Item	80	4	0	11	0	65	
E.L. Fudge	1 Item	53	2.3	1	8	0	33	
Stripes........................	1 Item	53	2.7	0	7	0	47	
(Mother's) W/Walnuts.....	1 Item	65	3.5	1	8	1	45	
(Nabisco):								
Snackwell's, Double								
FF..............................	1 Item	50	0	1	12	1	70	
Striped Shortbread.......	1 Item	53	2.7	1	7	0	47	
(Trolley Cake).................	1 Item	73	0.8	1	16	1	40	
(Westbrae) Marble..........	1 Item	100	4	1	16	1	125	
Ginger								
(Bakery Wagon)								
Snaps..........................	1 Item	32	1.4	0	4	0	28	
(Nabisco) Old-								
Fashioned	1 Item	30	0.6	0	6	0	43	
(Pepperidge Farm)								
Gingermans	1 Item	30	0.9	1	5	0	24	

	Serv.	K-Cal.	Fat	Prot.	Carb.	Fib.	Sod.	FAC
(Cookie cont.)								
(Sunshine) Snaps............	1 Item	19	0.6	0	3	0	21	
(Westbrae) Snaps	1 Item	44	2	1	3	1	10	
Gluten-Free								
(Ener-G):								
Almond Butter..............	1 Item	60	3.1	1	6	0	43	
Almond Orange...........	1 Item	74	3.7	2	9	1	39	
Biscotti, Chocolate								
Chip..............................	1 Item	122	5.1	1	17	0	136	
Biscotti, Plain	1 Item	81	3.3	1	11	0	96	
Chocolate Nut..............	1 Item	102	4.5	2	12	1	7	
Chocolate Walnut	1 Item	109	6.8	1	11	1	107	
Crisp Sugar..................	1 Item	93	3.1	3	14	2	218	
Date	1 Item	76	2.3	1	13	1	75	
French Almond	1 Item	104	3.6	2	17	1	31	
Ginger	1 Item	75	2.7	1	12	1	134	
Peanut Butter..............	1 Item	94	4.6	2	11	1	108	
Potato Chocolate								
Chip..............................	1 Item	91	3.9	1	12	0	34	
(Health Valley) *The*								
Great Wheat-Free.......	1 Item	40	1.5	1	7	2	18	
Graham								
(Keebler) Fudge Cov-								
ered, Deluxe	1 Item	47	2.3	0	6	0	35	
(Mother's)	1 Item	65	1.7	1	12	1	65	
(Nabisco):								
....	1 Item	15	0.4	0	3	0	23	
Chocolate....................	1 Item	53	2.7	1	7	0	30	
Chocolate, *Bugs*								
Bunny	1 Item	11	0.4	0	2	0	14	
Chocolate, *Teddy*								
Grahams	1 Item	6	0.2	0	1	0	6	
(Sunshine) Fudge-								
Dipped........................	1 Item	43	2.3	1	5	0	19	
(Westbrae) Cinnamon	1 Item	16	.6	0	2	0	8	
Lemon								
(Barbara's):								
Sandwich	1 Item	60	2.5	1	9	0	38	
W/Almonds..................	1 Item	23	1	0	3	0	23	
(Cookietree) Poppyseed,								
FF................................	1 Item	130	0	2	27	1	150	
(Keebler) Creme,								
Opera..........................	1 Item	80	3.5	1	12	0	70	
(Little Coobie) Creme								
Wafer	1 Item	100	5	1	13	0	25	
(Pepperidge Farm) Nut								
Crunch	1 Item	57	3	1	6	1	20	
(Sunshine) *Coolers*.........	1 Item	28	1.2	0	4	0	20	
(Westbrae) Snaps	1 Item	47	2	1	7	1	20	

	Serv.	K-Cal.	Fat	Prot.	Carb.	Flb.	Sod.	FAC
Marshmallow								
(Nabisco):								
Mallomars	1 Item	60	2.5	1	9	1	18	
Pinwheel	1 Item	130	5	1	21	1	35	
Puffs, Fudge	1 Item	90	4	1	14	0	45	
Twirl Fudge Cakes	1 Item	130	6	1	20	1	75	
Mint								
(Girl Scout)	1 Item	40	2.3	2	5	1	35	
(Nabisco) Mystic.............	1 Item	90	4	1	11	0	65	
(Sunshine) Patties..........	1 Item	65	3.5	1	8	0	30	
Molasses								
(Auburn Farms) FF	1 Item	40	0	1	10	1	20	
(Pepperidge Farm) Crisp	1 Item	30	1.2	0	4	0	28	
Oatmeal								
(Bakery Wagon) Soft......	1 Item	100	4	2	16	1	90	
(Entenmann's) Choco-								
late Chip, FF..............	1 Item	40	0	1	10	1	55	
(Grandma's) Big Spice...	1 Item	170	6	2	26	2	220	
(Keebler) Old-Fashioned	1 Item	80	3.5	1	10	0	75	
(Mother's)	1 Item	55	2.5	1	9	1	75	
(Nabisco) Family								
Favorites	1 Item	80	3	1	12	1	65	
(Pepperidge Farm):								
Irish	1 Item	43	2	1	6	1	23	
Santa Fe	1 Item	120	4.5	2	18	1	110	
W/Raisins.....................	1 Item	53	2	1	8	0	50	
(Sunshine) Country Style	1 Item	57	2.3	1	8	0	53	
(Westbrae) Snaps	1 Item	47	2	1	7	1	12	
Peach								
(Bakery Wagon) Cobbler								
W/Apricot, FF..............	1 Item	70	0	1	16	0	6	
(Health Valley)								
W/Apricot, FF..............	1 Item	35	0	1	10	1	13	
(Pepperidge Farm) Tart .	1 Item	60	1.5	1	12	0	58	
Peanut Butter								
(Cookietree).....................	1 Item	132	6.5	3	17	2	178	
Chocolate....................	1 Item	120	6	2	16	1	150	
(Grandma's) Big	1 Item	190	9	4	22	1	180	
Chocolate Chip, Bigs..	1 Item	190	10	4	23	1	170	
(Keebler) Fudgebutters..	1 Item	65	3.5	1	7	0	45	
Old-Fashioned.............	1 Item	80	4.5	1	9	0	80	
(Little Coobie) Bar..........	1 Item	270	15	4	32	1	190	
(Mother's) Gaucho								
Sandwich	1 Item	85	5	2	11	1	100	
(Pepperidge Farm)								
Cheyenne.....................	1 Item	110	6	4	13	NV	80	
(Pitter Patter) Creme......	1 Item	90	4	2	12	1	115	
(Nabisco) Sandwich	1 Item	65	3	2	10	1	55	

	Serv.	K-Cal.	Fat	Prot.	Carb.	Fib.	Sod.	FAC
(Cookie cont.)								
(Sunshine) Wafer	1 Item	43	2.3	1	5	0	19	
(Westbrae) W/Nuts.........	1 Item	110	3.5	2	17	0	110	
Pecan								
(Keebler) Sandies,								
RF................................	1 Item	70	3	1	10	0	50	
Sandies, Bite Size	1 Item	21	1.3	0	2	0	12	
(Nabisco) Passion								
Shortbread	1 Item	90	5	1	9	0	35	
(Pepperidge Farm)								
Shortbread	1 Item	70	4.5	1	7	1	43	
Raisin								
(Auburn Farms) *Jam-*								
mers, FF	1 Item	40	0.3	1	10	1	35	
(Barbara's) Mini,								
FF	1 Item	18	0	0	4	0	18	
(Cookietree):								
Oatmeal	1 Item	110	3.5	1	18	1	95	
Oatmeal, FF...............	1 Item	120	0	2	27	1	110	
(Entenmann's):								
FF...............................	1 Item	40	0	1	9	0	60	
Oatmeal, FF...............	1 Item	40	0	1	9	0	60	
(Health Valley):								
Jumbo, FF	1 Item	80	0	2	19	3	35	
Oatmeal, FF...............	1 Item	30	0	1	8	1	17	
(Keebler) *Soft Batch*.......	1 Item	70	3	1	10	NV	65	
(Nabisco) *Snackwell's*....	1 Item	55	1.3	1	10	1	68	
(Wt Watchers):								
W/Rasins....................	1 Item	60	1	1	11	1	45	
Oatmeal	1 Item	120	2	2	22	1	90	
(Westbrae)......................	1 Item	100	2	2	18	1	110	
Raspberry								
(Barbara's):								
Creme, Choc/Rasp	1 Item	60	2.5	1	9	0	40	
Creme, Van/Rasp	1 Item	60	2.5	1	9	0	38	
(Health Valley):								
Center, FF...................	1 Item	70	0	2	18	2	20	
Jumbo, FF	1 Item	80	0	2	19	3	35	
W/Apple, FF...............	1 Item	33	0	1	8	1	17	
(Nabisco):								
Newton......................	1 Item	80	2	1	15	NV	70	
Newton, FF................	1 Item	50	0	1	12	0	58	
(Pepperidge Farm):								
Chantilly.....................	1 Item	80	3	1	12	1	50	
Linzer.........................	1 Item	100	4	1	15	1	65	
(Wt Watchers) Fruit-								
Filled, FF....................	1 Item	70	0	1	16	0	45	

	Serv.	K-Cal.	Fat	Prot.	Carb.	Fib.	Sod.	FAC
Shortbread								
(Keebler):								
Animal, Iced	1 Item	23	0.8	0	4	0	22	
Fudge 'N Caramel	1 Item	60	3	0	8	0	28	
Pecan Sandies	1 Item	80	5	1	9	1	75	
Toffee Sandies	1 Item	80	4.5	1	10	0	55	
(Nabisco) *Lorna Doone*	1 Item	35	1.8	1	5	0	33	
(Pepperidge Farm)	1 Item	70	3.5	1	8	0	53	
(Sunshine) Striped	1 Item	53	3	1	7	0	28	
(Wt Watchers)	1 Item	27	0.7	0	4	0	32	
Strawberry								
(Health Valley) Fruit								
Center, FF	1 Item	35	0	1	10	1	13	
(Little Coobie) FF	1 Item	130	0	1	33	1	105	
(Nabisco) *Newton*, FF	1 Item	50	0	1	12	0	58	
(Pepperidge Farm)	1 Item	47	1.7	1	7	0	35	
Sugar								
(Keebler):								
Fiber-enriched	1 Item	70	3	0	9	1	60	
Old-Fashioned	1 Item	80	4	1	10	0	45	
Wafer, *Krisp*								
Kreem	1 Item	28	1.4	0	4	0	10	
(Mother's)	1 Item	70	3	1	10	1	37	
(Pepperidge Farm)	1 Item	47	2	1	7	0	30	
Wafer, Chocolate								
(Sunshine)	1 Item	43	2.3	1	6	0	10	
Wafer, Vanilla (Sunshine)	1 Item	43	2	0	6	0	7	
Wafers, *Biscos*								
(Nabisco)	1 Item	18	0.8	0	3	0	5	
Toffee								
(Cookietree)	1 Item	130	7	1	17	0	150	
(Pepperidge Farm)								
Charleston	1 Item	130	7	1	16	1	100	
Tofu								
The Great Tofu (Health								
Valley)	1 Item	45	1.5	1	7	1	15	
Vanilla								
(Fiber Classic) Original	1 Item	210	8	3	37	0	280	
(Nabisco):								
Nilla	1 Item	18	0.6	0	3	0	12	
Nilla, RF	1 Item	15	0.3	0	3	0	13	
Sandwich, *Family*								
Favorite	1 Item	57	2.7	1	8	0	40	
Sandwich, RF	1 Item	55	1.3	1	11	1	48	
(Keebler) Wafer	1 Item	19	0.9	0	3	0	15	
(Pepperidge Farm) Tart								
W/Raspberry	1 Item	60	1.5	1	12	0	58	
(Sunshine) Wafer	1 Item	21	1	0	3	0	16	

	Serv.	K-Cal.	Fat	Prot.	Carb.	Fib.	Sod.	FAC
(Cookie cont.)								
(Ultra Slim-Fast) Sandwich Creme	1 Item	43	1	0	8	0	40	
(Wt Watchers) Sandwich	1 Item	70	1.5	1	13	1	40	
(Westbrae):								
	1 Item	16	0.6	0	2	0	10	
W/Raspberry	1 Item	110	4	1	17	0	135	
White Chocolate								
(Auburn Farms) *Jammer*, WW P'Nutty Crisp	1 Item	45	0.3	1	10	1	45	
(Cookietree):								
Chunk, LF	1 Item	140	2	2	28	0	85	
W/Macadamia	1 Item	130	6	2	18	0	90	
W/Pecan	1 Item	120	5	2	18	0	100	
(Nabisco) *Oreo*, Fudge-covered	1 Item	100	6	1	14	1	70	

Cookie Dough, Prepared

	Serv.	K-Cal.	Fat	Prot.	Carb.	Fib.	Sod.	FAC
(Mrs. Fields):								
Chocolate Chips	1 Item	240	11	2	33	1	135	
Chocolate Chips W/Walnuts	1 Item	250	13	3	31	2	125	
Oatmeal/Raisin/Nut	1 Item	240	11	3	34	2	180	
(Pillsbury):								
Chocolate Chip	1 Oz	130	6	1	17	0	85	
Sugar	1 Oz	130	5	1	19	0	125	
White Chocolate Chunk	1 Oz	130	6	1	17	0	100	
(Nestlé):								
Tollhouse, Chocolate Chip	1 Oz	140	6	2	20	1	100	
Tollhouse, Sugar	1 Oz	170	5	1	18	0	130	

Cooking Sprays

	Serv.	K-Cal.	Fat	Prot.	Carb.	Fib.	Sod.	FAC
(Pam):								
Butter-flavored	1 Spray	0	0	0	0	0	0	
Olive Oil Flavor	1 Spray	0	0	0	0	0	0	
Unflavored	1 Spray	0	0	0	0	0	0	
(Wt Watchers) Buttery Spray	1 Spray	0	0	0	0	0	0	
(Wesson);								
Butter Flavor	1 Spray	2	0.2	0	0	0	0	
Nonstick	1 Spray	2	0.2	0	0	0	0	

Cool Whip (See Cream, Nondairy Alternative, Frozen)

Coriander, Leaf—Chinese Parsley (Also See Cilantro)

	Serv.	K-Cal.	Fat	Prot.	Carb.	Fib.	Sod.	FAC
Fresh	1 Oz	6	0.1	1	1	1	9	
Dried	1 Tsp	2	0.1	0	0	1	1	

	Serv.	K-Cal.	Fat	Prot.	Carb.	Flb.	Sod.	FAC
Coriander Seed								
Ground (McCormick)	1 Tsp	12	0.4	0	2	2	1	
Whole (Durkee)	1 Tsp	8	0.1	0	0	0	0	
Corn								
Fresh								
Raw	1 LB	140	1.9	5	31	5	25	FA
Kernels, Boiled, Drained	1 Ear	83	1	3	19	2	13	
Fresh, Cooked	1 Cup	166	2	5	40	4	26	FA
Canned								
Creamed (Green Giant)	1 Cup	200	1	4	44	2	960	FA
Creamed (S & W)	1 Cup	200	2	4	48	2	680	FA
Golden (Del Monte)	1 Cup	120	2	4	22	6	720	FA
Niblets (Green Giant)	1 Cup	210	0	6	15	6	690	FA
White (Del Monte)	1 Cup	160	0	4	34	4	720	FA
Whole Kernel (S & W)	1 Cup	180	2	4	28	4	680	FA
Frozen, Kernels								
(Green Giant):								
Creamed	1 Cup	220	2	4	46	4	660	FA
Niblets	1 Cup	120	0.8	5	26	5	90	FA
Niblets W/Butter	1 Cup	195	4.5	5	35	5	525	FA
(Health Valley)	1 Cup	152	0	4	34	3	8	FA
Boiled	1 Cup	160	2	6	2	4	8	FA
Frozen, on the Cob								
(Birds Eye)	1 Item	120	1	4	20	NV	0	FA
(Flav R Pac)	1 Item	140	1.5	5	34	2	20	FA
(Green Giant) Extra Sweet	1 Item	120	2	4	22	3	0	FA
(Green Giant) Niblets	1 Item	160	1.5	4	32	3	10	FA
Corn Bran								
Crude	1 Cup	168	0.7	6	64	64	5	
Cornbread								
Mix								
(Marie Callender's)	¼ Cup	150	3.5	2	26	1	310	
(Dromedary)	¼ Cup	130	2	2	26	1	340	
(General Mills) *Gold Medal*	1 Oz	110	1	2	24	0	210	
(Jiffy)	¼ Cup	160	4	2	28	1	320	
Mix, Prepared								
(Aunt Jemima) Easy Mix	1 Piece	196	6.3	4	33	1	679	
(General Mills) *Gold Medal*	⅙ Pan	150	5	4	22	NV	490	
(Pillsbury) *Ballard*	1 Piece	130	2.5	4	23	2	520	
(Robin Hood) *Gold*	1 Piece	120	3	2	21	NV	470	

	Serv.	K-Cal.	Fat	Prot.	Carb.	Fib.	Sod.	FAC
(*Cornbread cont.*)								
(Martha White)								
Buttermilk	⅙ Pan	110	2	2	21	NV	360	

Corn Cake, Popcorn
	Serv.	K-Cal.	Fat	Prot.	Carb.	Fib.	Sod.	FAC
(Chico San):								
Butter	1 Item	40	0	1	8	0	45	
Cheddar	1 Item	50	2	1	10	0	65	
White Cheddar............	1 Item	35	0	1	8	NV	130	
(Orville):								
Apple Cinn, Mini	1 Item	9	0	0	2	0	4	
Butter	1 Item	38	0.7	1	9	2	64	
Butter, Mini	1 Item	8	0.1	0	2	0	13	
Caramel	1 Item	42	0.1	1	11	2	15	
Caramel, Mini	1 Item	9	0	0	2	0	3	
Honey Nut, Mini..........	1 Item	9	0	0	2	0	3	
White Cheddar............	1 Item	37	0.6	1	9	2	37	
White Cheddar, Mini...	1 Item	8	0.1	0	2	0	8	
(Quaker):								
Caramel	1 Item	50	0	1	12	0	30	
Nacho..........................	1 Item	40	0	1	8	0	80	
White Cheddar............	1 Item	40	0	1	8	0	100	
(Snack Lovers):								
Butter	1 Item	50	0	1	11	0	55	
Caramel	1 Item	60	0	1	13	0	10	
White Cheddar............	1 Item	50	0	1	11	0	45	

Corn Chips (Also See Tortilla Chips)
	Serv.	K-Cal.	Fat	Prot.	Carb.	Fib.	Sod.	FAC
(Barbara's):								
Blue Corn....................	1 Chip	9	0.5	0	1	0	3	
Blue Corn, *Amazing*								
Bakes..........................	1 Chip	4	0	0	1	0	3	
Pinta Blue	1 Chip	9	0.5	0	1	0	7	
Pinta Blue, *Picante*	1 Chip	10	0.5	0	1	0	19	
Pinta Nacho	1 Chip	11	0.5	0	2	0	15	
Pinta Salsa	1 Chip	11	0.5	0	2	0	18	
(Bearitos):								
Pizza	1 Oz	120	4	2	20	NV	220	
Ranch..........................	1 Oz	120	4	2	20	NV	270	
(Bugles):								
Nacho..........................	1 Cup	120	6.8	2	14	0	225	
Original........................	1 Cup	120	6.8	2	14	0	233	
Ranch..........................	1 Cup	120	6.8	2	14	0	233	
(Frito-Lay):								
BBQ, *Fritos*.................	1 Chip	5	0.3	0	1	0	10	
Cheddar & Sour								
Cream, *Fritos*..............	1 Chip	6	0.3	0	1	0	9	
Choice, *Fritos*	1 Chip	9	0.6	0	1	0	12	
Mesquite Grill, *Fritos*..	1 Chip	13	0.8	0	1	0	13	

	Serv.	K-Cal.	Fat	Prot.	Carb.	Fib.	Sod.	FAC
Nacho, *Doritos*	1 Oz	140	7	2	18	0	150	
Original, *Fritos*	1 Chip	5	0.3	0	0	0	5	
Ranch, *Fritos*	1 Chip	15	0.9	0	2	0	14	
Sour Cream & Onion, *Fritos*	1 Chip	6	0.4	0	1	0	6	
Wild N' Mild, *Fritos*	1 Oz	160	10	2	15	1	170	
(Keebler) *Hooplas*, Original	1 Oz	140	8	2	18	1	210	
(Wt Watchers) Ranch	1 Oz	120	4	2	18	NV	340	
(Wise) Twists	1 Oz	160	10	2	15	NV	125	

Corn Dog

	Serv.	K-Cal.	Fat	Prot.	Carb.	Fib.	Sod.	FAC
(Foster Farm) Chicken	1 Item	180	10	7	15	1	490	
(Hormel)	1 Item	220	11	6	25	1	520	
Mini	5 Item	250	15	6	23	1	570	

Corn Dog, Alternative

	Serv.	K-Cal.	Fat	Prot.	Carb.	Fib.	Sod.	FAC
(Loma Linda)	1 Item	204	9.5	10	19	3	237	

Corned Beef (See Beef, Corned)

Corn Flour

	Serv.	K-Cal.	Fat	Prot.	Carb.	Fib.	Sod.	FAC
Harina, Preparada Para Tortillas (Quaker)	1 Cup	480	12	12	81	3	1,201	C
Masa Harina, Enriched (Quaker)	1 Cup	440	4	12	100	8	0	C
Masa, Sifted	1 Cup	415	4.3	12	86	11	6	C
Whole Grain	1 Cup	422	4.5	8	90	16	6	
Yellow, Whole Grain, Dry	2 Cups	884	8.6	20	186	18	85	FA
Yellow, Whole Grain (Arrowhead Mills)	2 Oz	210	2	4	43	7	1	

Corn Grit (See Grits)

Cornish Hen

	Serv.	K-Cal.	Fat	Prot.	Carb.	Fib.	Sod.	FAC
Meat Only, Cooked	9 Oz	470	18.3	72	0	0	788	
Meat and Skin, Roasted	11 Oz	727	41.4	83	0	0	957	

Cornmeal

	Serv.	K-Cal.	Fat	Prot.	Carb.	Fib.	Sod.	FAC
(Aunt Jemima):								
White, Bolted	1 Tbsp	27	0.2	1	6	0	113	
White, Bolted	1 Cup	480	2.7	11	107	5	920	C
White, Bolted, Enriched	1 Tbsp	30	0.2	1	7	0	120	
White, Buttermilk	1 Tbsp	27	0.2	1	6	0	147	
White, Degermed, Enriched	1 Tbsp	30	0.2	1	7	0	120	
Yellow Mix	1 Tbsp	27	0.2	1	6	80	103	

	Serv.	K-Cal.	Fat	Prot.	Carb.	Fib.	Sod.	FAC
(Cornmeal cont.)								
(Arrowhead Mills) Blue...	1 Cup	480	4	12	108	12	0	

Corn Nuts
Barbecue	1 Oz	124	4.1	3	20	2	277	
Nacho Cheese	1 Oz	124	4	3	20	2	180	
Plain................................	1 Oz	124	4	2	21	2	156	

Corn Oil
(Mazola)..........................	1 Tbsp	120	14	0	0	0	0	A
(Spectrum)......................	1 Tbsp	120	14	0	0	0	0	A

Corn Snack
(Health Valley) Puffs:
Apple Caramel............	1 Cup	110	0	2	24	2	60	
Caramel/Peanut..........	1 Cup	100	1	1	22	NV	75	
Caramel Original.........	1 Cup	110	0	2	24	2	60	

Cornstarch
(Argo)...............................	1 Tbsp	30	0	0	7	0	0	

Corn Syrup
(Chiefly Corn)	1 Cup	955	0	0	247	0	224	
(Karo) Dark....................	2 Tbsp	120	0	0	30	0	45	
Light	2 Tbsp	120	0	0	30	0	35	

Cottage Cheese (See Cheese, Cottage)

Cottonseed Oil
(Wesson)	1 Tbsp	122	13.6	0	0	0	0	

Couscous
Dry
(Fantastic)......................	1 Cup	840	0	28	172	12	20	
Whole Wheat	1 Cup	880	4	32	180	28	0	

Prepared from Mix
(Casbah):
Almond Chicken	10.6 Oz	160	1.5	5	29	1	470	AC
Asparagus Au Gratin, Original....................	10.6 Oz	150	2	14	28	1	400	A
Cheddar Broccoli........	10.6 Oz	130	2	11	23	1	470	A
Couscous Pilaf............	1 Cup	293	0.7	11	53	1	640	A
Hearty Harvest, Original....................	10.6 Oz	180	1	6	36	2	460	
Tomato Parmesan	10.6 Oz	170	1.5	7	34	2	460	A
WW	1 Cup	240	0.7	7	56	7	13	

(Fantastic):
Black Bean Salsa, Cup..........................	10 Oz	220	1.5	11	46	8	450	A
Creole Vegetable, Cup..........................	10 Oz	220	1.5	10	41	6	590	A

	Serv.	K-Cal.	Fat	Prot.	Carb.	Fib.	Sod.	FAC
Savory	1 Cup	240	1	9	50	4	450	A
Sweet Corn, Cup	10 Oz	180	1	7	36	6	510	A
W/Lentils	10 Oz	220	1	12	47	9	140	A
(Near East):	1 Cup	220	1	8	46	2	5	
	1 Cup	220	1	8	46	2	5	
W/Butter	1 Cup	250	4.5	8	46	2	90	
W/Margarine	1 Cup	250	6	8	46	2	65	
W/Oil	1 Cup	270	7	8	46	2	5	

Cowpea (See Bean, Black-eyed Pea)

Crab
Alaskan King
	Serv.	K-Cal.	Fat	Prot.	Carb.	Fib.	Sod.	FAC
Raw	3 Oz	71	0.5	16	0	0	711	F
Boiled	3 Oz	82	1.3	17	0	0	911	F
Canned	1 Cup	135	3.2	24	1	0	675	F

Blue
Raw	3 Oz	75	1.5	21	1	0	369	F
Boiled	1 Cup	140	2.4	28	0	0	382	F
Boiled	3 Oz	72	1	15	0	0	274	F
Canned	1 Cup	134	1.7	28	0	0	450	F

Dungeness
Raw	3 Oz	73	0.8	15	1	0	251	F
Boiled	3 Oz	94	1.1	19	1	0	321	F
Canned (S & W)	1 Cup	240	3	54	0	0	931	FC

Queen
Raw	3 Oz	77	1	16	0	0	459	F
Boiled	3 Oz	98	1.3	20	0	0	588	F

Softshell
Raw	3 Oz	75	1	15	0	0	250	F
Fried (4 Oz)	1 Item	334	17.9	11	31	NV	1,118	

Crab Alternative (See Surimi)

Crab Apple (See Apple, Crab)

Cracker
Cheese
(General Mills):
Cheddar Snacks	1 Item	8	0.4	0	1	0	13	
Snacks	1 Item	7	0.4	0	1	0	11	
(Keebler):								
American Cheese	1 Item	70	4	1	7	0	85	
Munch'ems	1 Item	5	0.2	0	1	0	13	
Touch of Cheddar								
Club	1 Item	18	0.6	0	2	0	45	
Wheatable, White								
Cheddar	1 Item	6	0.3	0	1	0	13	

	Serv.	K-Cal.	Fat	Prot.	Carb.	Fib.	Sod.	FAC
(*Cracker cont.*)								
(Nabisco):								
Better Cheddars	1 Item	7	0.4	0	1	0	13	
Nips.............................	1 Item	5	0.2	0	1	0	11	
Peanut Butter								
Sandwich..................	1 Item	32	1.7	1	4	0	65	
Ritz Bits, Sandwich	1 Item	11	0.7	0	1	0	21	
Swiss Cheese.............	1 Item	9	0.5	0	1	0	23	
(Pepperidge Farm)								
Goldfish.......................	1 Item	3	0.1	0	0	0	4	
(Snorels) Cheddar								
Snack	1 Item	3	0.1	0	0	0	4	
(Sunshine) *Krispy*, Mild								
Cheddar	1 Item	12	0.4	0	2	0	36	
Fat-Free or Reduced Fat								
(Auburn Farms):								
Grainers	1 Oz	120	0	2	24	2	220	
Salsa Chipolte	1 Oz	110	0	2	23	2	280	
Spicy Pizza, 7-Grainer	1 Oz	110	0	3	23	2	280	
(Health Valley):								
WW	1 Item	10	0	0	2	0	16	
WW Cheese	1 Item	10	0	0	2	0	16	
(Keebler):								
Cinnamon Crisp..........	1 Item	14	0.2	0	3	0	24	
Graham Honey	1 Item	13	0.2	0	3	0	23	
Wheatables.................	1 Item	4	0.1	0	1	0	11	
Zesta...........................	1 Item	10	0	0	2	0	18	
(Nabisco):								
Better Cheddars	1 Item	6	0.3	0	1	0	15	
Cracker Crumbs	1 Cup	400	0	12	92	4	0	
Premium Saltine	1 Item	10	0	0	2	0	23	
Snackwell's, Cheese ..	1 Item	3	0.1	0	1	0	9	
Snackwell's, Cinna-								
mon Graham	1 Item	6	0	0	1	0	5	
Snackwell's, Golden ...	1 Item	10	0.2	0	2	0	23	
Snackwell's, Wheat	1 Item	12	0	0	2	0	34	
Triscuit	1 Item	16	0.4	0	3	1	23	
Wheat Thins	1 Item	7	0.2	0	1	0	12	
Pretzel Chip (Mr.								
Phipps)	1 Item	6	0	0	1	0	39	
(Sunshine):								
Cheez-It	1 Item	5	0.2	0	1	0	10	
Hi-Ho............................	1 Item	14	0.5	0	2	0	28	
Krispy	1 Item	12	0	0	2	0	27	
Graham								
(Health Valley):								
Amaranth......................	1 Item	13	0	1	3	0	4	
Oat Bran	1 Item	13	0	1	3	0	4	

	Serv.	K-Cal.	Fat	Prot.	Carb.	Fib.	Sod.	FAC
(Honey Maid):								
Cinnamon....................	1 Item	14	0.3	0	3	0	21	
Honey........................	1 Item	15	0.4	0	3	0	23	
(Keebler):								
Apple Cinnamon.........	1 Item	16	0.5	0	3	0	25	
Honey Fiber	1 Item	30	0.7	0	6	1	48	
Honey, Old-Fashioned	1 Item	19	0.8	0	3	0	18	
Kitchen Rich	1 Item	30	1.3	0	5	0	28	
Old-Fashioned	1 Item	16	0.4	0	3	0	17	
(Sunshine):								
Cinnamon....................	1 Item	70	2.3	1	12	1	70	
Honey........................	1 Item	60	1.5	1	11	1	75	
Crumbs	1 Tbsp	27	0.7	1	4	0	50	
Low Sodium or No Salt								
(Barbara's) *Wheatine*	1 Item	15	0.5	1	2	NV	11	
(Devonsheer) Melba,								
Wheat...........................	1 Item	17	0.2	1	3	0	0	
(Health Valley)								
WW Veg	1 Item	10	0	0	2	0	3	
(Keebler):								
Saltine, *Zesta*..............	1 Item	13	0.5	0	2	0	18	
Townhouse	1 Item	16	0.9	0	2	0	15	
Waldorf.......................	1 Item	15	0.5	0	3	0	1	
Wheatables.................	1 Item	6	0.3	0	1	0	6	
(Nabisco):								
Better Cheddars	1 Item	7	0.3	0	1	0	3	
Ritz..............................	1 Item	16	0.8	0	2	0	7	
Saltine, *Premium*	1 Item	12	0.2	0	2	0	7	
Tops, Premium	1 Item	12	0.3	0	2	0	27	
Triscuit	1 Item	21	0.9	0	3	0	7	
Wheat Thins	1 Item	9	0.4	0	1	0	5	
(Mr. Phipps) Pretzel								
Chip.............................	1 Item	8	0.2	0	1	0	26	
(Sunshine):								
Cheez-It	1 Item	6	0.3	0	1	0	3	
Hi-Ho...........................	1 Item	18	1	0	2	0	15	
Krispy	1 Item	12	0.3	0	2	0	24	
Melba								
(Devonsheer)..................	1 Item	17	0.2	1	3	0	0	
(Keebler)........................	1 Item	13	0.1	1	2	0	15	
(Old London)	1 Item	16	0.4	1	3	0	30	
Oyster								
(Keebler)........................	1 Item	3	0.1	0	0	0	8	
(Nabisco):								
....	1 Item	3	0.1	0	0	0	10	
Oysterettes...................	1 Item	3	0.1	0	1	0	8	
(Ralston)	1 Item	2	0.1	0	0	0	4	
(Sunshine) Biscuits	1 Item	4	0.1	0	1	0	12	

	Serv.	K-Cal.	Fat	Prot.	Carb.	Fib.	Sod.	FAC
(Cracker cont.)								
Rye								
(Auburn Farms) 7-								
Grainers	1 Oz	120	0	2	24	2	210	
(Finn Crisp) Hi-Fiber	1 Item	40	0	1	10	NV	95	
(Keebler) Toasted	1 Item	15	0.8	0	2	0	30	
(Ralston):								
Rykrisp	1 Item	30	0	1	7	2	38	
Rykrisp, Sesame	1 Item	30	0.8	1	6	2	40	
Snacks	1 Item	9	0.4	0	1	0	14	
(Ryvita):								
Crisp Bread	1 Item	37	0.1	1	8	2	26	
Crisp Bread, Dark	1 Item	26	0.5	1	6	1	35	
(Wasa) *Crisp Bread,*								
Golden	1 Item	35	0	1	7	1	55	
Saltine								
(Keebler) *Zesta*	1 Item	13	0.5	0	2	0	40	
(Nabisco) Multigrain	1 Item	12	0.4	0	2	NV	34	
Premium	1 Item	12	0.3	0	2	0	36	
(Sunshine) Krispy	1 Item	12	0.2	0	2	NV	42	
Sesame								
(Health Valley) Stoned								
Wheat	1 Oz	18	0.6	1	3	4	60	
(Keebler) *Toasted*								
Complements	1 Item	16	0.7	0	2	0	36	
(Nabisco) *Twigs* W/								
Cheese	1 Item	10	0.5	0	1	0	20	
(Pepperidge Farm)								
Distinctive	1 Item	20	1	1	2	1	35	
(Ralston) Wheat	1 Item	9	0.4	0	1	0	8	
(Sunshine) *American*								
Heritage	1 Item	18	1	0	2	0	33	
(Wasa) *Crisp Bread*	1 Item	30	1	2	4	2	40	
Vegetable								
(Auburn Farms) 7-								
Grainers	1 Oz	120	0	4	24	2	210	
(Hain)	1 Item	10	0	0	2	NV	22	
(Nabisco):								
Garden Crisps	1 Item	9	0.2	0	1	0	19	
Thins	1 Item	11	0.6	0	1	0	22	
Wheat								
(American Classic)								
Cracked Wheat	1 Item	70	4	1	8	1	140	
(Barbara's) *Wheatine,*								
Pepper	1 Item	50	1.5	1	10	1	110	
(Health Valley) WW								
Onion	1 Item	10	0	0	2	0	16	

	Serv.	K-Cal.	Fat	Prot.	Carb.	Fib.	Sod.	FAC
(Keebler):								
Harvest Wheats..........	1 Item	15	0.8	0	2	1	24	
Sun-Toasted	1 Item	7	0.4	0	1	0	11	
Toasteds								
Complements..............	1 Item	16	0.7	0	2	0	30	
Wheatables, Ranch	1 Item	6	0.3	0	1	0	12	
Whole Grain................	1 Item	18	0.8	0	3	0	25	
(Nabisco):								
Multigrain Thins	1 Item	8	0.2	0	1	0	17	
Nutty Thins	1 Item	10	0.6	0	1	NV	24	
Original Thins	1 Item	9	0.4	0	1	0	11	
Triscuits.....................	1 Item	20	0.7	0	3	1	24	
Triscuits W/Bran	1 Item	20	0.7	0	3	1	24	
Wheatsworth...............	1 Item	16	0.7	0	2	0	27	
(Pepperidge Farm)								
Flutters......................	1 Oz	147	6.7	3	17	NV	227	
(Sunshine):								
American Heritage W/								
Bran........................	1 Item	16	0.8	0	2	0	31	
Krispy.......................	1 Item	12	0.3	0	2	0	26	

Cranberry

	Serv.	K-Cal.	Fat	Prot.	Carb.	Fib.	Sod.	FAC
Raw, Chopped	4 Oz	54	0.2	0	14	5	1	A
Raw, (Ocean Spray)	3 Oz	37	0	0	9	NV	0	A
Low Bush, Lingenberry..	1 Cup	74	0.8	1	18	NV	NV	A

Cranberry Bean Borlotti Bean (See Bean, Cranberry)

Cranberry Juice

	Serv.	K-Cal.	Fat	Prot.	Carb.	Fib.	Sod.	FAC
(Mighty Mott's)								
Cocktail	1 Cup	150	0	0	36	0	20	A
(Ocean Spray):								
Cocktail	1 Cup	140	0	0	34	0	35	A
Crantastic....................	1 Cup	150	0	0	37	0	35	A
Reduced Calorie.........	1 Cup	50	0	0	13	0	35	A

Cranberry Juice, Blended

	Serv.	K-Cal.	Fat	Prot.	Carb.	Fib.	Sod.	FAC
(Fruitopia) W/Lemonade								
Vision	1 Cup	117	0	0	29	0	26	A
(Minute Maid) W/Apple								
Cocktail	1 Cup	170	0	0	42	NV	26	A
(Ocean Spray):								
Cran-Apple..................	1 Cup	160	0	0	41	1	35	A
Cran-Blueberry............	1 Cup	160	0	0	41	0	35	A
Cran-Grape.................	1 Cup	170	0	0	41	0	35	A
Cranicot......................	1 Cup	160	0	0	40	0	35	A

	Serv.	K-Cal.	Fat	Prot.	Carb.	Fib.	Sod.	FAC
Cranberry Sauce								
Jellied (S & W)	1 Cup	400	0	0	104	4	60	
Jellied (Ocean Spray)	¼ Cup	110	0	0	28	1	35	
Whole Berry (S & W)	1 Cup	400	0	0	104	4	60	
Whole Berry (Ocean Spray)	¼ Cup	110	0	0	28	1	10	
Crayfish								
Farmed, Raw	1 Item	2	0	1	0	0	2	
Farmed, Boiled	3 Oz	75	1	15	0	0	78	
Wild, Raw	1 Item	3	0	1	0	0	2	
Wild, Boiled	3 Oz	75	1	15	0	0	75	
Cream								
15% Butterfat	1 Tbsp	24	2.3	0	1	0	6	
18% Butterfat	1 Tbsp	28	2.7	0	1	0	6	
20% Butterfat	1 Cup	483	48	6	9	0	96	AC
20% Butterfat	1 Tbsp	30	3	0	1	0	6	
Half and Half	1 Tbsp	20	1.7	0	1	0	6	
Whipping, Heavy	1 Cup	821	88.1	5	7	0	90	A
Whipping, Heavy	1 Tbsp	51	5.5	0	0	0	6	
Whipping, Light	1 Cup	699	73.9	5	7	0	82	A
Whipping, Light	1 Tbsp	44	4.6	0	0	0	5	

Cream Cheese (See Cheese, Cream)

Cream, Nondairy Alternative
Frozen
(Birds Eye):

	Serv.	K-Cal.	Fat	Prot.	Carb.	Fib.	Sod.	FAC
Cool Whip	1 Tbsp	13	0.8	0	1	0	0	
Cool Whip, FF	1 Tbsp	8	0	0	2	0	3	
Cool Whip, LT	1 Tbsp	10	0.5	0	2	0	0	
(Dream Whip)	1 Tbsp	8	0.3	0	1	0	0	
(Dzerta) RF	1 Tbsp	5	0.5	0	1	0	5	
(Lucerne)	1 Tbsp	13	0.7	0	1	0	3	

Liquid
(Carnation):

	Serv.	K-Cal.	Fat	Prot.	Carb.	Fib.	Sod.	FAC
	1 Tsp	10	0.5	0	1	0	0	
FF	1 Tsp	10	0	0	2	0	0	
LT	1 Tsp	10	0	0	2	0	0	
(Coffee-Mate):								
	1 Tbsp	20	1	0	2	0	0	
FF	1 Tbsp	10	0	0	2	0	0	
Flavored	1 Tbsp	40	2	0	5	0	5	
Flavored, FF	1 Tbsp	25	0	0	5	0	0	
LT	1 Tbsp	10	0.5	0	1	0	5	
(Mocha Mix):								
FF	1 Tbsp	9	0.4	0	1	0	5	

	Serv.	K-Cal.	Fat	Prot.	Carb.	Fib.	Sod.	FAC
LT	1 Tbsp	10	0.9	0	1	0	4	
Original	1 Tbsp	21	1.8	0	1	0	7.5	
(Westsoy) Soy Milk	1 Tbsp	10	0.2	0	2	NV	10	

Powder
(Coffee-Mate):

	1 Tsp	10	0.5	0	1	0	0	
FF	1 Tsp	10	0	0	2	0	0	
Flavored	1 Tsp	15	0.7	0	2	0	4	
LT	1 Tsp	10	0	0	2	0	0	

Cream, Sour

	Serv.	K-Cal.	Fat	Prot.	Carb.	Fib.	Sod.	FAC
FF (Land O Lakes)	1 Tbsp	15	0	1	3	0	18	
FF (Naturally Yours)	2 Tbsp	20	0	1	3	0	50	
Half and Half	1 Tbsp	20	1.8	0	1	0	6	

(Lucerne):

	2 Tbsp	60	6	1	2	0	15	
FF	2 Tbsp	20	0	2	3	0	45	
LT	2 Tbsp	30	2	1	3	0	50	

(R.W. Kundsen):

Free, FF	1 Tbsp	18	0	1	3	0	13	
Hampshire	2 Tbsp	60	6	1	1	0	15	
Light, LT	1 Tbsp	20	1.3	1	1	0	10	

Cream, Sour—Alternative

(Imo)	1 Tbsp	30	3	0	0	0	15	
(Molly McButter)	1 Gram	3	0.1	0	1	0	61	
(Soymage)	1 Tbsp	20	1.5	1	2	0	15	
(Tofutti) *Soy Supreme*	1 Tbsp	25	2.5	1	1	NV	60	

Cream of Tartar

	1 Tsp	8	0	0	2	0	0	

Cream, Whipped—Pressurized Can

(Reddiwip) FF	2 Tbsp	10	0	0	2	0	0	
Original	2 Tbsp	20	2	0	0	0	0	

Cress, Garden (Also See Watercress)

Raw	1 Cup	16	0.4	1	3	1	7	FA
Boiled	1 Cup	31	0.8	3	5	1	11	FA

Croissant

Apple	2 Oz	145	5	4	21	1	156	
Butter	2 Oz	231	12	5	26	1	424	
Cheese	2 Oz	236	11.9	5	27	1	316	
Chocolate	2 Oz	233	14	5	23	2	257	
Original (Sara Lee)	1.5 Oz	170	8	4	20	1	200	
Plain	1 Oz	115	6.1	3	13	0	15	
Plain (Pepperidge Farm)	1.5 Oz	170	7	4	22	0	250	

	Serv.	K-Cal.	Fat	Prot.	Carb.	Flb.	Sod.	FAC
Crouton								
(Brownberry) Seasoned .	2 Tbsp	30	1	1	4	0	70	
(Marie Callender's):								
FF	2 Tbsp	25	0	0	5	0	100	
Original	2 Tbsp	30	1	1	5	0	75	
(Ener-G):								
Italian, Gluten-Free	1 Cup	241	12.5	4	31	4	305	
Plain, Gluten-Free	1 Cup	125	7	1	17	3	135	
(Parisian) Parmesan &								
Herb	4 Pieces	30	1	1	4	0	105	
(Pepperidge Farm):								
Cheddar & Romano	1 Piece	3	0.1	0	0	0	11	
Cheese & Garlic	1 Piece	4	0.2	0	0	0	9	
Onion & Garlic	1 Piece	3	0.1	0	1	0	9	
Seasoned	1 Piece	4	0.2	0	0	0	9	
Cucumber								
Raw (10 Oz)	1 Item	32	0.4	2	7	1	7	
Raw, Sliced	1 Cup	14	0.1	1	3	1	2	
Cumin								
Black	1 Oz	99	4.2	4	12	4	6	C
Ground (McCormick)	1 Tsp	11	0.4	0	1	1	5	
White	1 Oz	73	3.8	3	6	10	4	C
Cupcake								
Assorted, FF								
(Entenmann's)	1 Item	190	0	2	48	NV	115	
Devil's Food (Hostess)	1 Item	180	6	2	31	1	290	
Devil's Food, LT								
(Hostess)	1 Item	140	1.5	2	28	1	180	
Currants								
European Black, Raw	1 Cup	71	0.5	2	17	5	2	A
Red and White, Raw	1 Cup	63	0.2	2	16	5	1	A
Zante, Dried	1 Cup	408	0.4	6	107	10	12	F
Curry								
Leaf	1 Oz	32	0.5	3	4	3	3	AC
Powder	1 Tsp	7	0.3	0	1	1	10	F
Custard (See Pudding)								
Cuttlefish								
Raw	3 Oz	67	0.6	14	1	0	315	
Boiled	3 Oz	132	1.2	27	1	0	633	
Dried	1 Oz	85	0.8	17	2	0	294	

D

	Serv.	K-Cal.	Fat	Prot.	Carb.	Fib.	Sod.	FAC
Daikon—Chinese Radish								
Raw	1 Cup	16	0	1	4	1	18	**A**
Raw	1 Oz	4	0	0	1	0	15	
Sliced, Boiled	1 Cup	25	0.4	1	5	2	19	**A**
Dandelion								
Raw, Chopped	1 Oz	13	0.2	1	26	1	22	**A**
Raw, Chopped	1 Cup	25	0.4	1	5	2	42	**A**
Boiled	1 Cup	35	0.6	2	7	3	46	**A**
Danish Pastry (See Pastry, Danish)								
Date, Pitted								
Domestic, Chopped (Dole)	1 Cup	560	0	10	124	0	0	
Domestic, Whole	10 Dates	228	0.4	2	61	4	2	
Imported, Chopped (Dromedary)	1 Cup	520	0	4	124	0	0	
Imported, Whole (Dromedary)	10 Dates	200	0	2	46	0	0	
Deer (See Venison)								
Dhal								
Orange	1 Oz	101	0.4	8	17	0	5	
Red	1 Oz	96	0	6	18	0	14	
Yellow	1 Oz	95	0.1	5	18	0	10	
Diet Bar (Also See Breakfast Bar; Snack Bar; Sport Bar)								
(Ener-G) Granola, Gluten-Free	1 Item	335	21.3	7	29	4	115	
(Health Valley) Fruit Fitness, FF	1 Item	110	0	2	27	1	35	
(Pillsbury):								
Caramel, *Figurines*	1 Item	110	5.5	3	12	1	65	**FA**
Chocolate, *Figurines*	1 Item	110	5.5	3	12	1	55	**FA**

	Serv.	K-Cal.	Fat	Prot.	Carb.	Fib.	Sod.	FAC
(Diet Bar cont.)								
Peanut Butter, *Figurines*	1 Item	110	5.5	3	12	1	55	**FA**
S'mores, *Figurines*	1 Item	110	5.5	2	13	0	58	**FA**
Vanilla, *Figurines*	1 Item	110	5.5	2	13	0	58	**FA**
(Sweet Success):								
Chocolate Chip	1 Item	120	4	2	23	3	40	**FA**
Chocolate Brownie	1 Item	120	4	2	23	3	45	**FA**
Chocolate Peanut Butter	1 Item	120	4	2	23	3	35	**FA**
Oatmeal	1 Item	120	4	2	23	3	30	**FA**
(Ultra Slim-Fast):								
Apple, FF	1 Item	160	0	2	38	1	250	**FA**
Blueberry, FF	1 Item	170	0	1	39	2	170	**FA**
Brownie	1 Item	120	4	2	20	1	45	**FA**
Chewy Caramel Crunch	1 Item	120	3.5	1	22	2	45	**FA**
Cocoa Almond Crunch	1 Item	120	4	2	20	1	35	**FA**
Peanut Butter Crunch	1 Item	120	4	2	19	2	45	**FA**
Peanut Caramel Crunch	1 Item	120	4	1	22	2	35	**FA**
Strawberry, FF	1 Item	170	0	2	39	2	190	**FA**
Vanilla Crunch	1 Item	120	4	2	20	1	30	**FA**

Diet Drink (Also see Nutritional Drink, Sport Beverage)
Mix, prepared

	Serv.	K-Cal.	Fat	Prot.	Carb.	Fib.	Sod.	FAC
(Sweet Success)								
Chocolate Mocha W/ Skim Milk	1 Cup	160	1.4	13	27	5	298	**FAC**
Vanilla Delight W/Skim Milk	1 Cup	160	0.6	13	29	5	278	**FAC**
(Ultra Slim-Fast):								
Chocolate Fudge W/ NF Milk	1 Cup	200	2.6	14	36	5	216	**FAC**
Chocolate Malt W/ Skim Milk	1 Cup	200	1.3	14	36	5	216	**FAC**
Chocolate Royale W/ NF Milk	1 Cup	200	1.3	14	36	6	264	**FAC**
Chocolate W/Skim Milk	1 Cup	190	1.3	14	33	2	240	**FAC**
Milk Chocolate W/NF Milk	1 Cup	210	1.3	13	36	6	240	**FAC**
Strawberry W/NF Milk	1 Cup	200	1.3	14	36	4	264	**FAC**
Strawberry W/Skim Milk	1 Cup	190	1.3	14	33	2	264	**FAC**

	Serv.	K-Cal.	Fat	Prot.	Carb.	Fib.	Sod.	FAC
(Shaklee) Vanilla, *Slim*								
Plan	1 Cup	420	6	30	66	8	740	FAC
Ready-to-drink								
Nutra Start:								
Chocolate,	12 Oz	210	2.5	10	40	5	370	FAC
Vanilla,	12 Oz	210	2.5	10	38	5	350	FAC
(Shaklee) Vanilla, *Slim*								
Plan	8 Oz	420	6	30	66	8	740	FAC
(Ultra Slim-Fast):								
Chocolate Fudge	12 Oz	220	3	10	42	5	180	FAC
Chocolate Royale	12 Oz	220	3	10	38	5	330	FAC
Coffee	12 Oz	220	3	10	38	5	300	FAC
Milk Chocolate	12 Oz	220	3	10	42	5	330	FAC
Strawberry	12 Oz	220	3	10	42	5	460	FAC
Dill								
Seed (McCormick)	1 Tsp	13	0.4	0	2	2	1	
Weed (McCormick)	1 Tsp	4	0	0	0	0	10	
Weed, Fresh	1 Cup	4	0.1	0	1	0	5	
Dip (Also See Salsa)								
(Chili Con Queso) Pep-								
per, Cheese	1 Tbsp	28	2.7	0	1	0	25	
(Durkee) Sour Cream	1 Tbsp	38	0.8	2	3	0	300	
(Frito-Lay):								
Cheddar Cheese	1 Tbsp	25	1.5	1	2	0	120	
Cheese N' Salsa,								
Doritos	1 Tbsp	20	1	1	3	0	325	
French Onion	1 Tbsp	30	2.5	1	2	0	115	
Hot Bean	1 Tbsp	18	0.5	1	3	1	110	
Jalapeño & Cheddar								
Cheese	1 Tbsp	25	1.5	1	2	0	140	
Jalapeño Bean	1 Tbsp	20	0.5	1	3	0	70	
(Guiltless Gourmet):								
Black Bean, BBQ, FF.	1 Tbsp	18	0	1	3	1	63	
Nacho, Spicy, FF	1 Tbsp	13	0	1	3	0	75	
Pinto Bean, FF	1 Tbsp	18	0	1	3	1	50	
(Kraft):								
Bacon & Horseradish.	1 Tbsp	30	2.5	1	2	0	110	
Buttermilk	1 Tbsp	40	3.5	1	1	NV	135	
Clam	1 Tbsp	30	2	1	2	0	125	
French Onion	1 Tbsp	30	2	1	2	0	115	
Garlic	1 Tbsp	30	2	1	2	NV	80	
Green Onion	1 Tbsp	30	2	1	2	0	95	
Guacamole	1 Tbsp	25	2	1	2	NV	108	
(Old El Paso) Black								
Bean FF	1 Tbsp	10	0	1	2	1	75	
(Tostitos) Black Bean,								
FF	1 Tbsp	13	0	1	3	1	95	

	Serv.	K-Cal.	Fat	Prot.	Carb.	Fib.	Sod.	FAC
Donut (See Doughnut)								
Doughnut								
Cake, Plain, Glazed	1 Item	192	10.3	2	23	1	181	
Cake, Wheat, Glazed	1 Item	162	8.7	3	19	1	160	
Chocolate, Glazed	1 Item	175	8.4	2	24	1	143	
Chocolate Icing	1 Item	204	13.3	2	21	1	184	
Holes, Gluten-Free	1 Item	17	0.6	1	2	0	69	
Pumpkin, Gluten-Free	1 Item	128	5.9	0	18	NV	7	
Yeast, Creme Filling	1 Item	307	20.8	5	26	1	263	
Yeast, Glazed	1 Item	242	13.7	4	27	1	205	
Yeast, Jelly Filling	1 Item	289	15.9	5	33	1	249	
(Entenmann's):								
Crumb	1 Item	260	13	3	34	0	230	
Devil's Food	1 Item	250	12	3	33	1	240	
Frosted, Mini	1 Item	135	10	1	11	1	90	
Glazed Buttermilk	1 Item	270	13	3	36	0	280	
French Cruller, Glazed	1 Item	169	7.5	1	24	0	141	
(Hostess):								
Cinnamon	1 Item	110	5	2	15	0	140	
Frosted	1 Item	180	11	2	20	1	170	
Glazed, Old Fashioned	1 Item	250	12	3	33	0	230	
Plain	1 Item	140	7	2	16	0	190	
Powdered	1 Item	110	6	1	15	0	135	
Raspberry Filled, Powdered	1 Item	230	10	3	35	0	230	
Duck								
Breast								
Meat Only, Roasted	3 Oz	112	1.8	23	1	0	89	
Meat Only, Wild, Raw	3 Oz	104	3.6	17	0	0	48	
Meat/Skin, Roasted	3 Oz	164	8.9	21	0	0	71	
Meat/Skin, Wild, Raw	3 Oz	182	13.1	14	0	0	48	
Leg								
Meat Only, Roasted	3 Oz	138	4.6	15	0	0	90	
Meat/Skin, Roasted	3 Oz	175	9.4	23	0	0	95	
Liver								
Raw	3 Oz	120	4	17	3	0	122	FA
Duck, Chinese Pressed								
	3 Oz	158	7.8	6	16	1	173	
Duck Fat								
	1 Tbsp	115	12.8	0	0	0	0	
Duck Sauce								
(La Choy)	1 Tbsp	31	0.1	0	7	0	64	
Dulse (See Seaweed, Dried)								

$$\lceil$$

	Serv.	K-Cal.	Fat	Prot.	Carb.	Fib.	Sod.	FAC
Eel								
Raw	3 Oz	156	9.9	16	0	0	43	**A**
Smoked	3 Oz	276	24	15	0	0	90	**A**
Steamed	3 Oz	190	12	20	0	0	49	**A**
Egg, Chicken (Also See Omelet)								
Whole								
Raw	1 Cup	362	24.3	30	3	0	306	**FA**
Raw	1 Lge	75	5	6	1	0	63	
Fried	1 Cup	366	27.6	25	3	0	649	**FA**
Hard-Boiled	1 Lge	78	5.3	6	1	0	62	
Hard-Boiled	1 Cup	211	14.4	17	2	0	169	**FA**
Poached	1 Lge	75	5	6	1	0	140	
Scrambled	1 Cup	365	26.9	24	5	0	156	**FA**
White								
Raw	1 Lge	17	0	4	0	0	55	
Raw	1 Cup	122	0	26	3	0	399	
Powdered	1 Tbsp	24	0	5	0	0	77	
Yolk								
Raw	1 Cup	870	75	41	4	0	333	**FAC**
Raw	1 Lge	59	5.1	3	0	0	7	
Raw	2 Oz	203	17	10	1	0	24	**FA**
Egg Alternative								
(Egg Beaters) *No Cholesterol*	1 Cup	120	0	24	4	0	400	
(Ener-G) *Replacer, Dry*	1 Tsp	10	0	0	3	0	85	
(Healthy Choice) *Cholest-Free*	1 Cup	100	0	24	2	0	380	
(Morningstar) *Better'n Eggs*	1 Cup	94	1.2	20	0	0	358	
Scramblers	1 Cup	148	1.6	25	9	1	388	
(Tofutti) *Egg Watchers*	1 Cup	120	0	24	4	0	320	

	Serv.	K-Cal.	Fat	Prot.	Carb.	Fib.	Sod.	FAC
Egg Dishes, Fast Food								
(Arby's) Egg Platter								
Breakfast....................	1 Item	575	30	12	56	0	1,146	
(Burger King):								
Croissant, Bacon/Egg/								
Cheese....................	1 Item	350	24	15	18	1	790	
Croissant, Egg &								
Cheese....................	1 Item	369	24.7	13	24	2	551	AC
Croissant, Egg/								
Cheese/Ham	1 Item	350	22	18	19	NV	1,390	
Croissant, Sausage/								
Egg/Cheese.............	1 Item	600	46	22	25	1	1,140	
(Hardee's):								
Big Country Bacon	1 Item	820	49	33	62	NV	1,870	C
Big Country Ham........	1 Item	620	33	28	51	NV	1,780	
Big Country Sausage .	1 Item	1,000	66	41	62	NV	2,310	C
Biscuit, Bacon, &								
Egg..........................	1 Item	530	30	19	45	NV	1,280	
Biscuit, Bacon, Egg &								
Cheese....................	1 Item	610	37	24	45	NV	1,630	FAC
Biscuit Ham & Egg.....	1 Item	370	19	15	35	1	1,050	FA
Biscuit, Ham, Egg &								
Cheese....................	1 Item	540	30	20	48	1	1,660	AC
(Jack In The Box):								
Scrambled Egg Platter	1 Item	560	32	18	50	0	1,060	
Scrambled Egg								
Pocket	1 Item	430	21	29	31	0	1,060	AC
(McDonald's):								
Bacon & Egg Biscuit ..	1 Item	440	26.4	18	33	1	1,230	
Bacon, Egg & Cheese								
Biscuit.....................	1 Item	450	27	17	33	1	1,340	
Egg McMuffin.............	1 Item	290	13	17	27	1	730	F
Sausage & Egg Biscuit	1 Item	520	35	16	33	1	1,220	F
Sausage McMuffin								
with Egg	1 Item	440	29	19	27	1	820	FA
Scrambled Eggs (2) ...	1 Item	170	12	13	1	0	190	A
Egg, Duck								
Whole	1 Item	130	9.6	9	1	0	102	
Yolk.............................	1 Oz	104	9.9	4	0	0	17	
Egg, Goose								
Cooked	1 Item	266	19	20	2	0	420	FA
Eggnog								
(Borden).........................	1 Cup	320	9	3	16	0	80	AC
(Darigold).......................	1 Cup	390	17	10	48	0	170	AC
Mix	1 Tsp	55	0.1	0	14	0	22	
Mix, Prep W/Whole Milk,								
2 Tsp Mix.....................	1 Cup	261	8.4	8	39	0	163	AC

	Serv.	K-Cal.	Fat	Prot.	Carb.	Fib.	Sod.	FAC
Egg Noodle (See Noodle, Egg)								
Eggplant								
Raw (3 Oz)	1 Cup	21	0.2	1	5	2	2	
Boiled	1 Cup	27	0.2	1	6	2	3	
Breaded Cutlets								
(Bernardi)	1 Cup	360	22	6	34	4	440	
Egg, Quail								
Whole	1 Oz	48	3.6	3	0	0	16	
Egg Roll								
Beef/Pork (2 Oz)	1 Item	114	6.2	5	9	1	304	
Chicken or Turkey (2 Oz)	1 Item	105	5.6	4	9	1	188	
(La Choy):								
Chicken, Sweet &								
Sour	1 Item	180	4	6	29	3	300	
Pork	1 Item	170	6	6	23	3	390	
Pork/Shrimp (1 Oz)	1 Item	64	2.4	3	9	1	189	
Shrimp	1 Item	150	4	6	24	3	420	
Vegetable (3 Oz)	1 Item	187	5.5	4	30	2	490	
(Worthington)								
Vegetarian	1 Item	181	8.5	6	20	2	384	
Egg Roll, Fast Food								
(Jack In The Box)	3 Item	440	24	3	54	4	960	
Egg Roll Wrapper								
(Azumaya)	1 Item	65	0	2	13	1	100	
(Nasoya)	1 Item	65	0	4	26	1	200	
Elderberry								
Fresh	1 Cup	106	0.7	1	27	NV	0	A
Elk								
Raw	3 Oz	94	1.2	20	0	0	50	
Roasted	3 Oz	124	1.6	26	0	0	52	
Enchilada, Frozen								
Bean								
(Amy's Kitchen) Black								
Bean & Veg	1 Item	130	4	4	20	2	390	
Beef								
(Banquet)	1 Item	380	12	15	54	10	1,330	
(Gebhardt)	1 Item	129	9.6	2	10	2	344	
(Swanson) Dinner	1 Item	470	17	20	60	10	1,790	A
Cheese								
(Amy's Kitchen)	1 Item	210	9	11	16	2	390	

	Serv.	K-Cal.	Fat	Prot.	Carb.	Fib.	Sod.	FAC
(Enchilada, Frozen cont.)								
(Banquet)	1 Item	340	6	15	56	9	1,500	C
(Stouffer's) W/Rice	1 Item	370	14	12	48	5	890	AC
(Wt Watchers)	1 Item	250	6	10	38	5	520	AC
Chicken								
(Le Menu Healthy)	1 Item	280	8	21	32	NV	530	C
(Stouffer's) *Lean Cuisine,*								
Suiza	1 Item	290	5	12	48	5	530	
(Wt Watchers) Nacho	1 Item	290	8	15	42	4	560	AC
Suiza	1 Item	270	9	14	33	4	540	C
Tofu								
(Legume) Classic	1 Item	270	8	14	36	10	390	AC
Enchilada Sauce								
(Gebhardt)	1 Cup	139	8.2	3	14	2	872	
(Old El Paso) Green								
Chili	1 Cup	120	6	2	12	0	1,320	A
Mild	1 Cup	100	4	0	16	0	640	A
(Rosarita)	1 Cup	91	4.3	3	10	0	20	
(Rosarita)	1 Tbsp	6	0.3	NV	1	0	102	
(Santiago)	1 Cup	84	0.8	2	16	3	1,104	
Endive								
Raw, Chopped	1 Cup	9	0.1	1	2	2	11	F
Raw, Chopped	6 Oz	29	0.3	2	6	5	38	FA

English Muffin (See Muffin, Ready-To-Serve, English)

Escargot (See Snail)

F

	Serv.	K-Cal.	Fat	Prot.	Carb.	Fib.	Sod.	FAC
Fajita								
Beef	1 Item	290	12.4	12	33	3	603	**A**
Chicken	1 Item	287	9.3	15	36	3	311	**A**
Chicken, Fiesta (Healthy Choice)	1 Item	260	4	21	36	5	410	**A**
Fajita, Fast Food								
(McDonald's) Chicken	1 Item	190	8	11	20	NV	310	
(Mighty Taco) Chicken, SM	1 Item	195	7	16	16	1	538	
Steak, SM	1 Item	205	8.5	14	17	2	673	
Fajita, Frozen								
Chicken (Healthy Choice)	1 Item	260	4	21	36	5	410	**A**
Falafel—Falafil								
Mix								
(Casbah)	2 Tbsp	108	2	4	14	1	357	
(Telma)	2 Tbsp	110	1	5	19	4	45	
Prepared From Mix								
Patty	1 Oz	94	5	4	9	NV	84	
(Fantastic) (4 Oz)	1 Cup	250	4	15	42	11	610	
Farina (See Cereal, Hot)								
Fat Substitute								
(Bob's Red Mill) *Oatrim*	2 Tbsp	40	0.2	1	7	0	0	
(Fruitsource)	1 Tsp	15	0	0	4	0	0	
(Sunsweet)	2 Tbsp	70	0	0	18	0	0	
(Wonderslim)	2 Tbsp	17	0	1	5	2	5	

Fava Bean—Broad Bean—Horse Bean—Jack Bean (See Bean, Fava)

	Serv.	K-Cal.	Fat	Prot.	Carb.	Fib.	Sod.	FAC
Feijoa								
Raw, Puree	1 Cup	120	1.9	3	26	NV	10	F
Fennel—Finocchio								
Bulb, Raw, Sliced...........	1 Cup	27	0.2	1	6	3	45	
Leaves, Raw	1 Oz	8	0.1	1	1	NV	3	
Fennel Seeds (Also See Anise Seed)								
Whole	1 Tsp	7	0.3	0	1	1	2	
Fenugreek Seed								
Whole	1 Oz	91	1.6	7	12	3	17	
Whole	1 Tsp	12	0.2	1	2	1	2	
Fern, Fiddlehead								
Shoots, Flower	1 Cup	61	0.4	6	9	6	150	A
Greens, Frozen	1 Cup	18	0.3	2	3	NV	1	A

Fettuccine (See Pasta, Fettuccine; Pasta Entree, Frozen)

	Serv.	K-Cal.	Fat	Prot.	Carb.	Fib.	Sod.	FAC
Fig								
Fresh								
Raw	1 Oz	21	0	0	5	1	0	
Raw	1 Lb	335	1.4	3	87	15	4	A
Raw (Large)	1 Item	37	0.2	NV	10	2	1	
Canned W/								
Heavy Syrup..................	1 Cup	228	0.3	1	60	6	3	A
Light Syrup....................	1 Cup	174	0.3	1	45	5	3	A
Water Pack.....................	1 Cup	131	0.3	1	35	5	3	A
Dried								
Uncooked	1 Cup	507	2.3	6	130	19	22	AC
Cooked	1 Cup	280	1.3	3	71	12	13	A

Filbert (See Hazelnut)

Filo (See Phyllo Dough)

Finocchio (See Fennel)

Fish (See individual listings)

	Serv.	K-Cal.	Fat	Prot.	Carb.	Fib.	Sod.	FAC
Fish Dish, Alternative								
Fillets (Worthington)	1 Item	91	4.9	8	4	2	375	
Fish Dish, Fast Food								
(Burger King) Tenders ...	1 Item	267	16	12	18	1	870	C
(McDonald's) *Filet O*								
Fish	1 Item	360	16	14	41	1	690	

	Serv.		K-Cal.	Fat	Prot.	Carb.	Fib.	Sod.	FAC
(Long John Silver's):									
Catfish Fillet	1 Item		860	42	28	90	0	990	**FAC**
Fish and Fries	1 Item		610	37	27	52	NV	1,480	
Homestyle Fish, 6									
Pieces	1 Item		1,260	64	49	124	2	1,590	**F**
Seafood Platter	1 Item		970	46	30	109	5	1,540	**FA**
Shrimp & Fish Entree.	1 Item		1,140	65	40	108	NV	2,440	**C**
Shrimp, Fish &									
Chicken	1 Item		1,160	65	45	113	NV	2,590	**C**
Shrimp Scampi	1 Item		610	18	25	87	0	2,120	**AC**
10 Piece Shrimp	1 Item		840	47	18	88	NV	1,630	**C**

Fish Eggs—Roe
(1 Oz equals approximately 2 Tbsp)

	Serv.		K-Cal.	Fat	Prot.	Carb.	Fib.	Sod.	FAC
Roe	1	Oz	40	1.8	6	0	0	26	
Salmon	1	Oz	40	2.2	5	0	0	NV	
Whitefish Roe	1	Oz	26	1.5	2	1	0	NV	

Fish Entree, Frozen
(Serving size given in Oz to reflect weight of 1 serving)

	Serv.		K-Cal.	Fat	Prot.	Carb.	Fib.	Sod.	FAC
(Gorton's) Potato									
Crisp	2	Oz	150	9.5	6	10	0	160	
(Healthy Choice) Lemon									
Pepper	10.8 Oz		290	5	14	47	7	360	**A**
(Mrs. Paul's):									
Dijon, LT	10	Oz	230	5.7	24	19	NV	743	**C**
Florentine, LT	10	Oz	275	10	31	13	NV	1,030	**C**
Mornay, LT	10	Oz	256	11	27	13	NV	744	**AC**
(Stouffer's) Lean Cuisine:									
Divan	10	Oz	210	6	25	15	3	490	**A**
Florentine	9	Oz	240	9	26	13	NV	700	
Jardiniere	11.4 Oz		290	10	31	18	NV	840	**A**
(Swanson) Fish 'N Chips	10	Oz	480	20	19	55	5	1,050	
(Van De Kamps) Fish 'N									
Fries	6.6 Oz		380	18	13	41	2	370	**A**

Fish Fillet, Frozen
(Serving size given in Oz to reflect weight of 1 serving)

	Serv.		K-Cal.	Fat	Prot.	Carb.	Fib.	Sod.	FAC
(Gorton's):									
Crispy Batter	3.8 Oz		290	21	10	16	0	550	
Crunchy	2	Oz	125	7	6	11	0	240	
Crunchy, Breaded	3.8 Oz		270	17	12	17	0	480	
Crunchy, Microwave	2	Oz	150	10	6	10	NV	255	
(Healthy Choice)									
Breaded	1.7 Oz		80	2.5	6	8	NV	175	**A**
(Mrs. Paul's):									
Battered	2 Items		330	17	16	28	0	650	
Crispy Crunchy	2 Items		220	9	13	23	0	380	

	Serv.	K-Cal.	Fat	Prot.	Carb.	Fib.	Sod.	FAC
(Fish Fillet, Frozen cont.)								
Crispy Crunchy,								
Breaded..................	2 Items	230	15	10	14	0	300	
Crunchy.....................	2 Items	280	14	12	26	0	730	
(Van De Kamp's)								
Battered	2.7 Oz	180	11	8	12	0	340	
(Wt Watchers) Fried.......	7.7 Oz	230	8	15	25	2	450	
Fish Sticks, Frozen								
(Gorton's):								
....	.7 Oz	44	1.6	2	5	0	94	
Crispy Batter..............	.7 Oz	58	4	2	4	0	120	
Crunchy......................	.7 Oz	60	3.7	2	5	NV	115	
Potato Crisp.............	.6 Oz	45	2.7	2	4	0	45	
(Healthy Choice)								
Breaded	2.4 Oz	120	4	8	14	NV	250	
(Mrs. Paul's):								
Battered	4 Items	210	12	7	15	0	590	
Crispy Crunchy	4 Items	190	8	9	18	0	560	
Crispy Crunchy,								
Breaded	4 Items	140	6	7	14	0	340	
Flaxseed								
(Arrowhead Mills)	3 Tbsp	140	10	5	11	6	0	
Flaxseed Oil								
(Spectrum) Organic........	1 Tbsp	120	14	0	0	0	0	A
(Puritan).........................	1 Tbsp	120	14	0	0	0	0	A
Flounder								
Fresh								
Raw	3 Oz	77	1	16	0	0	70	
Broiled	3 Oz	99	1.3	21	0	0	89	
Frozen								
(Mrs. Paul's):								
Breaded, LT................	1 Item	240	10	16	20	0	450	
Crunchy Batter............	2 Items	220	9	12	23	0	560	
(Van De Kamp's)								
Natural	4 Oz	110	2	22	0	0	105	
Flour (See individual listings)								
Frankfurter								
(Serving size equals 1 frankfurter)								
Beef								
(Armour) Jumbo	2 Oz	90	6	6	3	0	440	A
(Ball Park):								
FF..................................	1.8 Oz	40	0	6	4	0	560	
LT..................................	2 Oz	110	8	7	4	0	730	

	Serv.	K-Cal.	Fat	Prot.	Carb.	Flb.	Sod.	FAC
(Healthy Choice):								
....	1.7 Oz	60	1.5	7	5	0	430	
Bun-Length	2 Oz	70	1.5	7	6	0	480	
Jumbo	2 Oz	70	1.5	7	6	0	480	
LF................................	2.7 Oz	100	3	11	7	0	480	
(Hebrew National)	1.7 Oz	149	14	6	1	0	497	
(Hormel) *Light & Lean* ..	1.6 Oz	45	1	6	2	0	390	
(Oscar Mayer):								
....	2 Oz	130	11	7	1	0	630	A
Bun-Length	2 Oz	180	17	6	1	0	570	
Deli Style	2.7 Oz	230	22	9	1	0	680	
LT................................	2 Oz	110	8	6	2	0	620	
Original........................	2.7 Oz	240	22	9	1	0	700	
Turkey								
(Butterball)	2 Oz	120	10	7	1	0	620	
(Louis Rich):								
....	1.6 Oz	80	6	5	1	0	500	
Bun-Length	2 Oz	110	8	7	3	0	630	
W/Cheese	1.6 Oz	90	7	5	2	0	420	
(Mr. Turkey):								
....	1.6 Oz	110	9	5	2	0	540	
W/Cheese	2 Oz	140	11.8	7	2	0	682	

Frankfurter, Alternative

	Serv.	K-Cal.	Fat	Prot.	Carb.	Flb.	Sod.	FAC
(La Loma) Sizzle............	1.2 Oz	85	6.5	5	2	NV	170	
(Light Life) Tofu Dogs....	1.5 Oz	60	2.5	8	2	0	140	
(Loma Linda)	1.8 Oz	100	6.7	10	2	2	243	
(Morningstar)	1.6 Oz	109	6.5	10	3	3	524	
(Natural Touch)	1.6 Oz	99	5.5	10	2	2	471	
(Smart Dogs)	1.5 Oz	45	0	9	1	0	170	
(White Wave)	1.6 Oz	90	1.5	13	6	0	350	
(Wildwood) Wild Dogs ...	2 Oz	60	0	12	2	0	490	
(Worthington) Fripats	2.3 Oz	132	6.3	15	4	4	323	
(Yves):								
Chili Dog......................	1.6 Oz	70	0	12	5	2	295	
Veggie Wiener.............	1.6 Oz	50	0	11	2	0	320	

French Bean—Haricot Vert (See Green Bean)

French Toast, Frozen

	Serv.	K-Cal.	Fat	Prot.	Carb.	Flb.	Sod.	FAC
(Aunt Jemima):								
....	1 Slice	120	3	5	19	1	180	
W/Cinnamon	1 Slice	120	3	5	19	1	165	
(Campbell's)	1 Slice	94	5	4	11	2	235	
(Krusteaz):								
Homestyle....................	1 Slice	115	2.5	5	18	2	270	
Sourdough	1 Slice	140	2	6	24	0	280	
W/Cinnamon	1 Slice	115	2.5	5	18	1	270	

	Serv.	K-Cal.	Fat	Prot.	Carb.	Fib.	Sod.	FAC
French Toast, Fast Food								
(Arby's) Toastix	1 Item	72	3.5	2	9	1	92	
(Burger King) Sticks	1 Serv	500	27	4	60	1	490	
(Carl's Jr) Dips	1 Item	82	5	1	8	1	76	
Frog Leg								
Raw	3 Oz	62	0.3	14	0	0	50	
Fried	3 Oz	247	16.9	15	7	1	421	
Frosting								
Mix								
(Betty Crocker) Creamy:								
Chocolate Fudge	1 Tbsp	37	0.5	0	8	0	5	
Coconut Pecan	1 Tbsp	40	1.3	0	7	0	2	
Vanilla	1 Tbsp	37	0.5	0	8	0	0	
Ready-to-serve								
(Betty Crocker) *Rich and Creamy:*								
Butter Pecan	1 Tbsp	75	3	0	13	0	23	
Cherry, *Creamy*								
Deluxe	1 Tbsp	70	2.5	0	12	0	20	
Chocolate Chip	1 Tbsp	80	3	0	13	0	13	
Chocolate	1 Tbsp	75	3	0	12	0	23	
Cream Cheese	1 Tbsp	70	2.5	0	12	0	33	
Lemon	1 Tbsp	70	2.5	0	12	0	33	
Milk Chocolate	1 Tbsp	75	3	0	12	0	23	
Rainbow Chip	1 Tbsp	80	3	0	13	0	13	
Sour Cream,								
Chocolate	1 Tbsp	75	3	0	12	0	43	
Sour Cream, White	1 Tbsp	75	3	0	13	0	23	
Vanilla	1 Tbsp	70	2.5	0	12	0	18	
Vanilla, Light	1 Tbsp	60	0.3	0	14	0	13	
(Duncan Hines):								
Butter Cream	1 Tbsp	70	2.5	0	11	0	30	
Caramel	1 Tbsp	70	2.5	0	11	0	30	
Chocolate	1 Tbsp	65	2.5	0	10	0	48	
Chocolate								
Buttercream	1 Tbsp	65	2.5	0	10	0	48	
Cream Cheese	1 Tbsp	70	2.5	0	11	0	30	
Kiwi Strawberry	1 Tbsp	70	2.5	0	11	0	30	
Lemon Cream	1 Tbsp	70	2.5	0	11	0	30	
Mango Tangerine	1 Tbsp	70	2.5	0	11	0	30	
Milk Chocolate	1 Tbsp	65	2.5	0	10	0	48	
Peaches 'N Cream	1 Tbsp	70	2.5	0	11	0	30	
Raspberries 'N Cream	1 Tbsp	70	2.5	0	11	0	30	
Strawberries 'N Cream	1 Tbsp	70	2.5	0	11	0	30	
Vanilla	1 Tbsp	70	2.5	0	11	0	30	
Wild Cherry Vanilla	1 Tbsp	70	2.5	0	11	0	30	

	Serv.	K-Cal.	Fat	Prot.	Carb.	Fib.	Sod.	FAC
(Pillsbury):								
Caramel Pecan..........	1 Tbsp	75	4	0	10	0	33	
Chocolate Fudge, LF..	1 Tbsp	70	1.8	0	13	0	43	
Chocolate Fudge Supreme..................	1 Tbsp	70	3	0	11	0	38	
Coconut Almond Supreme..................	1 Tbsp	80	4.5	0	9	0	30	
Coconut Pecan Supreme..................	1 Tbsp	80	5	0	9	0	30	
Cream Cheese Supreme..................	1 Tbsp	75	3	0	12	0	35	
Lemon Creme Supreme..................	1 Tbsp	75	3	0	12	0	38	
Milk Chocolate Fudge Swirl........................	1 Tbsp	70	3	0	11	0	30	
Milk Chocolate Supreme..................	1 Tbsp	70	3	0	11	0	30	
Pink Vanilla Funfetti ...	1 Tbsp	75	3	0	12	0	35	
Strawberry Supreme...	1 Tbsp	75	3	0	12	0	38	
Vanilla/Fudge Swirl.....	1 Tbsp	75	3	0	13	0	38	
Vanilla Funfetti............	1 Tbsp	80	3	0	13	0	38	
Vanilla Supreme	1 Tbsp	75	3	0	12	0	35	

Fruit (See individual listings)

Fruit Bar, Frozen

	Serv.	K-Cal.	Fat	Prot.	Carb.	Fib.	Sod.	FAC
(Dole) Grape	1 Item	45	0	0	11	0	0	A
Raspberry	1 Item	45	0	0	11	0	0	
(Dreyers):								
Coconut......................	1 Item	160	5	2	27	0	30	A
Lime	1 Item	90	0	0	23	0	0	A
Peach..........................	1 Item	140	0	0	35	0	0	A
Strawberry..................	1 Item	90	0	0	23	0	0	A
(Garden of Eatin') All Flavors	1 Item	60	0	0	15	0	15	
(Minute Maid) All Flavors	1 Item	50	0	0	12	0	0	
(Natural Nectar) Fruit.....	1 Item	70	1	1	16	NV	15	
(Popsicle) All Flavors	1 Item	50	0	0	12	0	0	
(Tropicana) Orange........	1 Item	60	0	0	16	0	0	A
(Welch's):								
Grape	1 Item	80	0	0	19	0	0	A
Strawberry..................	1 Item	25	0	0	6	0	0	
Tropical Blend..............	1 Item	45	0	0	11	0	0	

Fruit Cocktail W/

	Serv.	K-Cal.	Fat	Prot.	Carb.	Fib.	Sod.	FAC
Extra Heavy Syrup.........	1 Cup	229	0.2	1	60	3	16	
Extra Light Syrup	1 Cup	111	0.2	1	29	3	10	
Juice Pack.....................	1 Cup	114	0	1	29	2	10	

	Serv.	K-Cal.	Fat	Prot.	Carb.	Fib.	Sod.	FAC
(Fruit Cocktail W/ cont.)								
Light Syrup Pack............	1 Cup	146	0.2	1	38	3	15	
Tropical, Heavy								
Syrup......................	1 Cup	221	0.3	1	58	3	5	
Water Pack....................	1 Cup	78	0.1	1	21	2	10	
(Del Monte) Heavy								
Syrup......................	1 Cup	200	0	0	48	2	20	
(Hunt's)......................	1 Cup	180	0	0	46	2	30	
(Libby's) Fruit Juice........	1 Cup	120	0	0	30	2	20	
(S & W) Heavy Syrup....	1 Cup	180	0	0	46	2	30	
Natural Style..............	1 Cup	160	0	2	40	4	40	
(Townhouse) Heavy								
Syrup......................	1 Cup	180	0	0	46	2	30	

Fruit Juice (See individual listings)

Fruit Punch
(Hawaiian Punch)								
Tropical......................	1 Cup	120	0	0	29	0	40	
(HI-C)...........................	1 Cup	125	0	0	31	0	22	
(Minute Maid)................	1 Cup	120	0	0	32	0	5	
(Mott's)........................	1 Cup	100	0	0	25	0	0	A
(Ocean Spray)...............	1 Cup	130	0	0	32	0	0	A
(Tree Top)	1 Cup	120	0	0	30	0	24	
(Tropicana)	1 Cup	118	0	0	27	0	20	
(Welch's)......................	1 Cup	144	0	0	36	0	0	

Fruit Punch, Mix
(Prepared as indicated)								
(Crystal Light) Berry								
Blend.........................	1 Cup	4	0	0	0	0	0	
(Kool-Aid):								
Great Bluedini.............	1 Cup	60	0	0	16	0	0	
NSA...........................	1 Cup	5	0	0	0	0	10	
Purplesaurus Rex.......	1 Cup	60	0	0	16	0	0	

Fruit Salad (See Fruit Cocktail)

Fruit Snack
Animals (Grist Mill).........	1 Item	100	1.5	0	22	0	30	
(Betty Crocker):								
Fruit by the Foot.........	1 Item	80	1.5	0	17	1	40	
Gushers	1 Item	90	1	0	20	0	50	A
Roll-Ups	1 Item	55	0.5	0	12	0	55	A
Shark Bites	1 Item	90	1	0	21	0	25	
Squeezit	1 Item	110	0	0	28	0	0	
String Thing................	1 Item	80	1	0	17	0	45	A
(Stretch Island) Leather,								
Org.............................	1 Item	90	0	0	25	2	10	

	Serv.	K-Cal.	Fat	Prot.	Carb.	Fib.	Sod.	FAC
(Sunkist) Fruit Rolls	1 Item	70	0	0	17	2	20	**A**
(Wt Watchers)	1 Item	50	0	0	13	NV	75	

Fruit Spread
(Knott's Berry Farm) All

	Serv.	K-Cal.	Fat	Prot.	Carb.	Fib.	Sod.	FAC
Flavors	1 Tbsp	40	0	0	10	0	0	
(Polaner) All Flavors	1 Tbsp	40	0	0	10	0	0	
(Sorrell Ridge) All								
Flavors	1 Tbsp	36	0.9	0	9	0	0	
(Smucker's) LT...............	1 Tbsp	10	0	0	5	0	0	
Simply Fruit.................	1 Tbsp	40	0	0	10	0	0	

Fudge (See Candy, Fudge)

Fudge Topping (See Chocolate Syrup and Toppings)

G

	Serv.	K-Cal.	Fat	Prot.	Carb.	Fib.	Sod.	FAC
Galangal								
Raw	1 Oz	10	0.2	0	2	0	1	
Garam Masala								
Fresh	1 Tbsp	25	0.7	1	5	3	9	
Garbanzo Bean—Chickpea—Cece Beans (See Bean, Garbanzo)								
Garbanzo Flour—Chickpea Flour								
Toasted (Arrowhead Mills)	1 Cup	360	4	20	60	12	0	
Garlic								
Raw, Bulb	1 Oz	45	0	1	10	0	3	A
Raw, Clove	1 Item	4	0	0	1	0	1	
Garlic, Dried								
Powder (McCormick)	1 Tsp	10	0	0	2	1	2	
Salt (French's)	1 Tsp	4	0	0	1	NV	2,050	
Salt (Morton)	1 Tsp	0	0	0	1	NV	1,300	
Gefilte Fish								
(Manischewitz)	2.3 Oz	70	5	6	1	0	320	
(Mother's) *Old World*	1 Item	70	1	8	7	NV	NV	
(Rokeach)	2 Oz	60	3	6	3	1	240	
Gelatin Dessert								
(Prepared as indicated on package)								
(D-Zerta) All Flavors	1 Cup	16	0	4	0	0	0	
(Jell-O):								
Apricot	1 Cup	160	0	4	38	0	100	
Black Cherry	1 Cup	160	0	4	38	0	100	
Cherry	1 Cup	160	0	4	38	0	140	
Cherry, SF/LC	1 Cup	20	0	2	0	0	120	
Grape	1 Cup	160	0	4	38	0	90	

	Serv.	K-Cal.	Fat	Prot.	Carb.	Fib.	Sod.	FAC
Grape, SF/LC	1 Cup	20	0	2	0	0	100	
Lemon	1 Cup	160	0	4	38	0	150	
Lemon, SF/LC	1 Cup	20	0	2	0	0	110	
Lime	1 Cup	160	0	4	38	0	120	
Lime, SF/LC	1 Cup	20	0	2	0	0	120	
Mango	1 Cup	160	0	4	38	0	90	
Mixed Fruit	1 Cup	160	0	4	38	0	100	
Mixed Fruit, SF/LC	1 Cup	20	0	2	0	0	100	
Orange	1 Cup	160	0	4	38	0	100	
Orange, SF/LC	1 Cup	20	0	2	0	0	130	
(Royal):								
Apple	1 Cup	160	0	4	38	0	190	
Fruit Punch	1 Cup	160	0	4	38	0	180	
Lime, SF	1 Cup	16	0	2	2	0	200	
Mixed Fruit	1 Cup	160	0	4	38	0	180	

Gelatin, Rennet
(Prepared as indicated on package)
(Junket):

	Serv.	K-Cal.	Fat	Prot.	Carb.	Fib.	Sod.	FAC
Chocolate	1 Cup	240	8	10	30	NV	130	
Strawberry	1 Cup	240	8	8	32	NV	120	
Vanilla	1 Cup	240	8	8	32	NV	120	

Gelatin, Unflavored

	Serv.	K-Cal.	Fat	Prot.	Carb.	Fib.	Sod.	FAC
Dry	1 Tbsp	31	0	8	0	0	8	
Dry	1 Cup	491	0.2	126	0	0	132	
Dry, Envelope	1 Item	27	0	1	6	0	18	

Ghee (See Butter, Clarified)

Ginger Root

	Serv.	K-Cal.	Fat	Prot.	Carb.	Fib.	Sod.	FAC
Raw, Sliced	1 Oz	17	0.2	0	4	0	3	
Crystallized	1 Oz	96	0.1	0	25	NV	17	
Pickled	1 Oz	27	0.1	1	6	1	20	
Powder	1 Tsp	6	0.1	0	1	0	1	

Ginkgo Nut

	Serv.	K-Cal.	Fat	Prot.	Carb.	Fib.	Sod.	FAC
Raw	1 Oz	50	0.5	1	11	0	2	A
Canned	1 Cup	170	2.5	4	34	3	475	FA

Ginseng Juice

	Serv.	K-Cal.	Fat	Prot.	Carb.	Fib.	Sod.	FAC
(Odwalla)	1 Cup	50	0	0	12	0	3	
(R.W. Knudsen) Boost	1 Cup	110	0	0	27	0	20	

Gluten (See Wheat, Gluten)

Gnocchi—Potato

	Serv.	K-Cal.	Fat	Prot.	Carb.	Fib.	Sod.	FAC
(Bertagni)	1 Cup	165	0	4	37	2	310	
(Emilia)	1 Cup	260	0.5	5	59	3	590	

Goa Bean (See Bean, Winged)

	Serv.	K-Cal.	Fat	Prot.	Carb.	Fib.	Sod.	FAC
Goat								
Raw	3 Oz	93	1.9	18	0	0	70	
Baked	3 Oz	136	4.7	21	0	0	288	
Boiled	3 Oz	177	6.6	28	0	0	276	
Gobo (See Burdock Root)								
Goose								
Liver, Raw	3 Oz	113	3.6	14	5	0	119	**FA**
Meat and Skin, Raw	3 Oz	315	28.6	13	0	0	62	
Meat Only	3 Oz	137	6.1	19	0	0	74	
Meat and Skin, Roasted	3 Oz	259	18.6	21	0	0	60	
Gooseberry								
Raw	1 Cup	66	0.9	1	15	6	2	**A**
Raw	1 Lb	200	2.6	4	46	20	5	**A**
W/Heavy Syrup, Canned	1 Cup	184	0.5	2	47	6	5	**A**
Goose Fat								
	1 Tbsp	115	12.8	0	0	0	0	
Goose Liver Pâté (See Pâté, Canned)								
Gourd (Also See Bitter Melon; Loofah; Winter Melon)								
Calabash, Bottled	1 Oz	4	0	0	1	0	1	
Snake	1 Oz	5	0	0	1	0	2	
Strips, Dried	1 Cup	139	0.3	5	35	NV	8	
White Flowered, Boiled	1 Cup	22	0	1	5	2	3	**A**
Graham Crackers (See Cracker, Graham; Cookie, Graham)								
Granola (See Cereal, Ready-To-Serve, Multigrain)								
Granola Bar (See Snack Bar)								
Grape								
Fresh								
Concord	1 Cup	58	0.3	1	16	1	2	**A**
Flames	1 Lb	323	2.6	3	81	5	9	**A**
Thompson	1 Cup	114	0.9	1	28	2	3	**A**
Canned, Thompson W/								
Heavy Syrup (S & W)	1 Cup	200	0	1	46	1	40	
Water	1 Cup	98	0.3	1	25	2	15	
Grapefruit								
Fresh								
Whole, 4" Diameter	1 Item	88	0.2	2	21	3	0	**A**
Sections, W/Juice	1 Cup	85	0.2	1	22	3	2	**A**

	Serv.	K-Cal.	Fat	Prot.	Carb.	Fib.	Sod.	FAC
Sections, Drained............	1 Cup	69	0.2	1	18	3	0	A
Canned W/								
Juice	1 Cup	92	0.2	2	23	1	17	A
Light Syrup	1 Cup	152	0.3	1	39	1	5	A
Natural Style (S & W)	1 Cup	75	0	0	21	0	38	A
Water Pack....................	1 Cup	88	0.2	1	22	1	5	A

Grapefruit Juice

	Serv.	K-Cal.	Fat	Prot.	Carb.	Fib.	Sod.	FAC
Fresh	1 Cup	96	0.3	1	23	0	2	A
(Del Monte)	1 Cup	93	0	1	23	0	13	A
(Minute Maid)	1 Cup	96	0	0	23	0	26	A
(Odwalla)	1 Cup	88	0	2	20	0	5	A
(R.W. Knudsen).............	1 Cup	100	0	2	23	1	35	A
(Sunkist)	1 Cup	96	0.2	1	23	0	3	A
(Tree Top)	1 Cup	104	0	0	24	0	32	A
(Tropicana)	1 Cup	93	0	1	19	0	26	A

Grapefruit Peel

	Serv.	K-Cal.	Fat	Prot.	Carb.	Fib.	Sod.	FAC
Candied	1 Cup	536	0.5	1	137	4	0	

Grape Juice

	Serv.	K-Cal.	Fat	Prot.	Carb.	Fib.	Sod.	FAC
(Fruitopia)	1 Cup	127	0	0	32	0	26	
(Kraft) No Sugar.............	1 Cup	138	0	1	33	NV	0	
(Libby's) Juicy	1 Cup	130	0	1	32	0	10	
(Powerade)	1 Cup	73	0	0	45	0	32	
(R.W. Knudsen).............	1 Cup	150	0	1	37	NV	30	
Concord	1 Cup	160	0	0	40	NV	15	
(Tree Top) Juice Fizz	1 Cup	120	0	0	30	NV	25	
(Welch's) Concord..........	1 Cup	160	0	0	40	0	13	
White...........................	1 Cup	160	0	0	40	0	20	

Grape Juice, Frozen, Diluted

	Serv.	K-Cal.	Fat	Prot.	Carb.	Fib.	Sod.	FAC
(Minute Maid)	8 Oz	120	0	0	32	0	0	
(Sunkist)	8 Oz	92	0	0	23	0	4	
(Welch's).......................	8 Oz	133	0	0	33	0	0	

Grapeseed Oil

	Serv.	K-Cal.	Fat	Prot.	Carb.	Fib.	Sod.	FAC
....	1 Tbsp	120	13.6	0	0	0	0	A

Gravy
Canned/Bottled
(Franco-American):

	Serv.	K-Cal.	Fat	Prot.	Carb.	Fib.	Sod.	FAC
Au Jus.........................	1 Cup	40	2	4	8	0	1,240	
Beef.............................	1 Cup	120	8	4	16	0	1,200	
Chicken	1 Cup	180	16	4	12	0	1,080	
Chicken Giblet	1 Cup	120	8	4	12	0	1,240	
Cream	1 Cup	140	8	0	16	0	882	
Mushroom	1 Cup	80	4	4	8	0	1,200	
Pork, Golden...............	1 Cup	180	16	4	12	0	1,360	
Turkey.........................	1 Cup	100	4	2	12	0	1,160	

	Serv.	K-Cal.	Fat	Prot.	Carb.	Flb.	Sod.	FAC
(Gravy cont.)								
(Heinz) Turkey, FF.........	1 Cup	50	0	4	12	NV	1,120	
(Pepperidge Farm)								
Beef............................	1 Cup	100	4	4	16	NV	1,440	
Mix								
(Loma Linda):								
Brown, Quik...............	1 Tbsp	20	0.2	1	4	0	367	
Chicken, Quik, Veg	1 Tbsp	19	0.1	1	3	0	408	
Country, Quik, Veg.....	1 Tbsp	22	0.6	1	4	0	249	
Mushroom, Quik, Veg	1 Tbsp	16	0.3	1	3	1	304	
Onion, Quik, Veg, FF.	1 Tbsp	18	0	1	3	1	229	
(McCormick) Brown,								
Herb	1 Tsp	10	0.3	0	2	0	150	
Onion	1 Tsp	10	0.3	0	2	0	180	
(Pillsbury):								
Brown, FF...................	1 Tsp	5	0	0	2	0	135	
Chicken Style, FF.......	1 Tsp	5	0	0	2	0	125	
Homestyle, FF	1 Tsp	5	0	0	2	0	135	
Mix, prepared								
(Lawry's) Au Jus FF	¼ Cup	10	0	0	2	NV	390	
(Pillsbury):								
Brown, FF...................	1 Cup	40	0	0	12	0	1,080	
Chicken, FF	1 Cup	80	0	2	16	0	1,040	
Homestyle, FF	1 Cup	40	0	0	12	0	1,080	
(Schilling):								
Au Jus, FF..................	¼ Cup	5	0	0	1	NV	280	
Brown..........................	¼ Cup	20	0.5	<1	4	NV	340	
Chicken	1 Cup	88	1.6	3	14	NV	1,200	
Onion	¼ Cup	20	0.5	<1	4	NV	360	
(Wt Watchers) Brown FF	¼ Cup	10	0	1	2	NV	360	

Great Northern Bean (See Bean, Great Northern)

Green Bean—Snap Bean—String Bean—Asparagus—French Haricot Vert—Long Bean—Yard-Long (Also See Wax Bean)

	Serv.	K-Cal.	Fat	Prot.	Carb.	Flb.	Sod.	FAC
Fresh								
Raw	1 Cup	34	0.1	2	8	4	7	**FA**
Raw	1 Lb	123	0.5	7	29	8	23	**FA**
Raw, Yard-Long	1 Cup	43	0.4	3	8	NV	4	**FA**
Boiled............................	1 Cup	44	0.4	2	10	4	4	**FA**
Canned								
Cut (Green Giant)	1 Cup	40	0	2	8	2	800	F
Cut (S & W)	1 Cup	40	0	2	8	4	680	F
French Style (S & W)	1 Cup	40	0	2	8	4	680	F
LS (Del Monte)	1 Cup	40	0	2	8	4	20	F
Whole (Green Giant)......	1 Cup	50	0	2	10	4	660	F
Frozen								
Cut (Green Giant)	1 Cup	38	0	1	8	3	142	F
French (Flav R Pac)	1 Cup	25	0	1	4	2	10	F

	Serv.	K-Cal.	Fat	Prot.	Carb.	Fib.	Sod.	FAC
(Health Valley)................	1 Cup	50	2	2	8	2	18	FA
W/Butter (Green Giant)..	1 Cup	60	2	2	8	3	460	F

Green Onions (See Onion, Green)

Grenadine
(Rose's)	2 Tbsp	90	0	0	22	0	10	

Grits
Cooked	1 Cup	145	0.5	3	32	0	0	
Mix								
White	1 Tbsp	36	0.1	1	8	0	0	
White (Arrowhead Mills).	1 Tbsp	35	0	1	8	0	0	
Yellow.............................	1 Tbsp	36	0.1	1	8	0	0	
Yellow (Arrowhead Mills)............................	1 Tbsp	33	0	1	7	0	0	
Hominy, Canned								
(S & W) Golden, *Sun Vista*............................	1 Cup	140	0	4	38	6	1,080	
White, *Sun Vista*.........	1 Cup	130	1	4	36	6	1,060	
(Van Camp's) White.......	1 Cup	160	2	2	32	2	1,060	
Hominy, mix								
(Quaker):								
White, Quick	1 Cup	520	2	12	116	8	0	
Yellow, Quick..............	1 Cup	480	2	12	116	8	0	
Yellow, Regular	1 Cup	560	2	12	128	8	0	
Instant								
(Quaker):								
Bacon Bits	1 Oz	100	0.5	3	22	1	340	
Butter Flavor..............	1 Oz	100	1.5	2	21	1	320	
Cheddar Cheese	1 Oz	100	1.5	2	21	2	520	
Original.....................	1 Oz	100	0	2	22	1	300	
Sausage Bits	1 Oz	100	1	3	21	2	480	
Zesty Cheddar............	1 Oz	100	1.5	3	20	2	460	

Ground-Cherry (See Cape Gooseberry)

Ground Husk Tomato (See Tomatillo)

Grouper
Raw	3 Oz	78	0.9	17	0	0	45	
Broiled	3 Oz	100	1.1	21	0	0	45	

Guacamole
(Calavo)..........................	2 Tbsp	60	5	0	3	0	140	
(Kraft).............................	2 Tbsp	50	4	1	3	0	216	
(La Mexicana)	2 Tbsp	40	3	0	4	0	100	

	Serv.	K-Cal.	Fat	Prot.	Carb.	Fib.	Sod.	FAC
Guava								
Raw	1 Cup	84	1	1	20	9	5	A
Raw	1 Lb	208	0.9	5	45	31	105	FA
Guava Juice								
(Kern's) Nectar	1 Cup	150	0	0	36	0	5	A
(Libby's) Nectar	1 Cup	152	0	0	38	0	7	A
Nectar W/Banana	1 Cup	154	0	0	35	0	17	A
(Ocean Spray)	1 Cup	130	0	0	32	0	35	A
W/Mango	1 Cup	130	0	0	33	0	35	A
Guinea Hen								
Meat Only, Raw	3 Oz	93	2.1	18	0	0	0	
Meat/Skin, Raw	3 Oz	107	4.4	16	0	0	0	

H

	Serv.	K-Cal.	Fat	Prot.	Carb.	Fib.	Sod.	FAC
Haddock								
Raw	3 Oz	74	0.6	16	0	0	58	
Broiled	3 Oz	95	0.8	21	0	0	74	
Broiled	1 Cup	291	2.4	63	0	0	226	A
Fried, Breaded	3 Oz	199	9.7	17	11	1	393	
Smoked	3 Oz	99	0.8	21	0	0	649	
Frozen, Crispy Batter (Gorton's)	2 Oz	135	8.5	5	10	0	280	
Frozen, Crunchy Batter (Mrs. Paul's)	1 Item	95	2.5	7	11	0	290	
Halibut								
Atlantic or Pacific, Raw..	3 Oz	94	1.9	18	0	0	46	
Greenland, Raw	3 Oz	158	11.8	12	0	0	68	
Atlantic, Broiled	3 Oz	123	2.6	23	0	0	60	
Greenland, Broiled	3 Oz	203	15.1	16	0	0	88	
Halvah (See Candy, Halvah)								
Hamburger (Also See Beef, Ground)								
Cheese/Bacon	1 Lge	756	48.9	40	38	NV	1,739	
Cheese	1 Lge	609	33.0	30	47	NV	1,589	
Plain	1 Lge	426	22.9	23	32	NV	474	
Hamburger, Alternative								
(Amy's Kitchen)								
California	2.5 Oz	100	3	4	17	3	290	
(Fantastic):								
Black Bean	2.5 Oz	110	2	7	20	4	290	
Tofu	3.4 Oz	137	5	9	14	3	337	
(Garden Burger):								
FF	2.5 Oz	140	0	11	23	4	250	
LF	2.5 Oz	130	3	6	19	2	340	
Zesty Bean	2.5 Oz	120	2.5	6	18	3	340	
(Imagine Foods)	2.5 Oz	130	1	5	26	3	260	
(La Loma) Sizzle	2.5 Oz	220	12	17	10	NV	420	

	Serv.	K-Cal.	Fat	Prot.	Carb.	Fib.	Sod.	FAC
(Hamburger, Alternative cont.)								
(Morningstar):								
Garden Grille	2.5 Oz	120	2.5	6	18	4	280	
Garden Veggie	2.4 Oz	100	2.5	10	9	4	350	
Prime Patties	2.8 Oz	110	2	19	5	3	300	
Spicy Black Bean	2.8 Oz	110	1	11	16	20	470	
(Natural Touch):	2.2 Oz	136	6.3	15	4	4	317	
Black Bean	2.7 Oz	110	1	11	15	5	330	
Garden Vegetable	2.4 Oz	100	2.5	10	8	3	280	
Okara	2.3 Oz	160	12	11	4	3	360	
Vegan........................	2.7 Oz	70	0	11	6	3	370	
(Nature's Burger):								
Black Bean	2.5 Oz	110	2	7	20	4	290	
Red Pepper	2.5 Oz	110	2	7	20	3	290	
Orig, Fantastic	3 Oz	170	3	8	30	5	320	
(Worthington).................	1 Cup	242	7.6	35	9	4	1,076	

Hamburger, Cheese, Fast Food
(Burger King):

	Serv.	K-Cal.	Fat	Prot.	Carb.	Fib.	Sod.	FAC
....	1 Item	380	19	23	28	1	770	
Bacon BBQ,								
Double..........................	1 Item	536	31	32	31	1	795	
Bacon Double	1 Item	640	39	44	28	1	1,240	C
Double........................	1 Item	600	36	41	28	1	1,060	AC
Whopper	1 Item	730	46	33	46	3	1,350	C
Whopper, Double........	1 Item	960	63	52	46	3	1,420	C
(Carl's Jr):								
Bacon DBL, Western..	1 Item	970	57	56	58	2	1,810	C
Bacon, Western	1 Item	687	35	34	59	2	1,490	C
(Jack In The Box):	1 Item	320	15	16	32	0	670	
Bacon Bacon	1 Item	710	45	35	41	0	1,240	
Double..........................	1 Item	450	24	24	35	0	970	C
Jumbo Jack	1 Item	650	40	31	42	0	1,150	C
Ultimate......................	1 Item	1,030	79	50	30	0	1,200	C
(McDonald's):								
Cheeseburger	1 Item	320	14	15	36	2	750	
McLean Deluxe,								
Cheese....................	1 Item	400	17	27	38	2	1,040	
Quarter Pound								
Cheeseburger..........	1 Item	530	30	28	37	2	1,160	
(Wendy's):								
Bacon Jr	1 Item	410	21	22	34	2	910	
Deluxe Jr	1 Item	360	16	18	36	3	840	
Jr.................................	1 Item	320	13	17	34	2	770	
Kid's Meal..................	1 Item	320	13	17	33	2	770	
Single, Everything.......	1 Item	490	25	29	38	3	1,130	C

Hamburger Entree Mix
(Prepared as indicated on the box)

	Serv.	K-Cal.	Fat	Prot.	Carb.	Fib.	Sod.	FAC
(Betty Crocker) *Hamburger Helper:*								
Beef Roman................	1 Cup	290	11	20	28	1	930	
Beef Taco	1 Cup	310	11	20	30	1	920	
Burger Stew................	1 Cup	250	10	19	22	3	920	A
Cheddar N Bacon.......	1 Cup	350	16	24	28	1	890	
Cheesy Italian.............	1 Cup	330	14	22	29	1	920	
Chili Macaroni.............	1 Cup	290	10	19	30	1	870	A
Lasagne	1 Cup	280	10	19	30	0	950	
Nacho Cheese............	1 Cup	340	13	22	30	1	930	
Pizza Pasta.................	1 Cup	290	10	19	31	1	670	
Pot Au Grat	1 Cup	290	14	18	24	2	820	
Potato Stroganoff.......	1 Cup	270	12	18	25	2	870	
Rice Orient.................	1 Cup	310	10	19	35	0	1,050	
Spagetti......................	1 Cup	300	11	21	29	1	940	A
Stroganoff	1 Cup	350	14	23	33	1	960	
Zesty Italian	1 Cup	320	11	21	34	1	890	

Hamburger, Fast Food

	Serv.	K-Cal.	Fat	Prot.	Carb.	Fib.	Sod.	FAC
(Burger King):								
....	1 Item	330	15	20	28	1	530	
Double Whopper.........	1 Item	870	56	46	45	3	940	
Mushroom Swiss								
DBL	1 Item	473	27	31	27	NV	746	
Whopper	1 Item	640	39	27	45	3	870	
Whopper, Jr	1 Item	420	24	21	29	2	530	
(Carl's Jr):								
Big Burger..................	1 Item	470	20	25	46	2	810	
Famous Big Star	1 Item	610	38	26	42	2	890	
Super Star,								
Hamburger	1 Item	820	53	43	41	2	1,030	
(Hardee's):								
Big Twin.....................	1 Item	450	25	23	34	2	580	AC
Mushroom N Swiss	1 Item	610	36	41	31	NV	1,420	C
(Jack In The Box):								
....	1 Item	280	11	13	31	0	470	
Colossus	1 Item	940	60	52	48	0	1,670	C
Grilled Sourdough.......	1 Item	670	43	32	39	0	1,180	C
Jumbo Jack	1 Item	560	32	26	41	0	700	
¼ LB............................	1 Item	510	27	26	39	0	1,080	
(McDonald's):								
Big Mac Hamburger ...	1 Item	530	28	25	42	3	960	
Hamburger	1 Item	270	10	12	35	2	520	
McLean Deluxe...........	1 Item	350	12	24	37	2	800	FA
(Wendy's):								
Bacon, *Big Classic*	1 Item	610	33	36	45	3	1,510	
Big Classic..................	1 Item	580	30.5	34	45	3	1,385	AC
Jr................................	1 Item	270	10	15	34	2	560	
Kid's Meal..................	1 Item	270	10	15	33	2	560	

	Serv.	K-Cal.	Fat	Prot.	Carb.	Fib.	Sod.	FAC
(Hamburger, Fast Food cont.)								
Single, Plain................	1 Item	360	16	25	31	2	460	
Single W/Everything ...	1 Item	420	20	26	37	3	810	

Ham, Canned
(Armour):

	Serv.	K-Cal.	Fat	Prot.	Carb.	Fib.	Sod.	FAC
Chopped	3 Oz	190	7	20	0	0	1,245	
Goldstar	3 Oz	100	4	14	2	0	980	
(Bryan Foods) Pureed ...	1 Cup	480	36	33	0	0	225	
(Dubuque)........................	3 Oz	100	4	14	1	0	1,040	
(Hormel):								
Black Label................	3 Oz	100	5	15	0	0	970	
Chopped	3 Oz	240	21	12	1	0	1,062	
Cured	3 Oz	90	3	15	1	0	954	
Curemaster	3 Oz	84	3	14	0	0	940	
(Oscar Mayer)								
Jubilee........................	3 Oz	87	2.7	15	0	0	861	

Ham Entree, Frozen

	Serv.	K-Cal.	Fat	Prot.	Carb.	Fib.	Sod.	FAC
(Armour) Classics...........	10.8 Oz	270	7	15	36	0	1,300	
(Banquet)........................	8 Oz	210	4	12	32	3	980	
(Le Menu) Steak	10 Oz	300	11	19	31	NV	1,500	
(Stouffer's):								
W/Asparagus	9.6 Oz	520	36	16	32	2	1,040	
W/Cheese Crepes	7.5 Oz	410	25	25	23	NV	905	

Ham, Fresh
Leg, rump half

	Serv.	K-Cal.	Fat	Prot.	Carb.	Fib.	Sod.	FAC
Raw	3 Oz	120	4.5	18	0	0	60	
Roasted	3 Oz	175	6.9	26	0	0	55	
Roasted, Diced..............	1 Cup	278	11	42	0	0	88	
Leg, shank half								
Raw	3 Oz	120	4.5	6	0	0	16	
Roasted	3 Oz	183	8.9	24	0	0	54	
Roasted, Diced..............	1 Cup	290	14.2	38	0	0	86	

Ham, Luncheon Meat
(Healthy Choice):

	Serv.	K-Cal.	Fat	Prot.	Carb.	Fib.	Sod.	FAC
....	1 Slice	30	1	6	1	0	240	
Fresh-Trak	1 Slice	30	1	5	1	0	240	
Thin	1 Slice	10	0.3	2	0	0	78	
(Hormel):								
Light & Lean..............	1 Slice	25	1	4	0	0	340	
Prosciutto	1 Oz	60	3.5	8	0	0	540	
Baked								
(Healthy Choice):								
....	1 Slice	30	1	5	1	0	240	
Thin Slice....................	1 Slice	10	0.3	2	0	0	78	

	Serv.	K-Cal.	Fat	Prot.	Carb.	Fib.	Sod.	FAC
(Oscar Mayer):								
....	1 Slice	20	0.3	4	1	0	240	
FF..................................	1 Slice	13	0	2	1	0	187	
Healthy Favorites........	1 Slice	13	0.4	2	0	0	108	
(Louis Rich):								
Carving Board..............	1 Slice	25	0.8	4	1	0	275	
Dinner Slice	1 Slice	80	1.5	16	1	0	1,150	
Boiled								
(Oscar Mayer)	1 Slice	20	0.8	3	0	0	273	
Thin Slice....................	1 Slice	13	0.5	2	0	0	170	
W/Honey								
(Healthy Choice):								
....	1 Slice	35	0.8	5	2	0	195	
Fresh-Trak	1 Slice	30	1	5	1	0	240	
Thin	1 Slice	10	0.3	2	0	0	78	
Thin Slice....................	1 Slice	10	0.3	2	0	0	78	
(Hillshire Farm)...............	1 Slice	10	0.3	2	1	0	100	
(Oscar Mayer):	1 Slice	23	0.8	3	1	0	253	
FF..................................	1 Slice	13	0	2	1	0	187	
Healthy Favorites........	1 Slice	15	0.4	2	1	0	108	
Thin Slice....................	1 Slice	15	0.5	2	1	0	158	
(Louis Rich):								
Carving Board..............	1 Slice	25	0.8	4	1	0	280	
Carving Board, Thin ...	1 Slice	12	0.3	2	0	0	125	
Smoked								
(Healthy Choice):								
....	1 Slice	30	1	5	1	0	240	
Thin	1 Slice	10	0.3	2	0	0	78	
(Hillshire Farm)...............	1 Slice	10	0.3	2	1	0	95	
(Oscar Mayer):								
....	1 Slice	20	0.8	3	0	0	250	
FF..................................	1 Slice	12	0	2	0	0	187	
Healthy Favorites........	1 Slice	13	0.4	2	0	0	108	
Thin	1 Slice	13	0.5	2	0	0	155	
(Louis Rich) *Carving*								
Board	1 Slice	23	0.8	4	0	0	285	
Turkey Ham								
(Healthy Choice)	1 Oz	30	1	5	0	0	240	
(Mr. Turkey) Smoked	1 Oz	33	1.4	5	0	0	322	
(Louis Rich):								
Chopped	1 Oz	45	2.5	5	1	0	300	
Thin..............................	½ Oz	15	0.4	3	0	0	145	
W/Honey	1 Oz	30	1	5	1	0	290	
Ham Patty								
(Hormel).........................	2 Oz	180	17	7	1	0	550	
W/Cheese	2 Oz	190	17	7	0	0	470	

	Serv.	K-Cal.	Fat	Prot.	Carb.	Fib.	Sod.	FAC

Ham, Spread
(Hormel):

	Serv.	K-Cal.	Fat	Prot.	Carb.	Fib.	Sod.	FAC
Deviled	4 Tbsp	140	12	8	0	0	432	
Potted	4 Tbsp	100	8	7	0	0	610	
Spam	4 Tbsp	140	12	8	1	0	570	
(Libby's)	4 Tbsp	75	3	1	7	0	350	
(Underwood) Deviled	1 Oz	104	9	4	0	NV	202	

Haricot Vert—French Bean (See Green Bean)

Hash
(Dinty Moore) Corned

	Serv.	K-Cal.	Fat	Prot.	Carb.	Fib.	Sod.	FAC
Beef	1 Cup	350	22	19	19	2	850	
(Libby's) Corned Beef	1 Cup	490	38	18	25	8	1,510	
Roast Beef	1 Cup	460	33	19	23	3	1,390	
(Mary Kitchen):								
Corned Beef	1 Cup	410	27	21	22	2	1,020	
Roast Beef	1 Cup	390	24	21	22	2	790	
Roast Turkey	1 Cup	420	11	39	42	3	1,800	
Sausage	1 Cup	410	27	20	23	2	1,020	

Hazelnut—Filbert
(1 Cup weighs approximately 4 Oz)

	Serv.	K-Cal.	Fat	Prot.	Carb.	Fib.	Sod.	FAC
Dried, Chopped	1 Oz	182	18	4	4	2	1	
Dried, Chopped	1 Cup	727	72	15	18	7	3	FC
Dry-Roasted, Salted	1 Cup	953	95.5	14	26	12	1,123	FC
Dry-Roasted, Salted	1 Oz	238	24	4	6	3	281	
Oil-Roasted, Salted	1 Cup	950	91.6	21	28	13	1,132	FC
Whole, Natural								
(Oregon)	1 Oz	178	16.7	5	5	4	64	

Hazelnut Butter

	Serv.	K-Cal.	Fat	Prot.	Carb.	Fib.	Sod.	FAC
(Roaster Fresh)	1 Oz	188	19	4	5	0	1	

Hazelnut Oil

	Serv.	K-Cal.	Fat	Prot.	Carb.	Fib.	Sod.	FAC
	1 Tbsp	120	13.6	0	0	0	0	A

Hazelnut Spread

	Serv.	K-Cal.	Fat	Prot.	Carb.	Fib.	Sod.	FAC
Nutella	2 Tbsp	160	9	2	19	0	30	

Head Cheese

	Serv.	K-Cal.	Fat	Prot.	Carb.	Fib.	Sod.	FAC
(Columbus)	1 Oz	85	7	6	0	0	240	
(Oscar Mayer)	1 Oz	50	4	5	0	0	360	
(Saag's)	1 Oz	50	3	4	0	0	300	

Hearts of Palm (See Palm Heart)

Herring

	Serv.	K-Cal.	Fat	Prot.	Carb.	Fib.	Sod.	FAC
Atlantic, Raw	3 Oz	134	7.7	15	0	0	77	
Atlantic, Broiled	3 Oz	173	9.9	20	0	0	98	

	Serv.	K-Cal.	Fat	Prot.	Carb.	Fib.	Sod.	FAC
Kippered	3 Oz	184	10.5	15	0	0	74	
Pacific, Raw	3 Oz	165	11.7	14	0	0	63	
Pacific, Broiled	3 Oz	224	15.9	19	0	0	85	
Pickled	3 Oz	223	15.3	12	8	0	740	
Kippered W/Wine (Vita)	¼ Cup	120	5	9	10	0	480	
Kippered W/Sour Cream (Vita)	¼ Cup	120	7	7	8	0	600	

Hickory Nut

	Serv.	K-Cal.	Fat	Prot.	Carb.	Fib.	Sod.	FAC
Dried	1 Oz	187	18.3	4	5	2	0	
Dried	2 Oz	374	36	7	10	4	0	A

Hollandaise Sauce

	Serv.	K-Cal.	Fat	Prot.	Carb.	Fib.	Sod.	FAC
(Aunt Penny's)	2 Tbsp	45	4	1	2	0	350	
(Kraft) All Natural	2 Tbsp	160	14	2	6	0	360	

Hominy (See Grits, Hominy; Cereal, Hot)

Honey

	Serv.	K-Cal.	Fat	Prot.	Carb.	Fib.	Sod.	FAC
Strained/Extracted	1 Cup	1,016	0	1	275	1	17	
Strained/Extracted	1 Tbsp	64	0	0	17	0	1	
(Golden Blossom)	1 Oz	90	0	0	23	0	0	

Honeydew Melon

	Serv.	K-Cal.	Fat	Prot.	Carb.	Fib.	Sod.	FAC
Fresh	1 Cup	60	0.2	1	16	1	17	A
Fresh	1 Lb	160	0.5	2	42	3	45	A
Frozen, Balls	1 Cup	60	0	1	15	1	21	A

Horsebean (See Bean, Fava)

Horseradish (Also See Wasabi)
Raw

	Serv.	K-Cal.	Fat	Prot.	Carb.	Fib.	Sod.	FAC
Grated	1 Tbsp	13	0	1	3	0	1	AC

Prepared

	Serv.	K-Cal.	Fat	Prot.	Carb.	Fib.	Sod.	FAC
Cream Style (Kraft)	1 Tbsp	12	0	0	2	0	85	
White (Gold's)	1 Tbsp	12	1	1	1	0	165	

Hot Dog (See Frankfurter)

Hubbard Squash (See Squash, Winter)

Huckleberry

	Serv.	K-Cal.	Fat	Prot.	Carb.	Fib.	Sod.	FAC
Alaska, Wild	1 Cup	56	0.2	1	13	NV	15	

Hummus

	Serv.	K-Cal.	Fat	Prot.	Carb.	Fib.	Sod.	FAC
Fresh	1 Cup	421	20.8	12	50	13	600	FA
Fresh (Wildwood)	2 Tbsp	55	3.5	2	5	NV	105	
Dry (Fantastic)	1 Tbsp	30	1	2	5	1	110	

	Serv.	K-Cal.	Fat	Prot.	Carb.	Fib.	Sod.	FAC
(Hummus cont.)								
Prepared from Mix								
(Casbah)	1 Cup	640	32	20	56	4	720	**FA**

Hyacinth Bean (See Bean, Hyacinth)

I

	Serv.	K-Cal.	Fat	Prot.	Carb.	Fib.	Sod.	FAC
Ice Cream								
(Also see Fruit Bars, Frozen; Sorbet; Yogurt, Frozen)								
Almond								
(Baskin Robbins) Buttercrunch, LT	1 Cup	240	8	8	36	2	110	C
(Dreyer's) Praline	1 Cup	320	16	6	40	NV	170	
Apple								
(Baskin Robbins) Apple Pie, Truly Free	1 Cup	160	0	8	32	2	150	C
Banana								
(Baskin Robbins):								
Chunky Banana	1 Cup	180	3	6	32	0	110	C
Nut	1 Cup	300	20	4	30	0	80	
W/Strawberry	1 Cup	260	14	4	34	0	80	
(Ben & Jerry's) W/ Walnut	1 Cup	580	40	10	52	2	100	A
(Edy's) Split	1 Cup	340	20	6	38	NV	100	
(Healthy Choice) Foster	1 Cup	220	3	6	42	2	120	AC
Brownie								
(Edy's) Batter	1 Cup	300	16	6	36	NV	110	
Fudge, LT	1 Cup	220	8	6	36	NV	90	
(Häagen-Dazs) A La Mode	1 Cup	562	35.6	10	50	1	265	C
Butter Pecan								
(Baskin Robbins)	1 Cup	320	22	4	26	0	100	
(Ben & Jerry's)	1 Cup	620	50	10	40	2	250	AC
(Dreyer's)	1 Cup	320	18	6	32	NV	100	
(Edy's) LT	1 Cup	240	10	6	32	NV	90	
(Häagen-Dazs)	1 Cup	644	48.8	10	40	1	288	AC
(Healthy Choice)	1 Cup	240	4	6	44	2	120	C
Caramel								
(Baskin Robbins) Ban Surprise, FF	1 Cup	220	0	6	48	0	190	C
Chocolate Crunch	1 Cup	320	20	4	38	0	170	

	Serv.	K-Cal.	Fat	Prot.	Carb.	Fib.	Sod.	FAC
(Ice Cream cont.)								
Cheesecake								
(Baskin Robbins):								
Blueberry....................	1 Cup	300	14	4	40	0	160	
Cherry	1 Cup	300	14	4	40	0	150	
NY	1 Cup	300	18	4	34	0	150	
Pineapple, FF	1 Cup	220	0	6	48	0	200	C
(Edy's) Chunk, LT	1 Cup	240	10	6	32	NV	70	
Strawberry..................	1 Cup	300	16	6	36	NV	60	
(Häagen-Dazs)								
Strawberry..................	1 Cup	579	35.6	8	56	1	320	AC
Cherry								
(Baskin Robbins):								
Chunk A Cherry								
Burnin' Love............	1 Cup	280	16	4	32	0	90	
Cordial, NSA...............	1 Cup	200	4	6	38	0	110	C
Jubilee........................	1 Cup	280	14	4	32	0	80	
(Ben & Jerry's) *Cherry*								
Garcia	1 Cup	480	32	6	50	0	110	A
(Dreyers) W/Vanilla	1 Cup	200	6	6	30	NV	100	
W/Vanilla, FF	1 Cup	200	0	8	42	NV	140	
(Edy's) W/Chocolate								
Chip............................	1 Cup	300	16	6	36	NV	70	
(Healthy Choice) Cherry								
Choc Chunk................	1 Cup	220	4	6	38	1	110	C
Chocolate								
(Baskins Robbins):								
....	1 Cup	300	18	4	36	0	120	
Mousse	1 Cup	340	20	4	40	2	120	
Ribbon	1 Cup	280	16	4	34	0	90	
Truly FF	1 Cup	160	0	10	30	2	160	C
(Dreyers) NSA...............	1 Cup	200	8	6	26	NV	90	
(Edy's)	1 Cup	280	18	6	30	NV	60	
(Häagen-Dazs)	1 Cup	528	35.8	10	45	2	151	AC
(Wt Watchers) *Tornado* .	1 Cup	300	7	8	52	2	160	
Chocolate Chip								
(Baskin Robbins)............	1 Cup	300	20	4	30	0	90	
NSA............................	1 Cup	200	5	8	34	0	140	
(Dreyers)........................	1 Cup	320	16	6	34	NV	70	
NSA............................	1 Cup	200	10	6	28	NV	100	C
Chocolate Chocolate Chip								
(Baskin Robbins) NS	1 Cup	200	5	8	34	0	140	C
(Edy's)	1 Cup	320	20	4	34	NV	50	
(Häagen-Dazs)	1 Cup	598	39.6	10	53	4	138	AC
Chocolate Fudge								
(Baskin Robbins)............	1 Cup	320	18	4	40	0	150	
Here Comes the								
Fudge..........................	1 Cup	300	14	4	40	0	110	

	Serv.	K-Cal.	Fat	Prot.	Carb.	Fib.	Sod.	FAC
(Ben & Jerry's) Brownie.	1 Cup	520	26	8	64	4	160	A
Double..........................	1 Cup	520	30	10	66	6	110	AC
(Dreyers):								
....	1 Cup	280	14	6	34	NV	80	
FF..................................	1 Cup	200	0	8	48	NV	150	
Mousse, LT................	1 Cup	220	8	6	34	NV	80	
(Edy's):								
Brownie	1 Cup	320	18	4	38	NV	80	
Marble, NSA	1 Cup	200	6	6	32	NV	120	
Sundae.......................	1 Cup	340	20	6	36	NV	110	
(Healthy Choice)								
Swirl	1 Cup	240	4	6	42	2	100	C
Coconut								
(Baskin Robbins)............	1 Cup	320	22	4	28	2	100	
W/Fudge, NSA............	1 Cup	220	3	6	40	2	120	C
(Ben & Jerry's) W/								
Almonds	1 Cup	520	40	10	38	2	160	AC
W/Almond Fudge........	1 Cup	600	44	10	46	4	120	AC
Coffee								
(Ben & Jerry's):								
Aztec Harvest	1 Cup	460	32	8	44	0	110	AC
Toffee...........................	1 Cup	560	38	8	56	0	240	AC
W/Almond Fudge........	1 Cup	580	40	12	48	4	170	AC
(Edy's)	1 Cup	280	16	6	30	NV	70	
(Häagen-Dazs)	1 Cup	532	36	10	42	0	170	AC
Cappuccino	1 Cup	628	42.8	11	50	2	210	AC
(Healthy Choice) W/								
Mocha Fudge..............	1 Cup	240	4	6	46	2	100	C
Cookies and Cream								
(Baskin Robbins)............	1 Cup	340	20	4	34	0	194	
(Dreyers) LT..................	1 Cup	220	8	6	30	NV	110	
(Edy's)	1 Cup	300	16	6	36	NV	150	
(Häagen-Dazs)	1 Cup	539	34.7	9	46	1	228	AC
(Healthy Choice)	1 Cup	240	4	6	42	1	180	C
Cookie Dough								
(Baskin Robbins)............	1 Cup	340	18	4	40	0	140	A
(Ben & Jerry's)	1 Cup	540	30	6	60	0	170	
(Edy's)	1 Cup	340	18	6	40	NV	130	
LT................................	1 Cup	240	10	6	36	NV	120	
(Häagen-Dazs)								
Dynmo........................	1 Cup	614	38.7	9	57	1	276	AC
(Wt Watchers) *Craze*	1 Cup	280	7	6	48	2	170	C
Jamocha								
(Baskin Robbins):								
....	1 Cup	280	18	4	28	0	100	
Swirl, FF	1 Cup	220	0	6	46	0	210	C
W/Almond Fudge........	1 Cup	320	18	6	34	2	80	
W/Swiss Almond, NSA	1 Cup	200	5	6	32	0	130	C

	Serv.	K-Cal.	Fat	Prot.	Carb.	Flb.	Sod.	FAC
(Ice Cream cont.)								
Mint								
(Baskin Robbins) W/								
Choc Chip	1 Cup	300	20	4	30	0	90	
(Ben & Jerry's) W/Choc								
Cookie	1 Cup	520	34	8	54	2	240	AC
(Dreyers) W/Fudge, FF	1 Cup	200	0	6	46	NV	150	
W/Fudge, NSA	1 Cup	200	8	6	30	NV	110	
(Edy's) W/Choc Chips	1 Cup	320	18	6	34	NV	70	
W/Cookie & Cream, LT	1 Cup	220	8	6	30	NV	110	
LT	1 Cup	240	8	6	32	NV	70	
(Healthy Choice) W/								
Choc Chip	1 Cup	240	4	6	42	1	100	C
Mocha								
(Ben & Jerry's) W/								
Fudge	1 Cup	540	36	10	60	2	130	AC
(Dreyers) W/Almond								
Fudge	1 Cup	300	18	6	34	NY	80	
W/Almond Fudge,								
LT	1 Cup	220	8	6	32	NV	70	
(Edy's) W/Fudge,								
NSA	1 Cup	200	6	6	32	NV	120	
Peach								
(Baskins Robbins)	1 Cup	260	14	4	32	0	80	
FF	1 Cup	200	0	6	44	0	180	C
Peanut Butter								
(Baskin Robbins):								
	1 Cup	360	24	6	32	2	190	
Cream, FF	1 Cup	200	0	8	42	0	220	C
Reese's PB	1 Cup	360	22	12	34	0	140	
(Ben & Jerry's)	1 Cup	740	52	16	60	4	280	AC
(Dreyers) Peanut Butter								
Cup, LT	1 Cup	240	10	6	34	NV	90	
(Häagen-Dazs)	1 Cup	647	43.1	13	52	2	297	AC
(Healthy Choice) W/								
Fudge	1 Cup	240	4	6	44	1	120	C
Pistachio								
(Baskin Robbins) W/								
Almonds	1 Cup	340	24	6	26	2	90	
W/Chip, LT	1 Cup	240	8	8	34	0	110	C
Praline								
(Baskin Robbins) LT	1 Cup	240	8	6	36	0	130	C
(Edy's) W/Caramel,								
LT	1 Cup	240	8	6	36	NV	120	
(Healthy Choice) W/								
Caramel	1 Cup	260	4	6	50	1	140	C
W/Caramel Cluster	1 Cup	260	4	6	50	1	140	C
Crunch (Wt Watchers)	1 Cup	280	6	6	50	0	210	C

	Serv.	K-Cal.	Fat	Prot.	Carb.	Fib.	Sod.	FAC
Pumpkin								
(Baskin Robbins):								
Cheezer	1 Cup	300	16	4	34	0	140	
Patch	1 Cup	280	16	4	34	0	100	
Pie	1 Cup	260	12	4	34	0	100	
Raspberry								
(Baskin Robbins) *Reve-*								
lation, NSA	1 Cup	200	2	6	40	2	110	C
(Dreyers) Vanilla Swirl,								
FF, NSA	1 Cup	140	0	8	36	NV	90	
Rocky Road								
(Baskin Robbins)	1 Cup	340	20	6	38	0	120	
LT	1 Cup	260	8	8	38	2	110	C
(Edy's)	1 Cup	340	20	6	34	NV	60	
LT	1 Cup	240	8	6	32	NV	70	
(Healthy Choice)	1 Cup	280	4	6	56	4	120	C
(Wt Watchers)	1 Cup	280	6	8	46	2	150	C
Rum Raisin								
(Baskin Robbins)	1 Cup	280	14	4	36	0	80	
(Häagen-Dazs)	1 Cup	543	34	8	44	1	148	AC
Strawberry								
(Baskin Robbins)	1 Cup	240	12	4	32	0	90	A
Shortcake	1 Cup	320	18	4	36	0	140	
(Dreyers) NSA	1 Cup	200	6	6	30	NV	100	
(Edy's)	1 Cup	260	12	4	34	NV	50	
(Häagen-Dazs)	1 Cup	513	32.9	8	46	1	157	AC
Vanilla								
(Baskin Robbins)	1 Cup	280	16	6	28	0	80	C
Soft, FF	1 Cup	240	0	10	50	0	170	C
(Ben & Jerry's)	1 Cup	460	34	8	42	0	110	AC
(Dreyers):								
LF	1 Cup	200	4	6	38	NV	80	
LT	1 Cup	200	8	6	28	NV	70	
NSA, FF	1 Cup	160	0	8	36	NV	90	
(Edy's)	1 Cup	300	20	4	28	NV	60	
FF	1 Cup	180	0	8	40	NV	140	
(Häagen-Dazs)	1 Cup	534	36.3	10	42	0	170	AC
(Healthy Choice)	1 Cup	200	4	6	36	2	100	C
(Wt Watchers)	1 Cup	240	5	8	40	2	130	C
Vanilla Bean								
(Baskin Robbins) FF	1 Cup	200	0	8	40	0	220	C
(Ben & Jerry's)	1 Cup	460	34	8	42	0	110	AC
(Edy's)	1 Cup	300	18	4	30	NV	60	
Vanilla Combinations								
(Baskin Robbins)								
W/Swiss Almond	1 Cup	220	4	6	40	2	120	
(Ben & Jerry's) W/Cara-								
mel Fudge	1 Cup	560	34	8	66	2	150	AC

	Serv.	K-Cal.	Fat	Prot.	Carb.	Fib.	Sod.	FAC
(Ice Cream cont.)								
(Dreyers) W/Caramel,								
FF	1 Cup	160	0	6	40	NV	110	
W/Choc Swirl, FF	1 Cup	160	0	8	38	NV	90	
(Edy's) W/Choc								
Strawberry	1 Cup	260	14	6	30	NV	60	
(Häagen-Dazs) W/Fudge	1 Cup	568	36.5	9	50	0	214	AC
W/Swiss Almond	1 Cup	611	42.2	12	45	3	155	C
Vanilla, French								
(Baskin Robbins)	1 Cup	320	22	4	30	0	90	C
FF	1 Cup	160	0	8	30	2	150	
(Dreyers)	1 Cup	320	20	4	32	NV	60	

Ice Cream Alternative
Soy
(Tofutti):								
Chocolate	1 Cup	240	4	4	50	0	196	
Coffee	1 Cup	200	2	2	48	0	154	
Fruit, All Flavors, FF	1 Cup	200	0	4	40	NV	180	
Peach/Mango	1 Cup	200	2	2	46	0	204	
Strawberry/Banana	1 Cup	200	2	2	46	0	184	
Vanilla	1 Cup	380	22	4	40	0	420	
Vanilla Fudge	1 Cup	240	4	4	48	0	180	

Rice
(Rice Dream):								
Carob Almond	1 Cup	280	12	2	40	4	170	
Carob Chip	1 Cup	260	12	2	40	2	140	
Cocoa Fudge	1 Cup	260	12	2	42	2	150	
Fruit Flavors	1 Cup	260	10	2	34	NV	160	
Mint Carob Chip	1 Cup	260	12	2	40	2	140	
Peanut Fudge	1 Cup	260	12	4	42	2	150	
Swiss Almond	1 Cup	260	12	2	40	2	140	
Vanilla	1 Cup	260	10	2	38	2	140	
Vanilla Fudge	1 Cup	260	10	2	40	2	140	

Ice Cream Bar
(Baskin Robbins):								
Cappuccino Blast	1 Item	120	5	2	18	0	35	
Jamoca Almond Fudge	1 Item	280	17	5	28	0	60	
Mint Chip, *Tiny Toons*	1 Item	240	17	3	20	2	40	
Peanut Butter								
Chocolate	1 Item	340	27	7	22	2	115	
Pralines N Cream	1 Item	280	17	4	28	2	105	
Vanilla, *Tiny Toons*	1 Item	210	16	3	18	0	40	
(Ben & Jerry's):								
Choc Cookie Dough	1 Item	450	28	6	48	1	145	
Toffee Coffee	1 Item	390	26	5	39	1	150	
Vanilla Pop	1 Item	330	23	4	29	1	55	

	Serv.	K-Cal.	Fat	Prot.	Carb.	Fib.	Sod.	FAC
(Eskimo Pie) Bar............	1 Item	160	11	2	13	0	40	
(Häagen-Dazs):								
Cappuccino	1 Item	331	23.9	5	24	1	71	
Caramel Cone	1 Item	352	23.4	4	32	1	155	
Choc/Dark								
Chocolate	1 Item	389	26.7	5	33	4	87	
Coffee W/Almonds......	1 Item	367	26.3	5	27	1	87	
Cookie Dough.............	1 Item	374	24.6	5	34	1	123	
Triple Brownie.............	1 Item	374	27	5	28	1	111	
Vanilla/Almond	1 Item	372	27	6	26	1	81	
(M & M/Mars) Chocolate,								
Dove............................	1 Item	260	17	3	24	0	45	
(Nestlé):								
Crunch Bar	1 Item	200	14	2	16	0	40	
Crunch Bar, RF	1 Item	150	9	2	14	0	50	
(Wt Watchers):								
Berries 'N Creme........	1 Item	35	0.8	2	4	1	38	
Caramel Nut	1 Item	130	8	2	14	0	25	
Chocolate Dip	1 Item	100	1	3	21	1	150	
Chocolate W/Almond..	1 Item	130	7	2	13	1	50	
Praline W/Creme	1 Item	130	7	2	15	0	40	
Toffee Crunch.............	1 Item	120	7	2	12	0	25	

Ice Cream Bar Alternative
(Rice Dream):

	Serv.	K-Cal.	Fat	Prot.	Carb.	Fib.	Sod.	FAC
Chocolate....................	1 Item	270	15	2	32	2	95	
Chocolate Nutty	1 Item	260	18	4	28	2	55	
Strawberry...................	1 Item	250	13	1	31	1	80	
Vanilla	1 Item	270	14	1	33	1	95	
Vanilla Nutty	1 Item	260	18	4	23	2	55	

Ice Cream Cone

	Serv.	K-Cal.	Fat	Prot.	Carb.	Fib.	Sod.	FAC
Cake (Baskin Robbins)..	1 Item	16	0	0	4	0	35	
Large Cup (Keebler)	1 Item	15	0	0	4	0	20	
Sugar..............................	1 Item	40	0.4	1	8	0	32	
Sugar (Baskin Robbins).	1 Item	60	0	1	7	0	50	
Sugar (Keebler)..............	1 Item	50	0.5	1	11	0	35	
Waffle								
Bowl (Keebler)...............	1 Item	60	1.5	1	12	0	20	
Fresh-Baked (Baskin								
Robbins)......................	1 Item	146	2	1	30	1	5	
Large (Baskin Robbins) .	1 Item	120	7	0	14	0	55	
Large (Keebler)	1 Item	100	2	2	20	0	35	

Ice Cream Parfait

	Serv.	K-Cal.	Fat	Prot.	Carb.	Fib.	Sod.	FAC
(Pepperidge Farm)								
Peach, Lt	1 Item	150	5	3	24	NV	70	A
(Swiss Miss) Vanilla								
Chocolate....................	1 Item	164	6	3	25	0	196	

	Serv.	K-Cal.	Fat	Prot.	Carb.	Fib.	Sod.	FAC
(Ice Cream Parfait cont.)								
Vanilla Chocolate, FF.	1 Item	96	0.3	2	21	0	143	
(Wt Watchers):								
Double Fudge								
Brownie	1 Item	190	2.5	6	39	2	170	C
Praline Toffee	1 Item	190	3	5	40	2	140	C
Strawberry Royale	1 Item	180	2	5	35	0	100	C

Ice Cream Sandwich

	Serv.	K-Cal.	Fat	Prot.	Carb.	Fib.	Sod.	FAC
(Eskimo Pie) Sugar Free	I Item	170	6	4	26	NV	140	
(Good Humor):								
Chocolate Chip	4 Oz	246	10.5	3	35	NV	181	
Vanilla	3 Oz	191	5.7	4	31	NV	155	
(It's It)	1 Item	340	18	4	39	1	90	
(Klondike) Original	1 Item	290	20	3	24	0	65	
(Wt Watchers) Vanilla	1 Item	150	3	3	28	NV	170	

Iced Tea (See Tea, Iced)

J

	Serv.	K-Cal.	Fat	Prot.	Carb.	Fib.	Sod.	FAC
Jack Bean (See Bean, Fava)								
Jackfruit								
Raw	1 Oz	27	0	0	0	7	0	1
Jalapeño (See Pepper, Jalapeño, canned)								
Jam (Also See Fruit Spread; Jelly; Marmalade; Preserves)								
(Estee) All Flavors	1 Tsp	2	0	0	8	NV	10	
(Kraft) All Flavors	1 Tsp	17	0	0	4	NV	0	
(Smucker's) All Flavors, Natural	1 Tsp	18	0	0	4	NV	0	
(S & W) All Flavors, *Nutradiet*	1 Tsp	4	0	0	1	NV	0	
Jambolan (See Java Plum)								
Java Plum—Jambolan								
Raw	1 Cup	81	0.3	1	21	2	19	A
Jelly								
(Also See Fruit Spread; Jam; Marmalade; Preserves)								
(Bama) All Flavors	1 Tsp	25	1	1	3	NV	13	
(Estee) All Flavors	1 Tsp	2	0	0	0	0	10	
(Knott's Berry Farm) All Flavors, LT	1 Tsp	8	0	0	2	NV	0	
(Kraft) All Flavors	1 Tsp	17	0	0	4	0	0	
(Smucker's) All Flavors..	1 Tsp	18	0	0	4	NV	0	
All Flavors, *Slenderella*	1 Tsp	7	0	0	2	0	0	
Jellyfish								
Pickled	1 Cup	21	0.8	3	0	0	5,620	

	Serv.		K-Cal.	Fat	Prot.	Carb.	Fib.	Sod.	FAC
Jerky									
Pork	1	Item	21	1	3	0	0	144	
(Cajun Jerky) Vegetable	0.5	Oz	50	2	5	2	1	125	
(Garden of Eatin')									
Vegetable..................	0.75	Oz	60	0	8	7	0	300	
(Nobull Foods) BBQ Fib									
Rib...........................	1.25	Oz	100	2	10	11	1	190	
(Old Trapper) Beef.........	1	Oz	80	0.5	10	9	0	350	
(Rustler's Roundup)									
Beef...........................	1	Item	20	1.5	2	1	1	115	
(Turkey Jerky)	1	Oz	80	1	14	3	0	550	
Teriyaki	1	Oz	80	0.5	14	4	0	580	
Jerusalem Artichokes—Sunchoke									
Raw	1	Cup	114	0	3	26	2	6	
Jerusalem Artichoke Flour									
(Zumbro)........................	3.3	Oz	125	0.7	9	66	13	0	
Jicama—Chinese Yam									
Raw	1	Cup	57	0.1	1	13	7	6	A
Juice (See individual listings)									
Jujube—Chinese Date									
Raw	1	Oz	22	0.1	0	6	NV	1	A
Dried	1	Oz	82	0.3	1	21	NV	3	

Junket Mix (See Gelatin, Rennet)

K

	Serv.	K-Cal.	Fat	Prot.	Carb.	Fib.	Sod.	FAC
Kale—Borecole—Cole								
Raw	1 Cup	33	0.5	1	3	NV	12	**A**
Raw	1 Lb	137	1.9	9	28	NV	120	**FAC**
Boiled	1 Cup	42	0.5	2	7	3	30	**A**
Frozen, Boiled	1 Cup	39	0.6	4	7	3	20	**A**
Scotch, Boiled	1 Cup	36	0.5	2	7	2	59	**A**
Kale, Chinese (See Broccoli, Chinese)								
Kamut Flakes								
Rolled (Arrowhead Mills)	1 Cup	390	3	15	87	15	0	
Kamut Flour								
(Arrowhead Mills)	1 Cup	440	2	16	100	16	0	
Kamut Grain								
(Arrowhead Mills)	1 Cup	560	4	24	128	20	0	
Kasha (See Buckwheat Groats)								
Kefir								
(Alta Dena)	1 Cup	200	9	9	24	NV	120	**C**
(Lifeway) LF	1 Cup	120	5	8	11	0	130	**AC**
Kelp (See Seaweed, Dried)								
Ketchup—Catsup								
(Hain) No Salt	1 Tbsp	16	0	0	4	NV	5	
(Healthy Choice)	1 Tbsp	10	0	0	2	0	100	
(Heinz):								
LS	1 Tbsp	8	0	0	2	NV	90	
LT	1 Tbsp	10	0	0	3	0	95	
(Hunt's):								
	1 Tbsp	16	0.1	0	3	0	198	
No Salt	1 Tbsp	16	0.1	0	3	0	6	

	Serv.	K-Cal.	Fat	Prot.	Carb.	Fib.	Sod.	FAC
(Westbrae):								
No Salt	1 Tbsp	10	0	0	3	0	5	
Unsweetened	1 Tbsp	5	0	0	1	0	60	

Kidney Bean (See Bean, Kidney)

Kielbasa (See Sausage, Kielbasa)

Kimchi—Kimchee

	Serv.	K-Cal.	Fat	Prot.	Carb.	Fib.	Sod.	FAC
Cabbage	1 Cup	31	0.3	2	6	2	995	FA
Cucumber	1 Cup	32	0.2	2	7	2	1,532	F
Cabbage (Joe Kim's)	1 Oz	5	0	0	1	0	210	

Kiwifruit—Chinese Gooseberry

	Serv.	K-Cal.	Fat	Prot.	Carb.	Fib.	Sod.	FAC
Dried	1.5 Oz	130	1	2	28	3	5	A
W/O Skin	3 Oz	61	0.6	1	13	3	2	A
W/O Skin	1 Lb	208	1.8	4	45	5	18	A

Knackwurst (See Sausage, Knockwurst)

Knish

	Serv.	K-Cal.	Fat	Prot.	Carb.	Fib.	Sod.	FAC
Cheese	1 Item	208	11.8	6	19	1	204	
Meat	1 Item	174	10.6	7	13	1	174	
Potato	1 Item	201	11.4	4	20	1	219	

Kohlrabi

	Serv.	K-Cal.	Fat	Prot.	Carb.	Fib.	Sod.	FAC
Raw, Sliced	1 Cup	38	0.1	2	9	5	28	A
Boiled	1 Cup	48	0.2	3	11	2	35	A

Kumquat

	Serv.	K-Cal.	Fat	Prot.	Carb.	Fib.	Sod.	FAC
Raw	1 Item	12	0	0	3	1	1	
Raw	3 Oz	54	0	1	14	6	5	A

L

	Serv.	K-Cal.	Fat	Prot.	Carb.	Fib.	Sod.	FAC
Lamb								
(Trimmed = All Separable Fat Removed After Cooking; Untrimmed = No Fat Removed After Cooking.)								
Chop, Rib								
Lean and Fat, Broiled....	3 Oz	307	25.2	19	0	0	65	
Lean Only, Broiled	3 Oz	200	11	24	0	0	72	
Foreshank								
Trimmed, Braised...........	3 Oz	159	5.1	26	0	0	63	
Untrimmed, Braised	3 Oz	207	11.4	24	0	0	61	
Ground								
Raw	3 Oz	240	20	14	0	0	50	
Broiled	3 Oz	241	16.7	21	0	0	69	
Leg, Shank Half								
Trimmed, Roasted..........	3 Oz	153	5.7	24	0	0	56	
Untrimmed, Roasted	3 Oz	191	10.6	22	0	0	55	
Leg, Sirloin								
Trimmed, Roasted..........	3 Oz	173	7.8	24	0	0	60	
Untrimmed, Roasted	3 Oz	248	17.6	21	0	0	58	
Leg, Whole								
Trimmed, Roasted..........	3 Oz	162	6.6	24	0	0	58	
Untrimmed, Roasted	3 Oz	219	14	22	0	0	56	
Liver								
Raw	3 Oz	117	42	17	2	0	59	**FA**
Braised	3 Oz	187	7.5	26	2	0	48	**FA**
Loin								
Lean and Fat, Roasted..	3 Oz	263	20.1	19	0	0	54	
Lean Only, Roasted	3 Oz	172	8.3	23	0	0	56	
Rib								
Lean and Fat, Roasted..	3 Oz	305	25.3	18	0	0	62	
Lean Only, Roasted	3 Oz	197	11.3	22	0	0	69	
Shoulder Arm								
Lean and Fat, Roasted..	3 Oz	237	17.2	19	0	0	55	
Lean Only, Roasted	3 Oz	163	7.9	22	0	0	57	
Shoulder Blade								
Lean and Fat, Roasted..	3 Oz	239	17.5	19	0	0	56	
Lean Only, Roasted	3 Oz	178	9.8	21	0	0	58	

	Serv.	K-Cal.	Fat	Prot.	Carb.	Fib.	Sod.	FAC
Lamb Alternative								
Leanies (Worthington)....	1 Item	106	7.8	7	2	1	425	
Linketts (Loma Linda)	1 Item	72	4.5	7	1	2	160	
Little Links (Loma Linda)	1 Item	47	2.8	4	1	1	113	
Lamb's-Quarter								
Raw	3 Oz	37	0.7	4	6	3	37	AC
Cooked	1 Cup	5.7	1.3	6	9	4	52	AC
Lasagna, Canned								
(Chef Boyardee).............	1 Cup	270	8	10	41	3	680	
(Libby's).........................	1 Cup	200	7	9	25	3	860	

Lasagna Entree and Dinner, Frozen
(Serving size given in Oz to reflect weight of 1 serving)
Cheese

	Serv.	K-Cal.	Fat	Prot.	Carb.	Fib.	Sod.	FAC
(Budget Gourmet):								
Light W/Vegetables	10.5 Oz	290	9	15	36	5	780	FAC
Three Cheese.............	10.5 Oz	370	16	20	38	5	870	AC
(Stouffer's) *Lean Cuisine*:								
Casserole....................	9.5 Oz	270	7	14	38	5	590	AC
Classic	11.5 Oz	290	6	20	38	5	560	AC
(Wt Watchers) Italian								
Cheese.......................	11 Oz	300	8	20	38	5	550	AC
Florentine								
(Light and Elegant)	11.2 Oz	280	5	24	34	NV	975	AC
(Wt Watchers)	10 Oz	200	2	10	34	6	590	AC
Meat Sauce								
(Budget Gourmet Light) .	9.5 Oz	250	7	15	31	3	690	C
(Le Menu) *Lightstyle*	10 Oz	290	8	19	36	NV	510	AC
(Stouffer's)	10.5 Oz	360	13	27	34	5	780	
(Stouffer's) *Lean Cuisine*	10.2 Oz	290	8	20	35	6	560	C
(Swanson)	10.5 Oz	410	15	24	45	5	1,080	
(Wt Watchers)	10.2 Oz	270	7	14	38	6	570	AC
Seafood								
(Stouffer's) *Lean Cuisine*,								
W/Tuna,								
Spinach Noodles	9.7 Oz	270	10	17	29	2	890	AC
Tofu								
(Amy's Kitchen)								
W/Vegetables..............	9.5 Oz	300	10	18	41	6	630	
(Legume) Classic	11 Oz	340	13	20	37	11	560	A
Vegetable								
(Amy's Kitchen)								
W/Cheese	9.5 Oz	300	10	15	39	5	680	
(Healthy Choice)								
W/Zucchini	13.5 Oz	330	1.5	20	58	11	310	AC
(Legume) W/Tofu	11 Oz	210	7	13	24	5	480	

	Serv.		K-Cal.	Fat	Prot.	Carb.	Fib.	Sod.	FAC
(Le Menu) *Lightstyle*									
Dinner	10.5	Oz	260	8	11	35	NV	500	**A**
(Stouffer's)	10	Oz	450	23	20	41	5	980	**AC**
(Stouffer's) *Lean Cuisine*,									
W/Zucchini	11	Oz	240	4	17	33	4	470	**AC**
(Wt Watchers) Garden...	11	Oz	270	7	14	36	5	4	**AC**

Lasagna Noodles (See Pasta, Lasagna)

Leek
Raw (4 Oz)....................	1 Item		76	0.4	2	18	2	25	**FA**
Raw, Chopped	1 Cup		64	0.4	2	15	1	20	**FA**

Lemon
W/O Peel (2 Oz)	1 Item		17	0.2	1	5	2	1	**A**

Lemonade
(Odwalla) Honey	1 Cup		70	0	0	26	NV	10	**A**
Strawberry..................	1 Cup		150	0	0	40	NV	35	**A**
(R.W. Knudsen) Natural.	1 Cup		120	0	0	29	NV	35	
Raspberry	1 Cup		120	0	0	29	NV	35	
(Santa Cruz) Strawberry	1 Cup		120	0	0	29	NV	35	
(Snapple)	1 Cup		110	0	0	29	NV	10	
Strawberry..................	1 Cup		120	0	0	29	NV	10	

Lemon Drink Mix
(Crystal Light)...............	1 Cup		5	0	0	0	0	0	
W/Lime........................	1 Cup		5	0	0	0	0	0	
(Kool-Aid)......................	1 Cup		108	0	0	28	0	31	

Lemongrass
....	1 Oz		17	0.2	0	4	1	1	

Lemon Juice
Raw	1 Cup		61	0	1	21	1	2	**A**
Raw	1 Tbsp		4	0	0	1	0	0	**A**
Canned and Bottled.......	1 Cup		51	0.7	1	16	1	51	**A**
Frozen (Sunkist).............	1 Oz		7	0.1	0	2	NV	0	**A**
Reconstituted									
(Realemon)	1 Oz		6	0	0	2	0	5	**A**

Lemon Peel
Raw	1 Tbsp		3	0	0	1	1	0	
Raw	1 Oz		13	0	0	5	3	2	**A**
Candied (S & W)	1 Oz		88	0.1	0	23	1	0	

Lentil
Canned, Organic									
(Westbrae)	1 Cup		260	0	12	26	10	280	**FA**

	Serv.	K-Cal.	Fat	Prot.	Carb.	Fib.	Sod.	FAC
(Lentil cont.)								
Cooked	1 Cup	230	0.8	18	40	16	4	**FA**
Dried (Arrowhead Mills)	1 Cup	600	0	44	108	28	60	**FA**
Sprouted	1 Cup	82	0.4	7	17	NV	8	**FA**

Lettuce
(Also See Salad Mix)

	Serv.	K-Cal.	Fat	Prot.	Carb.	Fib.	Sod.	FAC
Butterhead, Head	1 Item	21	0.4	2	4	2	8	**FA**
Butterhead, Leaves	1 Piece	1	0	0	0	0	0	
Iceberg	1 Oz	4	0.1	0	1	0	3	
Iceberg, Head	1 Item	65	1	5	11	8	49	**F**
Iceberg, Chopped	1 Cup	7	0.1	1	1	1	5	
Iceberg, Leaves	1 Piece	2	0	0	0	0	2	
Looseleaf, Shredded	1 Cup	10	0.2	1	2	1	5	
Romaine, Shredded	1 Cup	9	0.1	1	1	1	4	**FA**

Lima Bean—Butter Bean (See Bean, Lima)

Lime

	Serv.	K-Cal.	Fat	Prot.	Carb.	Fib.	Sod.	FAC
Sections	1 Oz	9	0.1	0	3	0	1	
W/Peel, 2" Diameter	1 Med	20	0.1	0	7	2	1	

Lime Drink
(Minute Maid) Prep from

	Serv.	K-Cal.	Fat	Prot.	Carb.	Fib.	Sod.	FAC
Frozen	1 Cup	93	0	0	25	0	0	
(Odwalla) Summertime	1 Cup	90	0	0	23	0	10	**A**
(R.W. Knudsen) Cactus								
Cooler	1 Cup	120	0	0	29	NV	35	

Lime Juice

	Serv.	K-Cal.	Fat	Prot.	Carb.	Fib.	Sod.	FAC
Fresh	1 Tbsp	4	0	0	1	0	0	
Fresh	1 Cup	66	0.3	1	22	1	2	**A**
Bottled	1 Cup	52	0.6	1	16	0	40	**A**
(Realime) Reconstituted	1 Oz	6	0	0	2	0	10	**A**
(Roses)	1 Oz	48	0	0	12	0	6	**A**

Lingcod

	Serv.	K-Cal.	Fat	Prot.	Carb.	Fib.	Sod.	FAC
Raw	3 Oz	72	0.9	11	0	0	50	
Broiled	3 Oz	94	0.7	21	0	0	147	

Litchi—Lychee

	Serv.	K-Cal.	Fat	Prot.	Carb.	Fib.	Sod.	FAC
Raw	1 Item	6	0	0	2	0	0	
Raw	1 Oz	19	0.1	0	5	0	0	**A**
Dried	1 Oz	79	0.3	1	20	1	1	**A**

Liver (See individual listings)

Liverwurst—Braunschweiger
(Farmer Jones):

	Serv.		K-Cal.	Fat	Prot.	Carb.	Fib.	Sod.	FAC
....	2	Oz	190	17	8	1	0	460	**FA**
LT................................	2	Oz	90	5	10	1	0	430	**FA**
Sliced	1.2	Oz	110	10	5	1	0	280	**FA**
(Oscar Mayer)	2	Oz	190	17	8	2	0	630	**FA**

Lobster

Raw	3	Oz	76	0.8	16	0	0	252	
Boiled...........................	3	Oz	83	0.5	17	1	0	324	
Boiled (5 Oz).................	1	Cup	142	0.9	30	2	0	551	
Paste, Canned	1	Tbsp	38	1.9	4	0	0	30	
Spiny, Boiled	3	Oz	121	1.6	22	3	0	193	
Spiny, Raw	3	Oz	95	1.2	18	2	0	150	

Loganberry

Fresh	1	Cup	90	0.9	1	22	4	1	**FA**
Fresh	1	Lb	281	2.7	5	67	3	0	**FA**
Frozen (5 Oz)................	1	Cup	81	0.5	2	19	7	1	**FA**

Long Bean (See Green Bean; Yard-Long Bean)

Loofah—Luffa—Silk Squash—Chinese Okra

Angled	1	Oz	6	0.1	0	1	0	13	
Smooth	1	Oz	6	0.1	0	1	0	8	

Loquat

Raw	1	Item	5	0	0	1	0	0	
Raw	1	Oz	13	0	0	3	1	0	
Raw	1	Lb	213	0.9	2	55	8	5	**FA**

Lotus Root

Raw (4 Oz)....................	1	Item	64	0.1	3	20	6	46	**A**
Boiled............................	1	Oz	19	0	0	5	1	13	

Lotus Seed

Dried.............................	40	Seeds	92	0.3	3	19	1	2	
Dried.............................	2	Oz	184	0.7	7	37	1	5	**F**
Dried.............................	1	Cup	106	0.6	5	21	1	2	

Lox (See Salmon, Smoked)

Luffa (See Loofah)

Luncheon Meat (See individual listings)

Luncheon Meat, Alternative (Also See individual listings)

(Loma Linda) Tender									
Rounds........................	1	Piece	15	0.6	2	1	0	41	
(Worthington):									
Prosage Roll...............	1	Oz	71	5.2	5	1	1	200	

	Serv.	K-Cal.	Fat	Prot.	Carb.	Fib.	Sod.	FAC
(Luncheon Meat, Alternative cont.)								
Wham........................	1 Oz	48	2.8	4	1	NV	375	

Luncheon Meat, Canned
(Armour):

Treet...........................	2 Oz	200	17	6	3	NV	840	
Treet, RS	2 Oz	190	16	6	3	NV	610	
(Hormel):								
Spam...........................	2 Oz	172	16	8	4	NV	743	
Spam, Lite	2 Oz	140	12	8	1	NV	560	
Spam, RS	2 Oz	176	15	8	1	NV	1,100	

Luncheon Meat Combination, Packaged
(Oscar Mayer) *Lunchables*:

Bologna/American.......	1 Item	470	35	17	22	1	1,640	C
Bologna/Cherry	1 Item	530	28	13	60	1	1,120	C
Ham/Punch	1 Item	440	20	15	54	1	1,270	C
Ham/Surf Cooler, LF ..	1 Item	390	11	17	58	1	1,350	C
Ham/Swiss	1 Item	340	20	21	20	1	1,790	C
Turkey/Cheddar	1 Item	350	20	20	22	1	1,760	C
Turkey/Jack.................	1 Item	350	21	20	20	1	1,690	C
Turkey/Pac Cooler,								
LF	1 Item	360	9	15	56	1	1,190	C
Turkey/Surf Cooler	1 Item	430	15	13	61	0	1,240	C

Lupine

Raw	1 Cup	668	17.5	65	73	NV	27	FC
Boiled..............................	1 Cup	198	4.9	26	16	5	7	F

Lychee (See Litchi)

M

	Serv.	K-Cal.	Fat	Prot.	Carb.	Fib.	Sod.	FAC
Macadamia Nut								
Dried	1 Cup	941	8.8	11	18	13	7	
Oil-Roasted	1 Cup	962	103	10	17	13	9	
Oil-Roasted, Salted	1 Cup	962	103	10	17	13	348	
Salted (Blue Diamond)...	1 Oz	190	18	3	3	3	140	
Macadamia Nut Butter								
(Maranatha)	2 Tbsp	230	24	3	5	3	0	
Macaroni (See Pasta, Macaroni)								
Macaroni Entree								
Canned								
(Chef Boyardee) W/								
Shells	1 Cup	150	1	6	31	2	930	
(Franco-American) W/								
Cheese	1 Cup	200	7	8	29	4	1,060	
(Libby's) W/Beef	1 Oz	28	1.2	1	4	1	98	
Prepared from Mix								
(Annie's) W/Cheddar	1 Cup	325	11.7	10	43	1	507	
(Fantastic) W/Cheddar...	1 Cup	200	1.5	8	40	5	550	
(Kraft) Original W/								
Cheese	1 Cup	390	17	11	48	1	730	
(Pacific Foods) W/								
Cheese, Kid's Cup	1 Cup	250	12	9	45	0	1,060	
Macaroni Entree and Dinner, Frozen								
Beef								
(Maria Callender's)	14 Oz	590	18	28	80	9	1,230	
(Stouffer's)	11.5 Oz	420	20	19	40	5	1,530	
(Stouffer's) *Lean Cuisine*	10 Oz	280	8	13	40	3	550	A
(Wt Watchers)	9.5 Oz	220	4.5	13	32	4	560	A
Frozen Entree, W/Cheese								
(Amy's Kitchen):								
	9 Oz	450	9	22	58	NV	430	
Soy	9 Oz	360	14	16	42	4	500	

	Serv.		K-Cal.	Fat	Prot.	Carb.	Fib.	Sod.	FAC
(Macaroni Entree and Dinner, Frozen cont.)									
(Banquet)	9.5	Oz	320	11	12	43	4	970	
(Green Giant)	9.2	Oz	220	8	10	27	2	480	
(Healthy Choice)	9	Oz	290	5	15	45	4	580	C
(Light and Elegant)	9	Oz	300	9	15	37	NV	1,015	C
(Lunch Express)	9.7	Oz	240	6	12	35	5	460	
(Stouffer's)	1	Cup	330	17	14	31	2	940	C
(Stouffer's) *Lean Cuisine*	9	Oz	270	7	13	39	2	550	C
(Swanson)	10	Oz	280	10	11	36	2	1,050	C
(Wt Watchers)	9	Oz	280	7	13	42	4	590	C

Mace

	Serv.		K-Cal.	Fat	Prot.	Carb.	Fib.	Sod.	FAC
Ground (McCormick)	1 Tsp		8	0.4	0	1	0	2	

Mackerel

	Serv.		K-Cal.	Fat	Prot.	Carb.	Fib.	Sod.	FAC
King, Raw	3 Oz		89	1.7	17	0	0	135	
King, Broiled	3 Oz		114	2.2	22	0	0	172	
Pacific/Jack, Raw	3 Oz		134	6.7	17	0	0	73	
Pacific/Jack, Broiled	3 Oz		171	8.6	22	0	0	94	
Spanish, Raw	3 Oz		118	5.4	16	0	0	50	
Spanish, Broiled	3 Oz		134	5.4	20	0	0	56	

Mahimahi

	Serv.		K-Cal.	Fat	Prot.	Carb.	Fib.	Sod.	FAC
Raw	3 Oz		72	0.6	16	0	0	75	
Broiled	3 Oz		93	0.8	20	0	0	96	

Malt

	Serv.		K-Cal.	Fat	Prot.	Carb.	Fib.	Sod.	FAC
Dry	1 Oz		104	0.5	4	22	0	23	
Dry, Extract	1 Oz		104	0	2	25	0	23	

Malted Milk (See Milk, Malted)

Malt Syrup

	Serv.		K-Cal.	Fat	Prot.	Carb.	Fib.	Sod.	FAC
Barley (Eden)	1 Tbsp		60	14	1	14	0	0	

Mandarin Orange
Fresh

	Serv.		K-Cal.	Fat	Prot.	Carb.	Fib.	Sod.	FAC
Whole (4 Oz)	1 Med		37	0.2	1	9	2	1	A
Peeled	1 Oz		13	0.1	0	3	0	1	
Sections, W/O Membrane	1 Cup		86	0.4	1	22	5	4	A
Canned W/									
LT Syrup (Geisha)	1 Cup		280	0	2	34	2	20	A
LT Syrup (S & W)	1 Cup		150	0	2	35	2	23	A
Natural (S & W)	1 Oz		13	0	0	3	0	0	

Mango

	Serv.		K-Cal.	Fat	Prot.	Carb.	Fib.	Sod.	FAC
Raw, Sliced	1 Cup		107	0.5	1	28	3	3	A
Raw (7 Oz)	1 Item		135	0.6	1	35	4	4	A

	Serv.	K-Cal.	Fat	Prot.	Carb.	Fib.	Sod.	FAC
Candied	1 Oz	91	0.1	0	22	0	57	A
Dried	3 Oz	314	0.8	1	82	6	6	A

Mango Juice

	Serv.	K-Cal.	Fat	Prot.	Carb.	Fib.	Sod.	FAC
(Kern's) Nectar	1 Cup	150	0	0	36	6	5	A
Nectar W/Orange	1 Cup	140	0	0	35	0	10	A
(Odwalla) Mango Tango	1 Cup	150	2.5	1	37	6	55	A
(R.W. Knudsen) W/ Peach	1 Cup	120	0	0	30	NV	50	A

Manicotti Entree, Frozen
Cheese

	Serv.	K-Cal.	Fat	Prot.	Carb.	Fib.	Sod.	FAC
(Bernardi)	3 Oz	170	8	8	16	1	230	
(Healthy Choice) 3 Cheeses	11 Oz	310	9	16	41	7	450	C
(Le Menu) 3 Cheeses Dinner	12 Oz	390	15	19	44	NV	870	AC
(Stouffer's)	9 Oz	340	16	18	32	7	810	AC
(Wt Watchers)	9 Oz	260	7	17	31	5	570	C
Tofu								
(Legume) Classic	11 Oz	360	13	23	40	10	510	A
Florentine	11 Oz	300	8	19	39	11	540	AC

Maple Syrup

	Serv.	K-Cal.	Fat	Prot.	Carb.	Fib.	Sod.	FAC
(Aunt Jemima):								
LT	¼ Cup	100	0	0	27	1	160	
Original	¼ Cup	210	0	0	53	0	120	
(Country Kitchen):								
	¼ Cup	200	0	0	53	0	115	
LT	¼ Cup	100	0	0	26	0	160	
(Log Cabin):								
	¼ Cup	200	0	0	53	0	110	
LT	¼ Cup	100	0	0	26	0	180	
(Mrs. Butterworth's):								
	¼ Cup	230	0	0	56	0	95	
LT	¼ Cup	100	0	0	24	0	100	
(Mrs. Richardson's):								
	¼ Cup	210	0	0	52	0	115	
LT	¼ Cup	100	0	0	51	0	160	
(S & W) LT	¼ Cup	60	0	0	15	0	105	

Margarine
Soft Spread, Whipped

	Serv.	K-Cal.	Fat	Prot.	Carb.	Fib.	Sod.	FAC
(Blue Bonnet) LT	1 Tbsp	45	4.5	0	0	0	95	
(Canola Harvest)	1 Tbsp	100	11	0	0	0	95	
(Country Crock) Churn Style	1 Tbsp	60	7	0	0	0	90	

	Serv.	K-Cal.	Fat	Prot.	Carb.	Fib.	Sod.	FAC
(Margarine cont.)								
(Fleischmann's):								
....	1 Tbsp	80	9	0	0	0	90	
Move Over Butter.......	1 Tbsp	90	10	0	0	0	100	
(I Can't Believe) LT........	1 Tbsp	50	6	0	0	0	90	
(Imperial) 40% Less Fat	1 Tbsp	60	7	0	0	0	90	
(Mazola) 40% Corn, LT .	1 Tbsp	50	6	0	0	0	100	
(Nucoa) *Heart Beat*........	1 Tbsp	25	3	0	0	0	110	
(Parkay)	1 Tbsp	100	11	0	0	0	105	
(Promise) Ultra FF	1 Tbsp	5	0	0	1	0	90	
Stick								
(Blue Bonnet)	1 Tbsp	70	7	0	0	0	95	
(Fleischmann's):								
....	1 Tbsp	90	10	0	0	0	100	
Lower Fat.....................	1 Tbsp	52	5.6	0	1	0	77	
(I Can't Believe) LT........	1 Tbsp	90	10	0	0	0	95	
(Imperial):								
....	1 Tbsp	90	10	0	0	0	110	
LT................................	1 Tbsp	70	7	0	0	0	110	
(Mazola):								
....	1 Tbsp	100	11	0	0	0	100	
Reduced Calories.......	1 Tbsp	50	5.5	0	0	0	135	
(Nucoa).............................	1 Tbsp	100	11	0	0	0	160	
(Parkay)	1 Tbsp	90	10	0	0	0	110	
(Promise):								
....	1 Tbsp	90	10	0	0	0	65	A
Extra Light	1 Tbsp	50	6	0	0	0	50	
(Saffola)	1 Tbsp	100	11	0	0	0	95	
(Willowrun)......................	1 Tbsp	100	11	0	0	0	160	

Marinara Sauce (See Pasta Sauce, Marinara)

Marjoram
Dried (McCormick)	1 Tsp	4	0	0	1	0	1	

Marmalade
(Bonne Maman) Orange	1 Tbsp	50	0	0	13	NV	0	
(Crosse & Blackwell)								
Lemon Pear.................	1 Tbsp	60	0	0	14	0	0	
Orange	1 Tbsp	50	0	0	13	0	0	
(Mary Ellen) Orange	1 Tbsp	50	0	0	13	NV	0	

Marmite (See Yeast Extract)

Marshmallow
(Campfire).......................	1 Item	20	0	0	5	0	5	
(Kraft) Miniature	1 Cup	200	0	1	50	0	60	
Jet Puffed	1 Item	22	0	0	5	0	8	

	Serv.	K-Cal.	Fat	Prot.	Carb.	Fib.	Sod.	FAC
Masa Harina (See Corn Flour)								
Mascarpone								
(Belgioioso)....................	1 Oz	124	13	2	1	0	16	
Matzo Meal								
(Manischewitz)...............	1 Cup	486	0.6	13	107	4	15	A
Matzo								
(Manischewitz):								
American.....................	1 Sheet	115	1.9	3	22	0	168	
Egg.............................	1 Sheet	111	0.6	4	22	NV	6	
Thin Tea	1 Sheet	100	0.3	3	22	0	3	
Whole Wheat W/Bran.	1 Sheet	110	0.6	4	21	1	1	
Mayonnaise								
(Best) LF	1 Tbsp	25	1	0	4	0	140	
(Estee)	1 Tbsp	20	1.5	0	2	0	40	
(Hellmann's):								
LT................................	1 Tbsp	50	5	0	1	0	115	
Real............................	1 Tbsp	100	11	0	0	0	80	
(Kraft):								
Cholesterol-Free	1 Tbsp	90	10	0	0	0	75	
FF...............................	1 Tbsp	10	0	0	2	0	105	
LT...............................	1 Tbsp	50	5	0	1	0	110	
Real............................	1 Tbsp	100	11	0	0	0	75	
(Nasoya) Soy,								
Nayonaise...................	1 Tbsp	35	3	0	1	0	105	
(Nucoa) *Heart Beat*........	1 Tbsp	40	4	0	1	0	110	
(Soymage) *Veganaise*....	1 Tbsp	90	9	0	1	0	80	
(Spectrum) Canola								
LT...............................	1 Tbsp	35	3	0	1	0	60	
(Wt Watchers) LS, LT....	1 Tbsp	25	2	0	1	0	40	
Meat (See individual listings)								
Meatloaf Entree, Frozen								
(Armour)	11.3 Oz	360	17	20	32	NV	1,170	
(Banquet)........................	9.5 Oz	280	16	13	22	3	1,020	
(Healthy Choice)								
Traditional	12 Oz	320	8	16	46	7	460	A
(Stouffer's) *Lean Cuisine*:								
Homestyle, W/Potato	10 Oz	390	24	20	24	3	910	
W/Macaroni & Cheese	9.5 Oz	270	10	10	24	4	530	
W/Whipped Potatoes..	9.5 Oz	250	7	22	25	5	570	
(Swanson)	11.2 Oz	380	16	16	44	5	1,160	A
Melba Toast (See Cracker, Melba)								

	Serv.	K-Cal.	Fat	Prot.	Carb.	Fib.	Sod.	FAC
Melon (See individual listings)								
Milk, Chocolate								
1% Fat	1 Cup	158	2.5	8	26	1	152	C
2% Fat	1 Cup	179	5	8	26	1	150	C
Whole	1 Cup	218	9.1	9	26	3	123	C
(Nestlé) *Quik*	1 Cup	266	9.8	8	36	4	177	AC
Quik LF	1 Cup	190	5	8	29	0	150	C
(Ovaltine)	1 Cup	225	8.7	9	29	NV	244	AC
Milk, Cow								
Fresh								
Nonfat	1 Cup	86	0.4	8	12	0	126	C
1% Fat, LF	1 Cup	120	2.6	8	12	0	123	C
2% Fat, Acidophilus	1 Cup	130	5	8	13	0	130	C
2% Fat, Lactose-Reduced	1 Cup	130	5	8	13	0	130	C
2% Fat, LF	1 Cup	130	5	8	13	0	122	C
3% Fat, Whole	1 Cup	150	8.2	8	11	0	120	C
Nonfat W/Calc, Lactose Reduced (Lactaid)	1 Cup	90	0.5	8	12	0	125	C
Buttermilk								
Bulgarian Culture	1 Cup	160	8	8	13	0	220	C
Cultured, Fluid, LF	1 Cup	99	2.2	8	12	0	257	C
Dried, Sweet Cream	1 Cup	464	6.9	41	59	0	621	FC
LF	1 Cup	110	2.5	9	14	0	240	
2% (R.W. Knudsen)	1 Cup	120	5	9	10	0	130	C
Condensed, Canned								
FF (Borden)	2 Tbsp	110	0	3	24	NV	40	
Whole	1 Cup	982	26.6	24	166	0	389	CA
Whole (Borden)	2 Tbsp	130	3	3	23	NV	40	
Whole (Carnation)	2 Tbsp	130	3	3	22	NV	45	
Evaporated, Canned								
(Carnation):								
FF	2 Tbsp	25	0	2	4	NV	40	
LF	2 Tbsp	25	0.5	2	3	NV	35	
Whole	2 Tbsp	40	2	2	3	NV	30	
Skim, 2% Fat	1 Cup	233	5.1	19	28	0	281	CA
Whole, 7.8% Butterfat	1 Cup	344	19.7	17	25	0	267	CA
Whole (Pet)	2 Tbsp	40	2	2	3	NV	30	
Powdered								
Nonfat, Low Lactose (Nutra Bal)	1 Cup	80	0.5	8	12	0	125	
Skim	1 Cup	244	0.5	24	36	0	373	
Whole	1 Cup	635	34.2	34	49	0	475	
Milkfish—Awa								
Raw	3 Oz	126	6	17	0	0	62	
Broiled	3 Oz	162	7.4	22	0	0	78	

	Serv.	K-Cal.	Fat	Prot.	Carb.	Fib.	Sod.	FAC
Milk, Goat								
Whole, Fluid	1 Cup	168	10.1	9	11	0	122	C
(Meyenberg)	1 Cup	140	7	8	11	0	115	C
Milk, Human								
Whole	1 Cup	171	10.8	3	17	0	42	A
Milk, Indian Buffalo								
Whole	1 Cup	236	16.8	9	13	0	127	C
Milk, Malted								
Mix								
Chocolate (Carnation)	3 Tbsp	90	1	1	18	NV	40	
Original (Carnation)	3 Tbsp	90	2	3	15	1	85	
Prepared								
Chocolate (Carnation)	1 Cup	228	9	9	30	0	172	C
Original (Carnation)	1 Cup	236	9.8	10	27	0	223	C
Milkshake								
(Alba) '77, Fit'N	6 Oz	346	2.5	26	56	NV	709	C
(Micromagic)	11.5 Oz	340	8	5	55	0	120	AC
(Wt Watchers) Dry Mix	1 Pkt	70	0	6	11	NV	210	
Milkshake, Fast Food								
(Arby's):								
Butterfinger Polar								
Swirl	12 Oz	457	18	15	62	0	318	C
Heath Polar Swirl	12 Oz	543	22	15	76	0	346	C
Jamocha Shake	12 Oz	384	10	15	62	0	262	C
(Burger King):								
Chocolate, Medium	11 Oz	320	7	9	54	3	230	C
Vanilla, Medium	10 Oz	300	6	9	53	1	230	C
(Carl's Jr) Vanilla	8 Oz	195	4.7	7	3	0	148	C
Milk, Sheep								
Whole	1 Cup	264	17.1	15	13	0	108	C
Milk Substitute (Also See Rice Beverage, Soy Beverage)								
Lacto-Free, Dry (Ener-G)	1 Gram	28	0.5	3	2	2	1	
Nondairy (Vitamite)	1 Cup	90	0	1	21	0	70	C
Millet								
Pearl, Cooked	1 Cup	286	2.4	8	57	3	5	F
Pearl, Raw	1 Cup	756	8.4	22	146	17	10	F

	Serv.	K-Cal.	Fat	Prot.	Carb.	Fib.	Sod.	FAC
(Millet cont.)								
Raw, Hulled (Arrowhead Mills)	1 Cup	600	6	20	136	12	0	F
Millet Flour								
(Arrowhead Mills)	1 Cup	440	4	16	104	8	0	F
Mincemeat								
(Comstock)	3.5 Oz	150	1	0	39	1	39	
(Crosse & Blackwell)	¼ Cup	180	0	0	43	0	230	
(S & W) Old-fashioned	4 Oz	234	2.3	1	56	NV	234	
Mint								
Fresh	1 Oz	12	0.2	0	2	NV	4	A
Dried, Spearmint	1 Tsp	2	0	0	0	0	2	
Miso								
Paste								
(Eden) Organic:								
Barley, Mugi	1 Tbsp	25	1	2	3	1	760	
Brown Rice, Gennmai	1 Tbsp	25	1	2	3	<1	810	
Rice, Kome	1 Tbsp	25	1	2	3	<1	850	
Rice, Shiro	1 Tbsp	35	1	2	5	1	410	
Soybean, Hacho	1 Tbsp	35	1.5	3	2	1	600	
(Westbrae):								
Barley, 2-Yr	1 Tsp	10	0	0	2	TR	310	
Brown Rice	1 Tsp	10	0	<1	<1	TR	250	
Red, 1-Yr	1 Tsp	15	0	<1	1	TR	300	
Soybean, Hacho	1 Tsp	15	0.5	1	1	TR	250	
Mochi								
(Grainaissance)								
	1.5 Oz	110	1	2	24	2	0	
W/Raisin	1.5 Oz	120	1	2	25	3	35	
Molasses								
Barbados	1 Tbsp	56	0	0	14	0	3	C
Blackstrap	1 Cup	699	0	0	180	0	315	C
(Brer Rabbit)	1 Tbsp	60	0	0	15	0	10	C
Cane, Blackstrap	1 Tbsp	47	0	0	12	0	11	C
Cane, Light	1 Tbsp	53	0	0	14	0	7	C
(Grandma's)	1 Tbsp	50	0	0	14	0	0	C
Mole Sauce								
(Faraon)	2 Tbsp	160	11	3	0	2	490	A
Monkfish								
Raw	3 Oz	64	1.3	12	0	0	15	
Broiled	3 Oz	83	1.7	16	0	0	20	

	Serv.	K-Cal.	Fat	Prot.	Carb.	Fib.	Sod.	FAC
Monosodium Glutamate—MSG								
(Accent)	1 Gram	0	0	0	0	0	640	
Moose								
Raw	3 Oz	87	0.6	19	0	0	55	
Roasted	3 Oz	114	0.8	25	0	0	59	
Mousse								
Frozen								
(Wt Watchers):								
Chocolate	2.7 Oz	190	5	6	31	3	150	
Chocolate Caramel	2.7 Oz	200	4	5	34	2	120	
Praline Pecan	2.7 Oz	170	3.5	4	31	0	140	
Mix, Prepared								
(Jell-O) Chocolate	1 Cup	300	12	10	42	NV	150	
Chocolate Fudge	1 Cup	280	12	10	40	NV	90	
(Lite Whip) Strawberry,								
W/Skim	1 Cup	120	4	4	18	NV	110	
MSG (See Monosodium Glutamate)								
Muffin, Mix								
(Prepared as indicated on the package)								
Apple W/Cinnamon								
(Betty Crocker)	1 Item	140	4	2	24	0	200	
(Krusteaz):								
	1 Item	160	4	2	29	1	260	
FF	1 Item	130	0	2	31	2	310	
(Robin Hood):								
	2 Oz	170	8	3	23	0	220	
Applesauce	1 Oz	140	4	2	25	NV	220	
Banana								
(Betty Crocker) W/Nuts	2 Oz	150	5	2	24	0	200	
(Krusteaz) FF	1 Item	140	0	2	34	2	350	
(Robin Hood) W/Nuts	2 Oz	170	8	3	21	0	190	
Blueberry								
(Betty Crocker) Wild	1 Item	170	5	2	29	0	220	
(Duncan Hines)	1.5 Oz	160	5	2	28	0	270	
(Krusteaz):								
	1 Item	180	6	3	29	<1	260	
FF	1 Item	130	0	2	31	2	330	
W/Bran	1 Item	190	6	4	28	3	330	
(Pillsbury) *Lovin Lite*	1 Oz	100	1	2	21	NV	150	
(Robin Hood)	2 Oz	160	6	3	24	0	220	
Bran								
(Arrowhead Mills)	1 Item	150	2	7	26	7	16	
(Bob's Red Mill):								
W/Date Nuts	1 Item	160	6	3	25	1	170	

	Serv.	K-Cal.	Fat	Prot.	Carb.	Fib.	Sod.	FAC
(Muffin, Mix cont.)								
W/Raisins...................	1 Item	160	5	3	25	1	170	
(Krusteaz) W/Honey.......	1 Item	160	4.5	4	26	3	320	
(Robin Hood) Gold W/								
Honey...........................	1 Oz	140	4	3	24	2	220	
Carrot								
Carrot.............................	2 Oz	177	6.7	4	26	1	251	A
Corn								
(Arrowhead Mills) Blue...	1 Item	110	4	4	15	3	NV	
(Flako)	1 Item	116	3.3	2	20	1	351	
(General Mills) *Gold*								
Medal	1 Item	170	6	2	25	1	270	
Home Recipe, Whole								
Milk..............................	2 Oz	183	7.4	4	25	1	333	
Oat Bran								
(Arrowhead Mills) W/								
Apple...........................	2.7 Oz	120	4	6	15	6	225	
(Bob's Red Mill):								
....	1 Item	210	6	5	33	2	160	
W/Date Nuts	1 Item	210	6	5	33	2	170	
(Krusteaz)	1 Item	190	5	4	31	2	310	
Poppyseed								
(Krusteaz) W/Almonds ...	1 Item	180	5	3	31	1	230	

Muffin, Ready-To-Serve

(Serving size given in Oz to reflect weight of 1 serving)

	Serv.	K-Cal.	Fat	Prot.	Carb.	Fib.	Sod.	FAC
Apple								
(Hostess) Streusel..........	1 Oz	100	1	1	23	1	160	
Banana								
(Hostess) W/Oat Bran,								
LF..............................	2.7 Oz	200	2.5	4	41	2	280	
(Otis Spunkmeyer)	4 Oz	480	24	6	60	1	380	
(Wt Watchers) W/Nuts ...	2.5 Oz	180	4	3	34	5	260	
Blueberry								
(Ener-G) Gluten-Free.....	1.7 Oz	51	1.9	1	8	0	54	
(Entenmann's) FF	2 Oz	120	0	2	26	1	220	
(Health Valley):								
Fancy Fruit..................	2 Oz	140	1	4	32	8	100	
Oat Bran	2 Oz	140	4	4	27	5	95	
(Natural Ovens) LF	2.5 Oz	145	1	6	32	2	190	F
(Otis Spunkmeyer)	4 Oz	420	22	6	48	1	400	
(Sara Lee):								
Free & Light................	2.2 Oz	120	0	3	28	1	140	
Hearty Fruit...............	2.2 Oz	220	11	3	27	1	170	
(Wt Watchers)	2.5 Oz	180	4	3	33	2	270	
Bran								
Honey Harvest								
(Wt Watchers)..............	2.5 Oz	220	4.5	3	42	5	180	

	Serv.	K-Cal.	Fat	Prot.	Carb.	Fib.	Sod.	FAC
Carrot								
(Health Valley) LF	2 Oz	130	1	4	30	5	110	**A**
(Natural Ovens) LF	2.5 Oz	140	2	4	30	2	200	**FA**
Corn								
(Thomas):								
....	1 Oz	110	3.5	2	19	1	180	
Banana Nut	1 Oz	110	4.5	2	16	1	170	
Blueberry	1 Oz	100	3	1	17	1	160	
Raisin Bran	1 Oz	90	3	2	17	1	170	
English								
(Oroweat):								
....	1 Item	170	3	6	30	2	220	
Cinnamon Raisin	1 Item	170	1	5	35	2	210	
Health Raisin	1 Item	180	3.5	6	33	3	200	
(Oatmeal Goodness) W/								
Honey	2 Oz	140	2	5	26	2	160	
(Pepperidge Farm):								
Plain	1 Item	140	1	8	27	NV	220	
Sourdough	1 Item	135	1	4	27	NV	260	
(Thomas):								
Sandwich Size	3.2 Oz	190	2	7	38	2	280	
Sour Dough	2 Oz	120	1	4	25	1	190	
Wheat-Sandwich Size	3.2 Oz	180	1.5	8	39	4	280	
W/Honey Wheat	2 Oz	110	1	5	24	3	190	
W/Oat Bran	2 Oz	120	1	4	26	2	210	**F**
W/Raisin Cinnamon	2 Oz	140	1	4	31	1	170	
Fat-Free								
(Unless specified, lowfat)								
(Entenmann's) Blueberry	2 Oz	120	0	2	26	1	220	
(Health Valley):								
Apple Spice	2 Oz	130	0	4	30	5	110	
Banana	2 Oz	130	0	4	29	5	110	
LF	2 Oz	130	1	4	30	5	110	**A**
Raisin Spice	2 Oz	130	0	4	32	5	110	
(Hostess) Banana Oat								
Bran, LF	2.7 Oz	200	2.5	4	41	2	280	
(Natural Ovens) Blue-								
berry, LF	2.5 Oz	145	1	6	32	2	190	**F**
Carrot, LF	2.5 Oz	140	2	4	30	2	200	**FA**
(Sara Lee) Blueberry	2.2 Oz	120	0	3	28	1	140	
Oat Bran								
(Arrowhead Mills) W/								
Apple	2.7 Oz	120	4	6	15	6	225	
(Health Valley)	2 Oz	140	3	5	31	5	100	
(Hostess) W/Banana, LF	2.7 Oz	200	2.5	4	41	2	280	
Mulberry								
Raw	1 Cup	60	0.6	2	14	2	14	**A**
Raw	1 Lb	195	1.7	7	44	8	45	**A**

	Serv.		K-Cal.	Fat	Prot.	Carb.	Fib.	Sod.	FAC
Mullet									
Raw	3	Oz	100	3.2	16	0	0	55	
Broiled	3	Oz	129	4.2	21	0	0	61	

Mung Bean (See Bean, Mung)

Mung Bean Noodle (See Noodle, Chinese)

	Serv.		K-Cal.	Fat	Prot.	Carb.	Fib.	Sod.	FAC
Mushroom									
Fresh									
Crimini, Raw	1	Oz	9	0	1	1	1	11	
Enoki, Raw	1	Item	1	0	0	0	0	0	
Oyster, Raw	1	Oz	11	0.2	1	1	1	2	
Portabella, Raw	1	Oz	10	0	1	1	1	3	
Shiitake, Cooked	1	Cup	80	0.3	2	21	3	6	
White, Raw	1	Oz	8	0.5	1	1	0	1	
White, Raw	1	Cup	18	0.4	1	3	1	2	
White, Boiled, Drained	1	Item	3	0.1	0	1	0	0	
Woodear, Raw	1	Oz	16	0	0	4	2	5	
Canned/Bottled									
(B & B) W/Butter	3	Oz	30	0.5	3	4	1	410	
(Green Giant):									
Sliced	1	Cup	60	0	6	8	4	880	
W/Garlic	4	Oz	70	1	6	8	2	820	
(Seneca):									
Marinated (5)	1	Oz	90	9	0	2	<1	190	
Shiitake	1	Cup	50	0	2	10	6	1,080	
Water-Packed	1	Cup	50	0	4	10	6	400	
(Townhouse) Button	1	Cup	50	0	4	8	2	960	
Dried									
Chinese Fungus	1	Cup	72	0.1	1	19	NV	17	
Chinese Fungus	1	Oz	63	0	2	14	9	33	
Shiitake	1	Item	11	0	0	3	0	0	
Shiitake	1	Oz	84	.3	3	21	3	4	
Frozen									
(Bird's Eye)	2.6	Oz	20	0	2	4	2	0	
(Green Giant) Creamy	9.6	Oz	220	11	6	29	4	860	

Muskmelon (See Cantaloupe)

	Serv.		K-Cal.	Fat	Prot.	Carb.	Fib.	Sod.	FAC
Mussel, Blue									
Raw	1	Cup	129	3.4	18	6	0	429	FA
Raw	3	Oz	98	2.4	17	2	0	408	F
Cooked, Steamed	3	Oz	146	3.8	20	6	0	314	F
Mustard Greens									
Fresh									
Raw	1	Cup	14	0.2	2	3	1	14	FA
Boiled	1	Cup	21	0.3	3	3	3	22	FA

	Serv.		K-Cal.	Fat	Prot.	Carb.	Fib.	Sod.	FAC
Chinese, Raw	1	Oz	8	0.2	1	1	0	3	FA
Indian, Raw	1	Oz	5	0.1	0	0	0	2	FA
Frozen									
Boiled	1	Cup	29	0.4	3	5	4	38	FA
Boiled	10	Oz	40	0.5	5	7	1	53	FA
Chopped (Seabrook)	3.3	Oz	20	0	2	3	1	20	FA

Mustard Oil

	1	Tbsp	124	14	0	0	0	0	

Mustard Powder

Ground	1	Tsp	19	0	0	0	0	0	
Ground	1	Oz	155	11.3	9	4	1	2	

Mustard, Prepared

Dijon (French)	1	Tsp	8	1	0	0	0	140	
Dijon (Grey Poupon)	1	Tsp	6	0.4	0	1	0	28	
Stone Ground (Hain)	1	Tbsp	14	1	1	1	NV	185	
Stone Ground (Westbrae)	1	Tbsp	16	1	1	1	NV	195	
Yellow	1	Cup	185	10.8	12	16	7	3,081	AC
Yellow	1	Tsp	5	0.2	0	0	0	63	
Yellow (Gulden's)	1	Oz	24	0	0	0	0	240	

Mustard Seed

Whole	1	Oz	133	8.2	7	10	1	1	
Whole (McCormick)	1	Tsp	17	0.8	1	1	0	0	

Mutton

Lean	3	Oz	110	4.5	17	0	0	77	

Mutton Tallow

	1	Tbsp	116	12.8	0	0	0	0	

N

	Serv.	K-Cal.	Fat	Prot.	Carb.	Fib.	Sod.	FAC
Nachos								
W/Beans and Cheese....	1 Cup	254	15.7	11	18	3	338	**FC**
W/Beans, No Cheese	1 Cup	208	10.1	6	24	4	249	**F**
W/Beef and Cheese.......	1 Cup	313	22	21	8	1	296	**C**
W/Beef/Beans/Cheese ..	1 Cup	417	27.6	22	20	3	476	**FC**
W/Chicken and Cheese .	1 Cup	270	17.1	20	8	1	302	**C**
W/Chili	1 Cup	222	11.2	8	26	5	690	**F**
Nachos, Fast Food								
(Taco Bell):								
....	1 Item	322	18.1	2	34	3	538	**A**
Bellgrande...................	1 Item	774	38.8	16	83	17	1,198	**AC**
Supreme	1 Item	453	23.5	12	43	9	723	**A**

Napa Cabbage (See Cabbage, Napa)

Navy Bean (See Bean, Navy)

Natto (See Soybean, Fermented)

Nectarine								
Raw (5 Oz).....................	1 Item	67	0.6	1	16	2	0	**A**
Raw, Sliced	1 Cup	68	0.6	1	16	2	0	**A**
Raw W/Skin....................	1 Lb	204	1.9	4	49	7	1	**A**

Noodle
(All Noodles Dry, unless indicated)
Chinese

Bifun (Eden)	2 Oz	200	0.5	5	44	0	5	
Chow Fun, Cooked........	1 Cup	139	0.5	2	30	1	3	
Chow Mein	1 Cup	237	13.8	4	26	2	198	
Chow Mein (Welpak)	2 Oz	200	1	7	41	0	120	
Crispy (La Choy)	1 Cup	296	16.5	5	32	2	578	
Rice (La Choy)...............	1 Cup	242	6.1	5	42	1	756	
Rice Stick	4 Oz	435	1	10	99	3	16	
Saifun (Mung Bean).......	1.7 Oz	170	0	0	42	0	10	

	Serv.	K-Cal.	Fat	Prot.	Carb.	Fib.	Sod.	FAC
Egg								
Cooked	1 Cup	213	2.4	8	40	2	11	
(Bernardi)	1 Cup	267	6	11	44	1	187	
(Golden Grain)	2 Oz	210	2.2	8	39	2	10	
(Mueller's)	1 Cup	145	1.6	5	27	1	8	
(Mueller's)	2 Oz	220	3	8	40	NV	10	
Spinach	2 Oz	218	2.6	8	40	4	41	
Spinach, Cooked	1 Cup	211	2.5	8	39	4	19	
(Zerega)	3 Oz	379	4.5	15	70	3	26	
Japanese								
Harusame	2 Oz	190	0	0	47	0	5	
Ramen	1 Cup	207	8.6	6	31	2	829	
Soba								
Buckwheat	1 Oz	96	0.2	4	21	1	226	
Buckwheat, Cooked	1 Cup	113	0.1	6	24	NV	68	
(Eden):								
Lotus Root	2 Oz	190	1	9	37	4	470	
Wild Yam	1 Oz	95	0.3	5	19	1	255	
40% Buckwheat	1 Oz	95	0.5	4	19	2	245	
100% Buckwheat	1 Oz	100	0.8	3	21	2	15	
Somen								
Wheat	1 Oz	101	0.2	3	21	1	524	
Wheat, Cooked	1 Cup	231	0.3	7	49	NV	283	
Organic (Eden)	2 Oz	200	1.5	8	38	3	80	
Udon								
(Eden)	2 Oz	555	1.5	8	37	3	660	
Brown Rice, Organic	2 Oz	200	2	8	38	3	80	
Noodle Entree								
W/Beef								
(Hunt's) *Homestyle*	1 Cup	151	3.9	10	22	5	1,241	A
(La Choy)	1 Cup	148	1.2	12	24	3	1,101	
W/Chicken								
(Hunt's) *Homestyle*	1 Cup	176	5.9	12	21	2	1,282	A
(La Choy)	1 Cup	161	3.8	11	23	4	1,163	
W/Vegetables								
(La Choy):								
	1 Cup	131	1.3	5	27	3	1,311	
W/Beef	1 Cup	156	3.5	7	27	3	1,332	
W/Chicken	1 Cup	163	3.3	10	24	1	858	
Noodle Entree, Mix								
(Westbrae):								
Ramen, Buckwheat	½ Pkg	140	1	5	30	2	750	
Ramen, Brown Rice	½ Pkg	140	1	5	30	2	750	
Ramen, Miso	½ Pkg	140	1	5	29	4	750	
Prepared from Mix								
(Farmhouse):								
Creamy Chicken	1 Cup	240	2	10	46	2	1,120	

	Serv.	K-Cal.	Fat	Prot.	Carb.	Fib.	Sod.	FAC
(Noodle Entree, Mix cont.)								
Creamy Garlic..............	1 Cup	260	3	10	48	2	780	
Fettuccine Alfredo.......	1 Cup	260	4	12	48	2	760	
Herb and Butter..........	1 Cup	240	2	10	46	1	930	
Parmesano..................	1 Cup	260	3	10	48	2	900	
Stroganoff	1 Cup	240	3	10	46	2	1,100	
(Lipton): Noodle & Sauce								
Butter	1 Cup	310	14	9	41	2	800	
Chicken	1 Cup	290	10.5	8	42	2	830	
Parmesan....................	1 Cup	330	15	10	37	2	850	
(Pasta Roni):								
Alfredo........................	1 Cup	470	26	13	48	2	1,110	
Broccoli Au Gratin	1 Cup	280	10	10	39	2	860	
Cheddar	1 Cup	290	22	10	39	1	890	
Chicken Sauce	1 Cup	320	13.5	10	41	2	1,020	
Romanoff	1 Cup	400	20	11	46	2	1,070	
Stroganoff	1 Cup	360	14	12	48	2	1,020	

Nopal (See Cactus)

Nori (See Seaweed, Dried)

Nutella (See Hazelnut Spread)

Nutmeg

	Serv.	K-Cal.	Fat	Prot.	Carb.	Fib.	Sod.	FAC
Fresh	1 Oz	145	10.3	2	11	1	1	
Ground (McCormick)......	1 Tsp	11	0.8	0	1	0	0	

Nutrasweet (See Sweetener, Alternative)

Nutritional Drink

(Also See Diet Drink; Sport Beverage)								
(Boost) All Flavors	1 Cup	240	4	10	40	0	130	**FAC**
(Ensure):								
Chocolate....................	1 Cup	250	6	9	40	0	200	**FAC**
Plus, Chocolate	1 Cup	360	13	13	47	0	250	**FA**
Vanilla, LT..................	1 Cup	200	3	10	33	0	200	**FAC**
Vanilla W/Fiber	1 Cup	250	6	9	44	4	200	**FAC**
(Resource):								
French Vanilla.............	1 Cup	250	6	9	40	0	220	**FAC**
Fruit, FF......................	1 Cup	180	0	9	36	0	70	**A**
(Savon):								
....	1 Cup	250	6	9	40	0	200	**FAC**
Plus............................	1 Cup	360	13	13	47	0	250	**FAC**

Nuts (See Individual Listings)

	Serv.	K-Cal.	Fat	Prot.	Carb.	Fib.	Sod.	FAC
Nuts, Mixed								
Dry-Roasted								
(Fisher)	1 Oz	170	14	6	7	NV	125	
(Planters)	1 Oz	160	14	5	7	NV	250	
W/O Salt	1 Cup	814	70.5	24	35	12	16	**FA**
Honey-Roasted								
(Fisher)	1 Cup	680	52	24	32	4	440	**FA**
(Planters)	1 Oz	170	12	5	9	NV	170	
Oil-Roasted								
(Fisher)	1 Cup	720	64	24	20	8	440	**FA**
(Planters):								
Deluxe	1 Oz	170	16	5	6	2	110	
Lightly Salted	1 Oz	170	15	6	6	3	55	
Unsalted	1 Oz	170	15	6	6	3	0	
W/O Peanuts	1 Cup	886	80.9	22	32	8	1,008	**FA**

O

	Serv.	K-Cal.	Fat	Prot.	Carb.	Fib.	Sod.	FAC
Oat								
(Also See Cereal, Hot, Oat)								
Dry	1 Oz	70	2	5	19	5	1	
Flakes, Rolled								
(Arrowhead Mills)	1 Cup	390	7.5	15	69	12	0	
Quick	1 Cup	311	5.1	13	54	9	3	
Quick, Cooked	1 Cup	145	2.3	6	25	4	2	
Steelcut (Arrowhead								
Mills)	1 Oz	110	2	5	19	1	1	
Whole Grain	1 Cup	607	2	26	103	NV	3	
Oat Beverage								
(Mill Milk)	1 Cup	110	2.5	2	19	2	29	
(Pacific) Naturally	1 Cup	110	1.5	4	21	0	110	
Oat Bran								
(Also See Cereal, Hot, Oat Bran)								
Raw	1 Cup	231	6.6	16	62	15	4	**F**
Oat Flour								
(Arrowhead Mills)	1 Cup	360	6	15	60	12	0	
(Ener-G) Breadmaker	1 Cup	477	9.3	21	79	11	11	
(General Mills) *Gold*								
Medal, Blend	1 Cup	390	3	14	81	4	0	
Oat Groats								
(Arrowhead Mills)	¼ Cup	160	3	6	29	4	0	
Oatmeal (See Cereal, Hot, Oatmeal)								
Oat Oil								
	1 Tbsp	120	13.6	0	0	0	0	
Ocean Perch—Redfish								
Raw	3 Oz	81	1.5	16	0	0	63	
Cooked	3 Oz	103	1.8	20	0	0	82	

	Serv.	K-Cal.	Fat	Prot.	Carb.	Fib.	Sod.	FAC
Frozen, Breaded								
(Gorton's)	5 Oz	140	3	25	2	0	100	
Octopus								
Raw	3 Oz	70	0.9	13	2	0	196	
Boiled	3 Oz	139	1.8	25	4	0	390	

Oil (See individual listings)

	Serv.	K-Cal.	Fat	Prot.	Carb.	Fib.	Sod.	FAC
Okra								
Raw, Sliced	1 Cup	38	0.2	2	8	3	8	FA
Batter-Dipped, Fried	1 Cup	175	13.4	3	12	2	137	FA
Boiled	1 Cup	51	0.3	3	12	4	8	FA
Frozen, Cut	1 Cup	33	0	3	5	4	20	FA
Olive, Canned/Bottled								
Black								
(S & W):								
Colossal, W/Pit	1 Item	15	1.5	0	1	0	80	
Jumbo, Pitted	1 Item	8	0.7	0	0	0	45	
Xtra Large, Pitted	1 Item	8	0.8	0	0	0	37	
Green								
Pickled	1 Cup	171	18.7	2	2	6	3,528	A
Pickled, Med Size	1 Item	4	0.5	0	0	0	78	
Ripe, Salted, Oil	1 Cup	456	48.3	3	12	NV	4,438	A
(S & W):								
Manzanilla, Stuffed	1 Item	8	0.7	0	0	0	80	
Queen	1 Item	10	1	0	1	0	110	
Stuffed, Large	1 Item	10	1	0	1	0	180	
Stuffed, Medium	1 Item	10	0.8	0	1	0	145	
Stuffed, Small	1 Item	8	0.8	0	1	0	125	
Varietal								
Ascolano, Pitted	1 Oz	23	1.9	0	2	1	255	
Greek, Pitted, Salt-cured, Oil-coated	1 Oz	96	10.2	1	3	NV	932	
Kalamata (Krinos)	1 Oz	90	8	0	4	0	540	
Manzanilla, Pitted, Pickled	1 Oz	33	3	0	2	1	247	
Mission, Pitted, Pickled	1 Oz	33	3	0	2	1	247	
Sevillano, Pitted, Pickled	1 Oz	23	1.9	0	2	1	255	
Olive Oil								
(Bertolli)	1 Tbsp	120	14	0	0	0	0	A
Omelet								
Western, 3 Eggs	8 Oz	348	25.2	25	4	0	785	
W/Cheese, 3 Eggs	8 Oz	432	33.7	28	3	0	1,076	
W/Ham, 3 Eggs	8 Oz	379	27.9	28	2	0	978	
W/Mushrooms, 3 Eggs	8 0z	289	21.3	20	4	0	500	

	Serv.	K-Cal.	Fat	Prot.	Carb.	Fib.	Sod.	FAC
(Omelet cont.)								
W/Sausage/Mushrooms, 3 Eggs	9 Oz	462	36.1	29	4	1	1,219	
W/Ham and Cheese, 2 Eggs	4 Oz	218	16.6	15	1	0	567	
Omelet, Frozen								
(Healthy Choice) Western W/Eng Muffin	5 Oz	200	3	16	29	NV	480	A
(Wt Watchers) Ham & Cheese	4 Oz	220	5	13	30	2	240	A
Onion								
Canned								
Cocktail, Large (S & W)	1 Item	1	0	0	0	0	38	
Cocktail, Spiced (Vlasic)	1 Oz	4	0	0	1	0	365	
Whole (Green Giant)	1 Cup	70	0	0	16	2	34	
Whole, Small (S & W)	1 Cup	80	0	0	16	2	820	
Frozen								
Chopped, Boiled	1 Cup	59	0.2	2	14	4	25	A
Diced	1 Cup	45	0	1	9	2	45	
Small, Whole	1 Cup	50	0	1	14	4	30	
Small (Bird's Eye)	4 Oz	40	0	1	10	2	10	
Whole (Seneca)	1 Cup	45	0	<1	11	5	0	
Green—Scallion								
Top and Bulb	1 Item	2	0	0	0	0	1	
Trimmed, Chopped	1 Tbsp	2	0.1	0	0	0	0	
Trimmed, Chopped	1 Cup	32	0.2	2	7	2	16	
Freeze-Dried (McCormick)	1 Tsp	4	0	0	1	0	3	
Varietal								
Raw, Red	1 Oz	11	0	0	2	0	1	
Cipolline (Frieda's)	3 Oz	30	0	1	7	2	0	
Maui (Frieda's)	1 Cup	30	0	0	9	3	0	
Yellow								
Raw	1 Oz	12	0	0	3	1	1	
Raw	8 Oz	96	0.2	3	20	4	9	FA
Raw, Chopped (6 Oz)	1 Cup	61	0.3	2	14	3	5	
Boiled	1 Cup	92	0.4	3	21	3	6	A
Onion, Dried								
Flakes	1 Tbsp	16	0	1	4	1	1	
Flakes	1 Oz	92	0.1	3	24	1	6	
Onion Powder								
(McCormick)	1 Tsp	10	0	0	2	0	2	
Onion Rings, Fast Food								
(Burger King)	1 Serv	310	14	4	41	6	810	
(Carl's Jr.)	1 Serv	520	26	8	63	3	940	

	Serv.	K-Cal.	Fat	Prot.	Carb.	Fib.	Sod.	FAC
(Jack In The Box)	1 Serv	380	23	5	38	NV	450	

Onion Rings, Frozen
(Bland Farms) *Vidalia*

O's....................	3 Oz	200	9	3	26	1	260	
(Mrs. Paul's)	3 Oz	228	14.4	2	23	1	275	
(Ore-Ida)	3 Oz	210	10.5	3	27	NV	285	

Orange (Also See Mandarin Orange)
All Varieties

Whole	1 Item	62	0.2	1	15	3	0	FA
Sections...........................	1 Cup	85	0.2	2	21	4	0	FA
Navel								
Peeled and Seeded	1 Oz	13	0	0	3	0	0	
Sections...........................	1 Cup	76	0.2	2	19	4	2	FA
Valencia								
Peeled and Seeded	1 Oz	14	0.1	0	3	0	0	
Sections...........................	1 Cup	88	0.5	2	21	5	0	FA

Orange Juice
Fresh

Freshly Squeezed	1 Cup	112	0.5	2	26	1	2	FA
(Odwalla)	1 Cup	110	0	2	24	1	24	FA
Canned/Bottled/Box								
(Hi-C) Box	8.45 Oz	130	0	0	33	NV	30	A
(R.W. Knudsen)...............	1 Cup	100	0	2	23	NV	35	A
(Kraft) NSA.....................	1 Cup	107	0	1	25	NV	0	A
(Minute Maid):								
....	1 Cup	124	0	0	32	NV	34	A
Box	8.45 Oz	120	0	0	28	NV	25	FA
(Mott's) Box	8.45 Oz	120	0	0	29	0	10	A
(Nutra/Balance)	1 Cup	100	0	0	24	NV	0	A
(Tree Top)	1 Cup	120	0	0	28	0	25	A
(Tropicana):								
....	1 Cup	110	0	1	27	NV	0	A
Plus Calcium...............	1 Cup	110	0	1	27	NV	0	AC
Plus Fiber	1 Cup	120	0	1	30	2	0	A
Plus Vitamins..............	1 Cup	110	0	1	27	NV	0	A
Frozen Concentrate								
Diluted (Flav R Pac)	1 Cup	120	0	1	29	0	0	A
Diluted (Minute Maid).....	1 Cup	110	0	0	27	0	0	A
Diluted (R.W. Knudsen) .	1 Cup	100	0	2	23	NV	35	A
Undiluted (Minute Maid).	1 Cup	440	0	0	108	0	0	FA
Mix, Prepared								
(Tang).............................	1 Cup	100	0	0	24	NV	0	A
(Tropicana)	1 Cup	110	0	0	26	NV	50	A
(Welchade)	1 Cup	140	0	0	34	NV	40	A

	Serv.	K-Cal.	Fat	Prot.	Carb.	Flb.	Sod.	FAC
Orange Juice, Blended								
(Kern's) W/Guava,								
Nectar	1 Cup	150	0	0	36	0	10	**A**
(R.W. Knudsen)								
W/Mango	1 Cup	120	0	0	30	NV	50	
(Ultra Slim-Fast)								
W/Pineapple	12 Oz	220	1.5	7	48	5	260	**FAC**
W/Strawberry/Banana.	12 Oz	220	1.5	7	47	5	240	**FAC**
Orange Peel								
Raw	1 Tbsp	6	0	0	2	1	0	
Candied (S & W)	1 Piece	1	0	0	0	0	1	
Orange Roughy								
Raw	3 Oz	59	0.6	13	0	0	54	
Broiled	3 Oz	75	0.8	16	0	0	69	
Oregano								
Fresh	1 Oz	19	0.6	1	3	NV	1	**A**
Ground (McCormick)	1 Tsp	6	0	0	1	1	1	
Oyster								
Canned								
(Chicken Of The Sea)	⅓ Cup	70	3	7	3	1	220	
(Geisha)	⅓ Cup	60	2.5	7	2	2	310	
Canned, Smoked								
(Chicken Of The Sea)	2.5 Oz	140	8	11	7	0	260	
(Crown Prince)	3 Oz	170	9	14	8	1	280	
Eastern, Farmed								
Raw	3 Oz	50	1.2	4	5	0	150	**A**
Cooked	3 Oz	91	6	6	3	0	138	**A**
Eastern, Wild								
Raw	1 Cup	169	6.1	18	10	0	523	**A**
Cooked	3 Oz	116	4.2	12	7	0	359	**A**
Cooked	1 Item	10	0.3	1	1	0	30	**A**
Pacific								
Raw	1 Item	41	1.2	5	2	0	53	**A**
Cooked (1 Oz)	1 Med	41	1.2	5	2	0	53	**A**

Oyster Plant
(See Salsify)

P

	Serv.	K-Cal.	Fat	Prot.	Carb.	Fib.	Sod.	FAC
Paella								
Marinara, W/Seafood	1 Cup	390	13.2	41	25	1	816	**A**
Valenciana Style	1 Cup	533	28.9	35	31	1	534	**A**
W/Seafood.......................	1 Cup	351	11.1	21	40	1	1,190	**A**
Pak Choi								
(See Bok Choy)								
Palm Heart—Hearts of Palm								
Cooked	1 Item	39	0.1	1	10	1	5	**A**
(Maria)	½ Cup	35	0	2	6	3	33	**A**
(Reese)..........................	½ Cup	23	0	3	4	3	55	**A**
(Roland).........................	½ Cup	25	0.5	2	4	2	450	**A**
Palm Kernel Oil								
....	1 Tbsp	117	13.6	0	0	0	0	**A**
Palm Oil								
....	1 Tbsp	120	13.6	0	0	0	0	**A**
Pam								
(See Cooking Spray)								
Pancake								
Dry Mix,								
Buttermilk								
(Aunt Jemima)................	1 Cup	571	6	18	114	6	1,441	**C**
(Betty Crocker)	1 Cup	601	7.5	15	117	3	1,622	
(Krusteaz):								
....	1 Cup	400	6	12	76	4	1,600	
FF..............................	1 Cup	380	0	10	94	12	880	
(Pillsbury):								
....	1 Cup	480	4.5	12	96	2	1,682	
Hungry Jack................	1 Cup	480	4.5	12	99	2	1,952	

	Serv.	K-Cal.	Fat	Prot.	Carb.	Fib.	Sod.	FAC
(Pancake cont.)								
Oat Bran								
(Arrowhead Mills)	1 Cup	420	4.5	21	75	18	480	
(Krusteaz) LT	1 Cup	280	2	12	68	16	860	
Original								
(Aunt Jemima)	1 Cup	450	1.5	12	102	3	1,862	
(Betty Crocker)	1 Cup	601	9	18	117	3	1,622	C
(Robin Hood)	1 Cup	541	9	15	93	3	1,532	
Specialty Grains								
(Arrowhead Mills):								
Blue Corn	1 Cup	450	6	12	84	9	390	
Kamut	1 Cup	520	4	28	104	16	1,320	
Wild Rice	1 Cup	420	3	9	90	0	195	
(Aunt Jemima)								
Buckwheat	1 Cup	480	4	20	112	16	2,240	C
(Bob's Red Mill)								
Cornmeal	1 Cup	420	2	12	84	0	1,240	
Whole Wheat								
(Arrowhead Mills)	1 Cup	480	2	20	96	16	1,040	
(Aunt Jemima)	1 Cup	520	2	24	112	12	2,240	FC
(Krusteaz) W/Honey	1 Cup	460	4	18	90	6	1,000	
Prepared From Mix								
(Serving size approximately one 4" diameter pancake)								
Blueberry								
Home Recipe	1 Item	84	3.5	2	11	0	157	
(Pillsbury) *Hungry Jack*	1 Item	170	1	3	38	1	780	
Buckwheat								
(Aunt Jemima)	1 Item	48	0.5	2	10	2	258	
(Bob's Red Mill)	1 Item	120	6	4	13	1	250	
Buttermilk								
(Aunt Jemima)	1 Item	41	0.2	1	9		233	
(Betty Crocker)	1 Item	70	1	2	14	NV	166	
(Bob's Red Mill)	1 Item	97	3	3	13		220	
(Pillsbury) *Hungry Jack*	1 Item	97	4.3	2	12	0	233	
Plain								
(Aunt Jemima) Original								
Complete	1 Item	84	1.2	2	17	1	203	
(Betty Crocker) *Bisquick*,								
Shake N Pour	1 Item	70	1.3	2	13	0	237	
Whole Wheat								
(Aunt Jemima)	1 Item	54	0.3	2	12	1	297	
(Betty Crocker) *Bisquick*	1 Item	67	1	2	13	0	227	
(Bob's Red Mill) 10-								
Grain	1 Item	93	3.3	4	12	1	220	
(Krusteaz)	1 Item	83	0.3	3	14	2	210	
Pancake, Fast Food								
(Carl's Jr.)	1 Serv	510	24	11	61	NV	950	
(Hardee's)	3 Items	280	2	8	56	1	890	

	Serv.	K-Cal.	Fat	Prot.	Carb.	Flb.	Sod.	FAC
(Jack In The Box) Platter	1 Serv	400	12	13	59	3	980	

Pancake, Frozen
(Aunt Jemima):
Blueberry	1 Item	70	1.2	2	13	1	223	
Buttermilk	1 Item	60	1	2	11	1	197	
Original	1 Item	67	1	2	13	7	233	
Original, LF	1 Item	43	0.5	1	11	3	193	
(Krusteaz) Blueberry	1 Item	85	1.5	3	16	1	215	
(Griddle Lite) Wheat-Free	1 Serv	130	2	4	24	5	180	

Pancake Syrup (See Maple Syrup)

Papaya
Raw	1 Cup	55	0.2	1	14	3	4	FA
Raw, Whole	1 Lb	247	0.6	2	59	8	29	FA
Dried	1 Oz	59	0.2	1	15	3	5	FA

Papaya Juice
(R.W. Knudsen)
| Creamed Conc | 1 Cup | 160 | 0 | 0 | 40 | NV | 40 | A |
| W/Lime | 1 Cup | 130 | 0 | 0 | 34 | NV | 35 | A |

Papaya Nectar
(After The Fall)	1 Cup	100	0	1	25	0	15	A
(Kern's)	1 Cup	208	0	1	51	0	10	A
(R.W. Knudsen)	1 Cup	130	0	0	34	NV	35	A

Paprika
| (McCormick) | 1 Tsp | 9 | 0.4 | 0 | 1 | 1 | 2 | |

Parfait (See Ice Cream Parfait)

Parsley
Fresh, Chopped	1 Oz	10	0.2	1	2	1	16	FA
Fresh, Chopped	1 Cup	22	0.5	2	4	2	34	FA
Fresh, Sprig	1 Piece	0	0	0	0	0	1	
Freeze-Dried	1 Cup	15	0.3	2	2	2	22	FA
Dried (McCormick)	1 Tsp	2	0	0	0	0	2	

Parsley Root
| Fresh | 1 Oz | 3 | 0.2 | 1 | 1 | 0 | 28 | |

Parsnip
Raw	1 Cup	100	0.4	2	24	7	14	FA
Boiled	1 Cup	126	0.5	2	31	6	16	FA
Boiled	1 Oz	23	0	0	6	1	3	

	Serv.		K-Cal.	Fat	Prot.	Carb.	Fib.	Sod.	FAC
Passion Fruit									
Purple, Raw	1	Item	18	0.1	0	4	2	5	
Purple, Raw	1	Oz	82	0.6	2	20	9	24	A
Passion Fruit Juice									
Fresh, Purple	1	Cup	126	0.1	1	34	0	15	
Fresh, Yellow	1	Cup	148	0.5	2	36	0	15	
Passion Supreme									
(Snapple)	1	Cup	128	0	0	31	NV	16	
W/Raspberry (R.W.									
Knudsen)	1	Cup	130	0	0	33	NV	35	
Pasta									
(All values for dry pasta unless indicated)									
(2 Oz dry pasta equal approximately 1 cup cooked)									
Amaranth									
(Health Valley)	2	Oz	170	1	7	33	9	10	A
Angel Hair									
(Contadina) Fresh	1	Cup	192	2.4	8	34	2	24	
(Delverde) Egg,									
Semolina	2	Oz	200	1.5	8	39	1	15	
(Trader Joe's) Durum									
Semolina	2	Oz	200	1	7	41	2	0	
(Westbrae) Corn	2	Oz	210	1.5	4	46	NV	15	
Bowties—Farfelle									
Egg (Mueller's)	2	Oz	220	3	8	38	1	10	
Wheat (Ronzoni)	2	Oz	210	1	7	42	NV	0	
Veggie (Westbrae)	1	Cup	380	3	18	80	10	10	
Egg									
Fresh	2	Oz	162	1.3	6	31	NV	15	
Spinach	2	Oz	216	2.6	8	40	4	41	F
(Mueller's)	2	Oz	220	3	8	38	1	10	
Fettuccini									
(Contadina):									
	1	Cup	240	3	9	46	2	16	
Fresh	1	Cup	200	2.8	8	36	2	24	
Spinach, Fresh	1	Cup	216	3.2	10	37	3	88	
(Ronzoni) Egg	2	Oz	220	3	8	42	NV	15	
Gluten-Free									
(Ener-G) Brown Rice	2	Oz	212	0.1	4	44	2	1	
Rice	2	Oz	214	0	4	42	2	1	
Lasagna									
(Bernard) Precooked	1	Piece	250	3	9	47	2	15	
(Health Valley) WW	2	Oz	170	1	9	40	7	10	
(Mueller's)	2	Oz	210	1	7	42	1	0	
(Westbrae):									
Spinach	1.8	Oz	180	2	9	35	5	20	
WW	1.8	Oz	200	1.5	8	36	7	10	

	Serv.	K-Cal.	Fat	Prot.	Carb.	Fib.	Sod.	FAC
Linguine								
(Contadina) Fresh	1 Cup	208	3.2	8	38	2	24	
(DiGiorno)	2 Oz	152	1.2	6	32	2	100	
Macaroni, Spirals/Elbows								
(Westbrae) WW	1 Cup	420	3	18	80	16	20	
Corn	1 Cup	440	3	8	94	0	30	
Plain	1 Cup	390	1.7	13	78	3	7	
Vegetable	1 Cup	308	0.9	11	63	4	36	
Mung Bean								
(Eden) Hursame	2 Oz	190	0	0	47	0	5	
Penne								
(De Cecco)	2 Oz	210	1	7	41	NV	0	
Rigatoni								
(Contadina) Fresh	1 Cup	200	3	9	34	NV	25	
(Ronzoni)	2 Oz	210	1	7	42	NV	0	
Rotini								
(Eden) Vegetable	2 Oz	210	1	7	42	2	10	
(Pasta Perfect)	1 Cup	140	0	5	28	1	0	
Shells								
(Eden) Vegetable,								
Organic	2 Oz	200	1	8	40	3	0	
(Mueller's)	2 Oz	210	1	7	42	1	0	
(Ronzoni) Wheat	2 Oz	210	1	9	41	NV	0	
(Westbrae) Corn	2 Oz	220	1.5	4	47	NV	15	
Spaghetti								
Plain	2 Oz	212	0.9	7	42	1	4	
(Eden) Organic	2 Oz	200	1	8	40	3	0	
Whole Grain, Organic.	2 Oz	210	1.5	10	40	6	0	
(Health Valley) Organic..	2 Oz	170	1	9	32	7	10	
(Westbrae):								
Corn	2 Oz	210	1.5	4	46	NV	15	
Spinach	2 Oz	180	2	9	38	6	20	
Whole Wheat	2 Oz	200	1.5	9	39	8	10	
Spinach, W/Egg								
Fresh	2 Oz	164	1.2	6	31	0	15	
Fresh, Cooked	1 Cup	208	1.5	8	40	6	10	
Enriched	1 Cup	145	1.7	6	27	3	27	F
Enriched, Cooked	1 Cup	211	2.5	8	39	6	19	F
Spinach, W/O Egg								
(Health Valley) Organic..	2 Oz	170	1	9	32	7	10	
(Westbrae)	2 Oz	180	2	9	38	9	20	
Spaghetti, Cooked	1 Cup	182	0.9	6	37	3	20	

Pasta Entree, Canned
(Serving size given in Oz to reflect weight of 1 serving)
(Chef Boyardee):

	Serv.	K-Cal.	Fat	Prot.	Carb.	Fib.	Sod.	FAC
ABC's & 123's W/								
Sauce	1 Cup	180	0	6	38	3	910	

	Serv.	K-Cal.	Fat	Prot.	Carb.	Flb.	Sod.	FAC
(Pasta Entree, Canned cont.)								
ABC's & 123's W/								
Meatballs..................	8.6 Oz	280	11	9	35	3	1,090	
Pac Man W/Meatballs	7.6 Oz	230	9	7	32	5	880	
Pac Man W/Tomato								
Sauce	7.6 Oz	150	1	6	30	NV	830	
Smurf	7.6 Oz	150	1	6	29	3	830	
Smurf Pasta/Meatballs	7.6 Oz	240	9	8	31	2	900	A
Tic Tac Toes/								
Meatballs..............	1 Cup	260	10	9	35	4	1,060	
*Zooroni/*Meatballs in								
Sauce	7.6 Oz	240	8	8	33	NV	970	
(Franco-American):								
Circuos's, W/Cheese								
Sauce	8 Oz	184	2	5	36	3	936	
Teddyo's W/Cheese								
Sauce	8 Oz	182	2.1	5	35	3	960	
(Libby's) *Spirals &*								
Chicken......................	7.7 Oz	130	4	8	16	4	980	

Pasta Entree, Frozen

(Serving size given in Oz to reflect weight of 1 serving)

	Serv.	K-Cal.	Fat	Prot.	Carb.	Flb.	Sod.	FAC
(Budget Gourmet Light)								
Linguini/Scallops/								
Clams......................	9.5 Oz	280	8	14	38	3	800	
(Green Giant):								
Creamy Cheddar	1 Cup	107	3.4	4	15	2	300	A
Dijon..........................	9.5 Oz	260	17	7	21	4	630	A
Florentine..................	1 Cup	155	4.5	7	22	3	455	A
Garden Herb..............	1 Cup	115	3.5	5	16	4	375	
Garlic Seasoning	1 Cup	130	5	4	18	3	320	A
Parmesan W/Peas......	5.7 Oz	160	5	9	21	3	420	
Primavera...................	1 Cup	142	5.3	6	18	3	222	
Rotini, Cheddar...........	9.5 Oz	230	10	9	32	5	570	A
(Healthy Choice):								
Fettucini Alfredo..........	8 Oz	250	5	11	39	3	480	
Fettucini Alfredo W/								
Chicken	8.5 Oz	260	4.5	22	35	3	410	
Linguini, Shrimp W/								
Tomato	9.5 Oz	230	2	12	40	4	390	
Pasta Italian................	12 Oz	350	5	16	59	NV	530	A
Pasta Primavera	11 Oz	280	3	11	51	2	360	
Shells, Marinara..........	12 Oz	370	4	25	59	5	390	C
(Legume) Shells,								
Stuffed, Tofu Sauce ...	11 Oz	240	11	13	23	6	660	
(Stouffer's):								
Carbonara..................	9.7 Oz	620	45	19	34	4	780	C
Casino........................	9.2 Oz	300	10	9	44	2	800	

	Serv.		K-Cal.	Fat	Prot.	Carb.	Fib.	Sod.	FAC
Cheese Shells W/									
Meat Sauce	9	Oz	320	14	19	30	2	1,310	
Fettucini Alfredo	10	Oz	580	39	14	42	4	810	C
Linguine/Clam Sauce	10.2	Oz	285	8	17	36	NV	1,010	
Mexicali	10	Oz	490	31	16	36	NV	1,020	C
Oriental	10	Oz	300	14	8	35	NV	760	A
Primavera	5.3	Oz	270	21	7	13	6	580	
Shells, Cheese W/									
Tomato	9.2	Oz	340	16	19	29	5	920	C
(Stouffer's) Lean Cuisine:									
Angel Hair	10	Oz	210	4	9	35	4	420	A
Cannelloni, Cheese	9	Oz	240	5	19	29	4	590	
Chicken Marinara	9	Oz	270	6	15	38	4	540	
Fettucini Alfredo	9	Oz	270	7	13	38	2	590	C
Linguine/Clam Sauce	9.7	Oz	280	8	17	36	NV	560	
Marinara Twist	10	Oz	240	3	10	42	4	440	A
(Ultra Slim-Fast)									
Primavera	12	Oz	340	9	18	52	4	730	A
(Wt Watchers):									
Angel Hair	9	Oz	170	2	8	29	7	520	A
Bowtie Pasta, Marsala	9.7	Oz	280	9	13	36	5	560	
Fettucini Alfredo W/									
Broccoli	8.5	Oz	230	6	10	34	3	450	C
Pasta Portofino	9.5	Oz	150	1	7	29	4	270	A
Penne, Dried Tomato	10	Oz	290	9	13	40	5	560	AC
Romanoff Supreme	9.5	Oz	240	8	12	30	6	570	

Pasta Entree, Mix

(Prepared as indicated on package)

	Serv.		K-Cal.	Fat	Prot.	Carb.	Fib.	Sod.	FAC
(Hain):									
Cheddar	1	Cup	380	22	14	38	7	680	C
Italian	1	Cup	340	20	14	36	8	700	C
Parmesan	1	Cup	320	14	14	40	6	800	
Primavera	1	Cup	360	20	12	38	5	720	AC
Swiss/Mixed Grain	1	Cup	360	18	14	40	7	780	
(Kraft):									
Herb & Garlic	1	Cup	360	16	12	38	1	1,100	
Parmesan	1	Cup	360	16	12	38	1	1,260	
(Noodle Roni):									
Four Cheese	1	Cup	410	18	13	49	2	1,040	A
Herb	1	Cup	320	13	9	42	2	850	
Herb & Butter	1	Cup	430	25	10	43	2	910	A
Parmesano	1	Cup	390	17	12	49	2	940	
Tomato Basil	1	Cup	240	9	6	35	2	690	A
White Cheddar	1	Cup	390	16	12	47	2	1,150	
(Pasta Perfect)									
Vegetables	1	Cup	260	2	12	50	NV	130	

	Serv.	K-Cal.	Fat	Prot.	Carb.	Fib.	Sod.	FAC
Pasta Salad Mix								
(Fantastic):								
Italian Herb	1 Cup	170	1.5	7	34	2	380	A
Spicy Oriental	1 Cup	200	3	7	37	3	420	A
(Kraft):								
Classic Ranch	1 Cup	480	30.7	9	40	3	667	
Garden Primavera	1 Cup	373	16	11	45	3	973	
Herb & Garlic	1 Cup	420	24	10	42	1	600	A
Homestyle	1 Cup	480	32	8	82	2	940	A
Italian, LT	1 Cup	253	2.7	11	45	3	880	
Rancher's Choice	1 Cup	480	32	10	42	1	1,080	A
(Suddenly Salad):								
Caesar	1 Cup	293	12	7	40	1	773	
Macaroni	1 Cup	427	26.7	7	40	3	720	
Macaroni, LF	1 Cup	280	2	7	40	3	773	
Pasta Primavera	1 Cup	360	18	8	40	NV	680	
Pasta Primavera, LF	1 Cup	280	8	8	42	NV	740	
Pasta Sauce—Spaghetti Sauce								
(Eden) Organic	1 Cup	160	5	6	24	6	640	A
(Healthy Choice)								
Traditional	1 Cup	100	0	4	22	4	780	A
(Hunt's):								
Homestyle	1 Cup	113	5.1	4	14	3	1,192	A
Old Country	1 Cup	105	5.3	4	14	5	1,084	A
Original	1 Cup	129	4.7	4	22	8	1,242	A
(Prego)	1 Cup	280	9	4	46	4	1,220	A
(Ragú) Traditional	1 Cup	160	7	4	20	6	1,640	A
Alfredo								
(Bernardi)	1 Cup	360	26	12	20	1	1,000	AC
(Contadina):								
Fresh	1 Cup	800	76	16	16	0	1,020	C
LT	1 Cup	380	26	8	20	0	1,100	C
(Five Brothers)	1 Cup	480	44	8	8	0	120	
(Kraft)	1 Cup	800	64	32	32	NV	2,720	
Cheese								
(Hunt's) Classic								
Parmesan	1 Cup	100	4.2	4	16	4	1,268	A
(Prego) Three Cheese	1 Cup	200	4	6	40	6	960	A
Chunky								
(Contadina) *Thick & Zesty*, FF	1 Cup	80	0	4	12	4	1,360	A
(Hunt's) W/Garlic	1 Cup	121	2	3	25	3	1,052	A
(Muir Glen) Organic	1 Cup	160	4	4	26	6	600	A
Clam								
(Contadina) Red	1 Cup	180	8	12	14	6	1,060	A
White	1 Cup	260	20	12	8	0	1,400	

	Serv.	K-Cal.	Fat	Prot.	Carb.	Fib.	Sod.	FAC
(Progresso) Red.............	1 Cup	160	6	12	16	2	1,240	
White......................	1 Cup	230	18	20	2	0	610	
Garden								
(Muir Glen) Original	1 Cup	140	4	4	20	4	720	A
(Prego)..........................	1 Cup	180	2	4	32	6	960	A
(Ragú):								
....	1 Cup	240	8	4	38	4	1,140	A
LT....................	1 Cup	100	0	4	22	6	780	A
Garlic and Onion								
(Healthy Choice) FF.......	1 Cup	80	0	4	18	4	780	A
(Hunt's)	1 Cup	126	5.5	5	18	7	1,044	A
(Muir Glen) Organic, FF	1 Cup	100	0	4	22	6	600	A
(Prego)..........................	1 Cup	220	6	4	38	6	840	A
(Ragú)..........................	1 Cup	260	10	6	38	6	1,060	A
Italian								
(Healthy Choice) FF.......	1 Cup	80	0	4	18	4	780	A
(Hunt's)	1 Cup	127	5.2	5	18	6	1,232	A
(Muir Glen) Organic, FF	1 Cup	120	0	4	26	4	600	A
Marinara								
(Bernardi).......................	1 Cup	240	8	4	40	4	960	A
(Contadina) Fresh	1 Cup	160	8	4	16	4	940	A
(Five Brothers)	1 Cup	160	8	4	18	4	960	A
(Hunt's):								
....	1 Cup	120	3.2	3	25	3	1,052	A
Angela Mia..................	1 Cup	95	0.6	4	18	8	1,006	A
(Prego)..........................	1 Cup	220	12	4	24	6	1,340	A
(Ragú)..........................	1 Cup	180	10	4	18	6	1,640	A
Meat								
(Del Monte)	1 Cup	140	4	6	26	6	1,020	A
(Healthy Choice)	1 Cup	100	2	4	16	4	780	A
(Hunt's)........................	1 Cup	129	4.7	4	22	4	1,208	A
(Prego)..........................	1 Cup	280	12	6	42	6	1,000	A
(Ragú):								
Hearty	1 Cup	260	9	8	38	6	1,160	A
Old World..................	1 Cup	180	10	6	18	6	1,640	A
Mushroom								
(Del Monte)	1 Cup	140	2	4	30	4	1,040	A
(Five Brothers)	1 Cup	180	8	4	20	6	920	A
(Healthy Choice)	1 Cup	100	0	4	22	4	780	A
(Hunt's) Homestyle..........	1 Cup	113	5.1	4	14	3	1,172	A
(Prego)..........................	1 Cup	300	10	4	46	6	1,340	A
(Progresso).....................	1 Cup	160	6	4	22	4	720	A
(Ragú):								
LT............................	1 Cup	100	0	6	22	4	780	A
Old World..................	1 Cup	160	7	4	20	6	1,640	A
Pesto								
(Armanino)	¼ Cup	190	18	4	3	1	370	A
(Candoni).......................	¼ Cup	170	17	3	2	2	700	A
(Contadina).....................	¼ Cup	290	24	6	5	3	580	AC

	Serv.	K-Cal.	Fat	Prot.	Carb.	Flb.	Sod.	FAC
Primavera								
(Five Brothers)	1 Cup	140	6	4	18	4	1,000	A
(Healthy Choice) FF	1 Cup	90	0	4	18	4	780	A
(Ragú)	1 Cup	220	8	4	34	8	960	A
Tomato and Basil								
(Five Brothers)	1 Cup	120	4	4	16	4	940	A
(Hunt's)	1 Cup	97	4.2	4	15	8	1,226	A
(Prego)	1 Cup	220	6	4	38	6	840	A
Pastrami								
(Serving size equals 1 slice)								
(Healthy Choice)	1 Oz	30	0.8	5	1	0	240	
(Hillshire Farm)	0.3 Oz	10	0.1	2	1	0	100	
(Oscar Mayer)	0.6 Oz	16	0.3	3	0	0	217	
Turkey								
(Louis Rich)	1 Oz	30	1	5	0	0	320	
Speciality	1 Oz	35	1	6	1	0	295	
(Mr. Turkey)	⅓ Oz	12	0.4	2	0	0	87	
Pastry								
Bun, Sweet								
(Entenmann's):								
Apple, FF	1 Item	150	0	3	33	1	140	
Blueberry Cheese, FF	1 Item	140	0	4	31	1	150	
Cheese, FF	1 Item	140	0	4	30	1	150	
Raisin, FF	1 Item	160	0	3	36	1	125	
Raspberry Cheese, FF	1 Item	160	0	4	36	1	135	
(Hostess):								
Honey-Glazed	1 Item	320	19	5	35	2	210	
Honey-Iced	1 Item	390	20	5	49	2	220	
(Little Debbie) Honey	1 Item	210	13	3	22	1	180	
Danish								
(Entenmann's):								
Apple Twist, FF	⅛ Item	200	0	4	47	NV	147	
Apricot Twist, FF	⅛ Pkg	150	0	3	34	1	110	
Cinnamon Apple Twist, FF	⅛ Pkg	150	0	3	35	1	110	
Lemon Twist, FF	⅛ Pkg	130	0	3	31	1	140	
Pecan Ring	1 Item	190	12	3	19	NV	130	
Raspberry Twist, FF	⅛ Pkg	140	0	8	33	2	125	
(Hostess):								
Apple	1 Item	400	22	4	47	2	340	
Apple Fruit Roll	1 Item	180	4	4	33	1	170	
Apple Twist	1 Item	220	4	4	42	0	270	
Caramel Pecan Swirl	1 Item	250	15	3	25	1	130	
(Pepperidge Farm):								
Apple	1 Item	220	8	2	35	NV	130	
Cheese	1 Item	240	14	3	25	NV	230	

	Serv.	K-Cal.	Fat	Prot.	Carb.	Flb.	Sod.	FAC
Cinnamon/Raisin.........	1 Item	250	11	3	35	NV	170	
Raspberry	1 Item	220	9	3	31	NV	140	
(Sara Lee):								
Apple, LT	1 Slice	130	0	2	30	NV	120	
Apple Streusel, LT......	1 Slice	170	2	1	36	NV	140	
Cheese....................	1 Item	130	8	2	13	0	130	
Cherry Streusel, FF/								
LT	1 Slice	160	2	2	34	1	140	
Cinnamon...................	⅛ Pkg	200	12	3	21	0	270	
(Wt Watchers):								
Apple Cinnamon	1 Item	160	2.5	3	30	1	170	
Cheese.......................	1 Item	160	3	4	29	1	200	
Raspberry	1 Item	160	2.5	4	30	1	170	
Puff								
(Pepperidge Farm):								
Dough Sheet...............	¼ Sheet	260	17	4	22	NV	290	
Shells	1 Item	210	15	3	16	NV	180	
Shells, Mini	1 Item	50	4	1	4	NV	40	
Toaster								
(Auburn Farms) *Jammer*	1 Item	180	0	3	42	4	200	
(Kellogg's) *Pop Tarts*:								
Blueberry....................	1 Item	210	7	2	36	1	210	F
Cherry	1 Item	200	5	2	37	1	220	F
Choc Fudge, Frosted .	1 Item	200	5	3	37	1	220	F
Chocolate Graham	1 Item	210	6	3	36	1	220	A
Frosted S'Mores	1 Item	200	5	3	37	1	200	F
Grape, Frosted	1 Item	200	5	2	38	1	200	
Raspberry, Frosted.....	1 Item	210	6	2	37	1	210	F
Strawberry...................	1 Item	200	5	2	37	1	180	F
Strawberry, Frosted....	1 Item	200	5	2	38	1	170	F
(Nabisco) *Toastettes*:								
Frosted Blueberry	1 Item	190	5	2	35	1	190	
Frosted Fudge	1 Item	190	5	2	34	1	280	
Strawberry...................	1 Item	190	5	2	35	1	200	
Toaster Strudel								
(Pillsbury):								
Apple..........................	1 Item	180	7	3	27	1	190	
Blueberry....................	1 Item	180	7	3	26	1	200	
Cinnamon...................	1 Item	190	8	3	26	1	200	
Strawberry...................	1 Item	180	7	3	26	1	200	
Turnover								
(Pepperidge Farm):								
Apple..........................	1 Item	300	17	3	34	NV	210	
Blueberry....................	1 Item	310	19	3	32	NV	230	
Peach.........................	1 Item	310	18	3	34	NV	260	A
Raspberry	1 Item	310	17	4	36	NV	260	A
(Pillsbury) Apple	1 Item	75	8.5	2	23	1	330	
Cherry	1 Item	180	8.5	2	24	0	325	

	Serv.	K-Cal.	Fat	Prot.	Carb.	Flb.	Sod.	FAC
Pâté, Canned								
Chicken..............................	1 Tbsp	26	1.7	2	1	0	50	F
Goose, Smoked	1 Tbsp	60	5.7	2	1	0	90	
(Mariel & Henri) W/Pork	2 Oz	240	23	6	1	0	310	A
W/Pork & Chicken	2 Oz	190	18	7	1	1	360	A
(Sells)	¼ Cup	160	14	7	3	1	380	A
Pea								
Fresh								
Raw	1 Lb	366	1.8	25	66	23	23	FA
Raw	1 Cup	117	0.6	8	21	7	7	FA
Boiled	1 Cup	134	0.4	9	25	9	5	FA
Snap Pea, Boiled	1 Cup	57	0.4	5	11	4	6	FA
Snap Pea, Raw..............	1 Cup	61	0.3	4	11	4	6	FA
Canned								
(Del Monte) Sweet	1 Cup	120	0	6	22	8	720	FA
(Green Giant) LS	1 Cup	120	0	8	22	6	380	
Sweet	1 Cup	120	0	8	22	8	780	
(S & W):								
Petit Pois	1 Cup	140	0	8	24	8	660	FA
Sun Vista, Early/June.	1 Cup	160	0	12	36	10	1,020	FA
Sweet...........................	1 Cup	140	0	8	24	8	660	FA
Frozen								
Baby								
(Flav R Pac)...................	1 Cup	105	0.8	8	18	6	157	FA
(Green Giant) *Le Sueur*.	1 Cup	105	0	6	20	6	330	FA
W/Butter	1 Cup	133	2.7	7	21	5	493	FA
Green, Sweet								
(Green Giant)	1 Cup	90	0	6	18	6	300	FA
W/Butter	1 Cup	133	2.7	5	21	7	533	FA
(Health Valley)................	1 Cup	160	2	8	22	6	140	FA
(Seneca)	1 Cup	120	0	7	21	9	45	FA
Snow								
(Flav R Pac)								
Chinese Pod..............	1 Cup	50	0	2	6	2	10	
Sugar Snap								
(Flav R Pac)...................	1 Cup	40	0	3	9	3	13	FA
(Green Giant)	1 Cup	75	0	5	15	5	142	FA
(Seneca)	1 Cup	67	0	3	12	4	0	FA
Pea, Combination								
Canned								
W/Carrots, LS.................	1 Cup	97	0.7	6	22	8	10	FA
(Green Giant)								
W/Carrots.....................	1 Cup	100	0	4	8	6	810	FA
(S & W) W/Carrots.........	1 Cup	100	0	6	20	6	660	FA
(S & W) W/Onions	1 Cup	80	0	6	22	6	1,060	FA

	Serv.	K-Cal.	Fat	Prot.	Carb.	Fib.	Sod.	FAC
Frozen								
W/Carrots, Boiled	1 Cup	77	0.7	5	16	5	109	FA
W/Carrots (Flav R Pac) .	1 Cup	75	0	5	14	5	112	FA
W/Onions, Boiled	1 Cup	81	0.4	5	16	4	67	FA
W/Pearl Onions								
(Flav R Pac)	1 Cup	105	0.8	6	18	6	142	FA
Peach								
Fresh								
Raw, Whole (3 Oz)	1 Item	37	0.1	1	10	2	0	A
Raw, W/O Skin	1 Oz	12	0.5	0	3	0	1	
Sliced	1 Cup	94	0.2	2	24	4	0	A
Sliced W/O Skin	1 Cup	73	0.2	1	19	3	0	A
Canned W/								
Extra Heavy Syrup	1 Cup	252	0.1	1	68	3	21	A
Extra Light Syrup	1 Cup	104	0.3	1	27	2	12	A
(Hunt's) Heavy Syrup	1 Cup	200	0	2	48	2	20	A
(S & W):								
Heavy Syrup	1 Cup	200	0	2	48	2	20	A
Juice	1 Cup	160	0	2	38	2	40	A
Water	1 Cup	160	0	1	38	0	30	A
Dried								
Cooked, Unsulfured,								
Sweetened	1 Cup	278	0.6	3	72	6	5	
Cooked, Sulfured,								
Unsweetened	1 Cup	199	0.7	3	51	7	5	
Uncooked, Sulfured	1 Cup	382	1.2	6	98	13	11	A
Frozen								
(Flav R Pac)	1 Cup	75	0	2	20	3	0	A
W/Syrup	1 Cup	150	0	2	38	2	0	A
Peach Juice								
(After The Fall)	1 Cup	100	0	1	27	NV	20	
(Odwalla) Big Red								
Peaches	1 Cup	140	0	1	33	4	10	A
(Santa Cruz Orchard)	1 Cup	110	0	1	28	NV	35	
(Snapple) Dixie Peach ...	1 Cup	112	0	0	31	NV	16	
Peach Nectar								
(Kern's)	1 Cup	146	0	1	36	0	3	A
W/Passion Fruit	1 Cup	153	0	1	37	1	3	A
(Libby's)	1 Cup	150	0	1	20	0	0	A
(R.W. Knudsen)	1 Cup	120	0	0	30	NV	25	A
Peanut								
(1 Oz equals approximately 35 peanuts)								
(1 cup equals approximately 5 Oz)								
Boiled, All types	1 Cup	200	13.9	9	13	6	473	FA

	Serv.	K-Cal.	Fat	Prot.	Carb.	Fib.	Sod.	FAC
(Peanut cont.)								
Boiled, All types	1 Oz	39	2.7	2	3	1	93	**FA**
Dried, All types	1 Cup	828	71.9	38	24	12	26	**FA**
Dried, All types	1 Oz	162	11.8	7	5	2	5	**FA**
Roasted								
Oil								
Salted	1 Oz	164	14	7	5	2	122	**FA**
Unsalted	1 Oz	164	14	7	5	2	1	**FA**
Lite Salt (Fisher)	1 Oz	170	15	7	5	NV	65	**FA**
Unsalted (Fisher)	1 Oz	133	11.8	6	5	1	102	**FA**
Dry								
All types	1 Oz	167	14.2	7	6	2	233	**FA**
(Fisher):								
BBQ	1 Cup	640	44	28	40	8	840	**FA**
Golden Roasted	1 Oz	125	9.4	5	8	1	173	**FA**
W/Honey	1 Oz	134	10	5	5	1	86	**FA**
Low Sodium	1 Oz	167	14.2	7	6	2	1	**FA**
Unsalted	1 Oz	170	14	7	6	NV	0	

Peanut Butter
Creamy

	Serv.	K-Cal.	Fat	Prot.	Carb.	Fib.	Sod.	FAC
(Health Valley)	1 Tbsp	85	7	4	3	1	1	
(Hershey's) *Reese's*	1 Tbsp	102	8.1	4	3	1	53	
(Jif):								
....	1 Tbsp	95	8	4	4	1	75	
....	¼ Cup	380	32	16	14	4	300	**FA**
RF	1 Tbsp	95	6	4	8	1	125	
Simply LS	1 Tbsp	95	8	4	3	1	33	
(Peter Pan):								
....	1 Tbsp	95	8	4	3	1	76	
LS	1 Tbsp	99	8.8	4	3	1	5	
Whipped	1 Tbsp	74	6.3	3	3	1	60	
(Skippy):								
....	1 Tbsp	95	8.5	4	3	1	75	
Honeynut	1 Tbsp	95	8.5	4	3	1	60	
RF	1 Tbsp	95	6.3	5	7	1	100	
Crunchy								
(Health Valley)	1 Tbsp	85	7	4	3	1	1	
(Jif)'								
Extra	1 Tbsp	95	8	4	4	1	65	
Simply LS	1 Tbsp	95	8	4	4	1	25	
(Laura Sludder's) Old-								
fashioned	1 Tbsp	95	8.1	4	3	1	75	
(Peter Pan):								
....	¼ Cup	376	32	17	13	4	240	**FA**
....	1 Tbsp	94	8	4	3	1	60	
Crunch	1 Tbsp	98	5.9	4	7	1	77	
LS	1 Tbsp	99	8.7	4	3	1	4	

	Serv.	K-Cal.	Fat	Prot.	Carb.	Fib.	Sod.	FAC
Whipped......................	1 Tbsp	74	6.3	3	2	1	47	
(Skippy):								
Honeynut, Super-								
chunk......................	1 Tbsp	95	8.5	4	3	1	60	
RF, Superchunk..........	1 Tbsp	90	6.2	4	6	1	85	
Superchunk.................	1 Tbsp	95	8.5	4	3	1	70	

Peanut Butter Topping

	Serv.	K-Cal.	Fat	Prot.	Carb.	Fib.	Sod.	FAC
(Smucker's)	2 Tbsp	150	2	3	29	0	120	

Peanut Flour

	Serv.	K-Cal.	Fat	Prot.	Carb.	Fib.	Sod.	FAC
Defatted..........................	1 Cup	196	0.3	31	21	9	108	F
Lowfat.............................	1 Cup	257	13.1	20	19	9	1	F

Peanut Oil

	Serv.	K-Cal.	Fat	Prot.	Carb.	Fib.	Sod.	FAC
(Planters).......................	1 Cup	1,920	224	0	0	0	0	A
(Spectrum)......................	1 Tbsp	120	14	0	0	0	0	
(Wesson)	1 Tbsp	122	14	0	0	0	0	

Peanut, Spanish

	Serv.	K-Cal.	Fat	Prot.	Carb.	Fib.	Sod.	FAC
Dried	1 Oz	163	14.1	7	5	3	7	FA
Oil-Roasted....................	1 Oz	170	14.2	8	5	3	127	FA
Oil-Roasted, LS.............	1 Oz	170	14.2	8	5	3	127	FA
Dry-Roasted (Fisher)......	1 Oz	141	12.5	4	5	2	102	FA

Peanut, Valencia

	Serv.	K-Cal.	Fat	Prot.	Carb.	Fib.	Sod.	FAC
Dried	1 Oz	163	13.5	7	6	3	0	FA
Oil-Roasted....................	1 Oz	166	14.5	8	5	3	218	FA
Oil-Roasted, unsalted.....	1 Oz	166	14.5	8	5	3	1	FA

Pear
Fresh

	Serv.	K-Cal.	Fat	Prot.	Carb.	Fib.	Sod.	FAC
Raw	1 Cup	140	1	1	36	7	0	
Raw	1 Lb	266	1.8	2	68	14	0	A
Asian.............................	1 Item	51	0.3	1	13	4	0	
Asian.............................	1 Lb	190	1	2	48	16	0	A
Bartlett..........................	1 Item	98	0.7	1	25	4	0	
Bartlett..........................	1 Lb	268	1.8	2	68	11	0	A
Bosc..............................	1 Item	85	1	1	21	4	0	
Bosc..............................	1 Lb	273	3.2	3	67	12	0	A
D'Anjou..........................	1 Item	120	1	1	30	5	0	
D'Anjou..........................	1 Lb	272	2.3	2	68	12	0	A

Canned W/

	Serv.	K-Cal.	Fat	Prot.	Carb.	Fib.	Sod.	FAC
Extra Heavy Syrup.........	1 Cup	253	0.3	1	66	4	13	
Extra Light Syrup	1 Cup	116	0.3	1	30	4	5	
Heavy Syrup (S & W)....	1 Cup	180	0	0	44	4	20	
Juice (S & W)	1 Cup	160	0	0	42	4	20	
Light Syrup Pack............	1 Cup	143	0.1	0	38	4	13	
Water Pack....................	1 Cup	71	0.1	0	19	4	5	

	Serv.	K-Cal.	Fat	Prot.	Carb.	Fib.	Sod.	FAC
(Pear cont.)								
Dried								
Cooked, Unsweetened...	1 Cup	324	0.8	2	86	16	8	A
Cooked, Sweetened.......	1 Cup	392	0.8	2	104	16	8	A
Uncooked	1 Cup	472	1.1	3	125	14	11	A
Pear Juice								
(Kern's) Nectar..............	1 Cup	152	0	0	38	2	3	A
(R.W. Knudsen)..............	1 Cup	120	0	0	30	NV	25	
(Tree Top) W/Apple	1 Cup	120	0	0	29	0	25	
Pecan								
(1 Cup equals approximately 4 Oz)								
Dried, Halves.................	1 Oz	189	19	2	5	2	0	FA
Dry-Roasted, Salted.......	1 Oz	187	18.4	2	6	2	222	FA
Oil-Roasted, Salted........	1 Oz	198	20.6	2	5	2	232	FA
Oil-Roasted, Unsalted....	1 Oz	198	20.6	2	5	2	0	FA
Pectin								
Fruit (Sure Jel)..............	1 Tsp	20	0	0	4	0	0	
Unsweetened, Dry..........	1 Oz	92	0	0	25	24	57	
Pepper, Bell (See Pepper, Sweet)								
Pepper, Cherry—Hot								
(Progresso).....................	½ Cup	190	20	0	3	1	130	
(Vlasic)............................	1 Oz	10	0	0	2	NV	425	
Pepper, Chile								
Fresh								
Raw, Green or Red	1 Cup	60	0.4	3	14	2	10	A
Raw, Green or Red	1 Oz	11	0.1	1	5	1	4	
Canned								
Chopped (Old El Paso) .	1 Tbsp	3	0	0	1	1	55	
Whole (Old El Paso)......	1 Tbsp	10	0	0	2	1	230	
Whole (Rosarita)	1 Tbsp	2	0	0	1	0	37	
Pepper, Dried								
Cayenne	1 Tsp	6	0.3	0	1	0	1	
Hot...................................	1 Tsp	6	0.2	0	1	0	7	
(McCormick):								
Black	1 Tsp	7	0	0	1	0	0	
Red	1 Tsp	10	0.4	0	1	1	1	
White............................	1 Tsp	8	0	0	2	0	0	
Pepper, Jalapeño, Canned								
Diced (Old El Paso).......	1 Oz	15	0	0	2	1	400	
Diced (Rosarita)	1 Tbsp	3	0.1	0	0	0	61	

	Serv.	K-Cal.	Fat	Prot.	Carb.	Fib.	Sod.	FAC
Whole (Old El Paso)	1 Item	3	0	0	1	0	190	
(Vlasic)	1 Cup	40	0	0	8	0	1,960	A

Pepperoni
(Hickory Farms)	1 Oz	140	13	6	1	0	580	
(Hormel)	1 Oz	140	13	5	0	0	500	
(Oscar Mayer)	1 Slice	9	0.9	0	0	0	37	
(Oscar Mayer)	1 Oz	132	12.3	6	0	0	520	

Pepper, Pimento, Canned
Chopped	1 Tbsp	3	0	0	1	0	2	
Whole (S & W)	1 Oz	9	0	0	1	0	80	

Pepper Sauce, Hot
(Crystal)	1 Tsp	0	0	0	0	0	135	
(Picka Peppa)	1 Tsp	5	0	0	1	0	40	
(Tabasco)	1 Tsp	0	0	0	0	0	36	
(Tapatio)	1 Tsp	0	0	0	0	0	110	
(Tico Pica)	1 Tsp	0	0	0	0	0	90	
(Tiger)	1 Tsp	10	0	0	2	0	140	

Pepper, Sweet
Fresh
Green Bell	1 Item	20	0.1	1	5	1	1	A
Green, Boiled	1 Oz	20	0.2	1	5	1	1	A
Green, Boiled	1 Cup	38	0.3	1	9	2	3	A
Green, Chopped (8 Oz)	1 Cup	28	0.2	1	6	2	2	A
Red Bell	1 Item	25	0.2	2	5	3	2	A
Red (Le Rouge Royale)	1 Item	50	0.5	3	11	5	7	A
Yellow Bell	1 Item	50	0.4	2	12	2	4	A

Frozen
Green (Seabrook)	1 Oz	6	0	0	1	NV	0	
(Seneca)	1 Cup	25	0	1	4	2	0	A

Red, Roasted, Bottled
(Mezzetta)	1 Oz	10	0	0	2	NV	110	A
(Peloponnese)	1 Oz	8	0	0	2	0	120	A

Perch
Raw, All Varieties	3 Oz	77	0.8	17	0	0	53	
Cooked, Dry Heat	3 Oz	103	1.8	20	0	0	82	
Fried, Breaded	3 Oz	187	9.9	17	7	0	324	

Persimmon
Raw	1 Oz	23	0	0	5	0	0	A
Dried	1 Oz	71	0.1	1	17	1	2	A
Hachiya	1 Lb	318	0.8	3	84	16	5	A
Hachiya, 6 oz.	1 Lge	118	0.3	1	31	6	2	A

Pesto Sauce (See Pasta Sauce, Pesto)

	Serv.	K-Cal.	Fat	Prot.	Carb.	Fib.	Sod.	FAC
Pheasant								
Breast Meat, Raw	3 Oz	113	2.8	21	0	0	28	
Leg, Meat Only, Raw	3 Oz	143	4.6	24	0	0	48	
Meat and Skin, Raw	3 Oz	153	7.9	19	0	0	34	
Meat Only, Raw	3 Oz	113	3.1	20	0	0	32	
Boneless, Cooked	3 Oz	162	8	21	0	0	180	
Phyllo Dough								
	1 Piece	57	1.1	1	10	0	92	
Physalis (See Cape Gooseberry)								
Pickle								
Bread and Butter								
(Claussen) Chips	1 Piece	5	0	0	1	0	43	
(Vlasic):								
Chunks	1 Oz	25	0	0	6	0	120	
Deli	1 Oz	25	0	0	6	0	120	
Sandwich	1 Oz	30	0	0	7	0	170	
Stixs	1 Oz	18	0	0	5	0	110	
Dill								
(Claussen):								
Hamburger	1 Piece	1	0	0	0	0	42	
Mini	1 Piece	5	0	0	1	0	300	
Sandwich Slice	1 Slice	3	0	0	1	0	195	
Whole	1 Oz	5	0	0	1	0	330	
(Del Monte):								
Hamburger	1 Oz	5	0	0	0	0	300	
Tiny Kosher	1 Oz	5	0	0	0	0	240	
Whole	1 Oz	5	0	0	0	0	370	
(Vlasic):								
Baby	1 Oz	4	0	0	1	0	210	
Crunchy	1 Oz	4	0	0	1	0	210	
Gherkins	1 Oz	4	0	0	1	0	210	
Halves, Deli	1 Oz	4	0	0	1	0	290	
Low Sodium	1 Oz	2	0	0	1	0	175	
Milwaukee	1 Oz	5	0	0	1	0	260	
Original	1 Oz	2	0	0	1	0	375	
Polish	1 Oz	5	0	0	1	0	280	
Sandwich	1 Oz	5	0	0	1	0	260	
Sno Garlic	1 Oz	4	0	0	1	NV	210	
Zesty, Crunchy	1 Oz	4	0	0	1	VN	375	
Sour								
(Claussen) Half Sours,								
NY Style	1 Oz	5	0	0	1	0	260	
(Heinz) Old-Fashioned	1 Oz	4	0	0	1	NV	280	
Sweet								
(Del Monte):								
Chips	1 Oz	40	0	0	0	0	210	

	Serv.	K-Cal.	Fat	Prot.	Carb.	Fib.	Sod.	FAC
Midget	1 Oz	40	0	0	0	0	210	
Whole	1 Oz	40	0	0	0	0	210	
Gherkins, Whole	1 Item	20	0	0	5	0	107	
(Vlasic):								
	1 Oz	40	0	0	10	0	170	
Chip, LS	1 Oz	30	0	0	7	0	80	

Pie (All pies frozen unless indicated fresh)

Apple

	Serv.	K-Cal.	Fat	Prot.	Carb.	Fib.	Sod.	FAC
(Amy's Kitchen)	8 Oz	280	12	4	42	NV	180	A
(Banquet)	⅕ Pie	300	13	3	41	2	370	
(Entenmann's) Beehive, FF, Fresh	⅛ Pie	169	0	1	41	1	206	A
(Mrs. Smith's):								
	⅛ Pie	310	14	2	44	1	380	
Crumb	⅛ Pie	350	14	3	53	1	300	
(Sara Lee) Dutch	⅛ Pie	350	15	3	53	2	320	

Banana Cream

	Serv.	K-Cal.	Fat	Prot.	Carb.	Fib.	Sod.	FAC
(Mrs. Smith's)	¼ Pie	290	15	2	38	1	190	A

Blueberry

	Serv.	K-Cal.	Fat	Prot.	Carb.	Fib.	Sod.	FAC
(Banquet)	⅙ Pie	270	11	3	40	NV	350	
(Mrs. Smith's)	⅛ Pie	220	9	2	32	NV	240	

Cherry

	Serv.	K-Cal.	Fat	Prot.	Carb.	Fib.	Sod.	FAC
(Banquet)	⅕ Pie	290	14	3	39	2	310	
(Entenmann's) Beehive, FF, Fresh	¹/₁₀ Pie	135	0	2	32	1	155	A
(Mrs. Smith's):								
	⅛ Pie	310	14	3	25	1	400	
Deep Dish W/Berry	¹/₁₀ Pie	360	10	3	53	1	400	
LF	4.5 Oz	250	8	2	44	1	310	A
(Sara Lee)	⅛ Pie	330	15	3	46	2	290	

Chocolate

	Serv.	K-Cal.	Fat	Prot.	Carb.	Fib.	Sod.	FAC
(Mrs. Smith's) Creme	¼ Pie	330	17	2	42	1	220	

Lemon

	Serv.	K-Cal.	Fat	Prot.	Carb.	Fib.	Sod.	FAC
(Banquet) Cream	⅙ Pie	170	9	2	23	NV	120	
(Mrs. Smith's) Meringue	⅛ Pie	210	5	2	38	NV	130	

Lime

	Serv.	K-Cal.	Fat	Prot.	Carb.	Fib.	Sod.	FAC
(Mrs. Smith's)	4.5 Oz	380	14	5	58	0	240	A

Mince

	Serv.	K-Cal.	Fat	Prot.	Carb.	Fib.	Sod.	FAC
(Mrs. Smith's)	4.5 Oz	300	11	2	48	2	400	A
(Sara Lee) Homestyle	¹/₁₀ Pie	300	13	3	43	NV	340	

Mississippi Mud

	Serv.	K-Cal.	Fat	Prot.	Carb.	Fib.	Sod.	FAC
(Pepperidge Farm)	1 Item	310	23	3	23	NV	45	
(Wt Watchers)	1 Item	160	5	4	24	0	120	

Peach

	Serv.	K-Cal.	Fat	Prot.	Carb.	Fib.	Sod.	FAC
(Banquet)	⅕ Pie	260	12	2	36	2	340	
(Mrs. Smith's)	⅙ Pie	260	11	2	38	1	310	

	Serv.	K-Cal.	Fat	Prot.	Carb.	Fib.	Sod.	FAC
Pecan								
(Mrs. Smith's)	1/8 Pie	330	13	3	51	NV	200	
(Sara Lee)	1/10 Pie	400	18	4	56	NV	290	
Pumpkin								
(Entenmann's) Fresh	1/5 Pie	250	10	5	37	2	350	A
(Mrs. Smith's) Custard	1/8 Pie	230	8	5	36	1	320	
(Sara Lee)	1/8 Pie	260	11	4	37	2	460	
Strawberry								
(Mrs. Smith's):								
	5 Oz	280	11	2	45	1	190	A
W/Rhubarb	4.5 Oz	280	11	2	44	0	380	A
Pie Crust								
Mix								
Dry Mix (Flako)	1 Cup	520	32	8	52	4	680	
Dry Mix (Pillsbury)	1 Tbsp	50	3	1	5	0	75	
Prepared (Betty Crocker)	1/8 Pie	110	8	1	9	0	150	
Prepared (Krusteaz)	1/8 Pie	90	5	1	10	1	100	
Ready-To-Fill								
(Keebler) Graham	1 Slice	100	5	1	13	1	130	
(Mrs. Smith's):								
	1/8 Pie	110	7	1	12	0	105	
RF	1/8 Pie	100	5	1	13	0	95	
(Nabisco) *Oreo*	1/6 Pie	140	7	1	18	1	180	
(Pet-Ritz):								
	1/8 Pie	80	4	1	9	0	65	
Deep-Dish	1/8 Pie	90	5	1	11	0	80	
Vegetable	1/8 Pie	80	4.5	1	10	0	70	
(Pillsbury):								
	1/8 Pie	110	7	1	12	0	140	
All Ready	1/8 Pie	120	7	1	13	0	100	
(Wonderslim)	1/8 Pie	70	0	1	16	1	120	
Pie Filling (Also See Pudding, Ready-To-Serve)								
Instant Mix, Prepared								
Banana Cream	1 Oz	38	1	1	7	NV	75	
Butterscotch	1 Oz	40	1	1	7	NV	75	
Chocolate	1 Oz	40	1	1	7	NV	80	
Coconut	1 Oz	40	1	1	7	NV	62	
Lemon	1 Oz	38	0.3	0	9	NV	43	
Vanilla	1 Oz	38	1	1	6	NV	40	
Canned								
(Comstock):								
Apple, More Fruit	1 Cup	240	0	0	60	3	120	
Blueberry, More Fruit	1 Cup	240	0	0	63	3	135	
Blueberry, Original	1 Cup	300	0	0	75	3	45	
Cherry, LT	1 Cup	180	0	0	45	3	45	
Cherry, Original	1 Cup	270	0	0	69	3	75	
(Oregon) Cherry, Bing	1 Cup	220	0	0	52	2	20	

	Serv.	K-Cal.	Fat	Prot.	Carb.	Flb.	Sod.	FAC

Pignolia (See Pine Nut)

Pike

	Serv.	K-Cal.	Fat	Prot.	Carb.	Flb.	Sod.	FAC
Northern, Raw	3 Oz	75	0.6	16	0	0	33	
Walleye, Raw	3 Oz	80	1	16	0	0	34	
Northern, Broiled	3 Oz	96	0.8	21	0	0	42	
Walleye, Broiled	3 Oz	101	1.3	21	0	0	55	

Pilaf, Prepared

(Prepared as indicated on the package)
(Casbah):

	Serv.	K-Cal.	Fat	Prot.	Carb.	Flb.	Sod.	FAC
	1 Cup	280	0.7	8	51	1	520	
Bulgur	1 Cup	320	1.3	13	48	5	613	A
Couscous	1 Cup	293	0.7	11	53	1	640	A
Lentil	1 Cup	320	0.7	12	51	3	533	A
Nutted	1 Cup	253	2.7	4	27	1	667	
Spanish	1 Cup	267	0.7	5	53	1	573	A
(Ener-G) Old World, Brown	1 Cup	364	3.1	9	76	6	418	A
(Fantastic) 3 Grain/Herb	1 Cup	240	2	7	49	8	570	
(Farmhouse) Chicken	1 Cup	190	2	5	41	3	720	
(Knorr):								
Chicken	1 Cup	210	1	5	45	2	1,000	
Lemon-Herb	1 Cup	260	2	6	55	0	790	
Spanish	1 Cup	230	1	5	50	1	1,120	
(Kraft) W/Cheddar	1 Cup	300	8	8	46	NV	1,300	
(Lundberg):								
Country Chicken	1 Cup	220	3	4	47	4	370	
Savory Mushroom	1 Cup	190	2.5	4	41	3	590	
Spanish Fiesta	1 Cup	190	2	5	43	3	750	A
(Rice-A-Roni):								
	1 Cup	310	9	6	53	1	1,100	
Long Grain/Wild	1 Cup	240	5.5	5	43	1	910	

Dry Mix

(Fantastic) Brown Rice,

	Serv.	K-Cal.	Fat	Prot.	Carb.	Flb.	Sod.	FAC
Miso	1 Cup	500	6	14	110	2	1,140	A
(Manischewitz):								
Lentil	1 Cup	160	0.5	5	34	5	410	
Rice	1 Cup	160	1	4	35	1	470	
Spanish	1 Cup	150	0.5	4	34	1	370	
Wheat	1 Cup	170	1	5	35	4	360	
(Rice-A-Roni)	1 Oz	120	0	4	26	NV	620	

Frozen

(Green Giant):

	Serv.	K-Cal.	Fat	Prot.	Carb.	Flb.	Sod.	FAC
	10 Oz	230	3	6	44	3	1,020	A
W/Asparagus	9 Oz	190	4	5	37	3	610	A
(Wt Watchers) Florentine	10 Oz	290	7	9	47	6	550	A

Pimento (See Pepper, Pimento, Canned)

	Serv.	K-Cal.	Fat	Prot.	Carb.	Fib.	Sod.	FAC
Pineapple								
Fresh								
Whole	1 Lb	260	0.5	2	62	5	22	FA
Diced	1 Oz	16	0	0	4	0	1	
Diced	1 Cup	76	0.7	1	19	2	2	A
Canned W/								
Extra Heavy Syrup	1 Cup	216	0.3	1	56	2	3	A
Heavy Syrup	1 Cup	199	0.3	1	52	2	3	A
Light Syrup	1 Cup	131	0.3	1	34	2	3	A
Heavy Syrup								
(Del Monte)	1 Cup	180	0	0	48	2	20	A
Water, Bits	1 Cup	79	0.2	1	20	2	2	A
(Dole) Juice	1 Cup	140	0	0	34	2	20	A
(S & W) Sliced	1 Piece	45	0	0	12	1	5	
Frozen								
Chunks	1 Cup	112	0	0	29	0	0	A
Pineapple, Dried								
Pieces	¼ Cup	130	0	2	32	0	0	A
Pineapple Juice								
Canned/Bottled								
(Del Monte)	1 Cup	110	0	1	29	2	15	A
(Dole)	1 Cup	110	0	1	29	2	10	A
(S & W)	1 Cup	120	0	0	31	2	14	A
Frozen								
Diluted (Dole)	1 Cup	110	0	0	27	0	0	A
Undiluted (Dole)	1 Cup	440	0	0	108	0	0	A
Pineapple Juice, Blended								
W/Apricot (Kern)	1 Cup	153	0	1	36	1	4	A
W/Banana (Kern)	1 Cup	153	0	1	36	NV	4	A
W/Coconut (R.W.								
Knudsen)	1 Cup	130	0	0	32	NV	50	
W/Orange (Kraft)	1 Cup	106	0	1	25	NV	0	A
W/Orange (Ultra Slim-								
Fast)	1 Cup	146	1	5	32	3	173	FA
W/Cranberry (Ocean								
Spray)	1 Cup	130	0	0	32	0	35	A
Pineapple Topping								
(Kraft)	1 Tbsp	50	0	0	13	0	0	
Pine Nut—Pignoli—Piñon								
Chopped, Dried	1 Tbsp	57	5.1	2	1	0	0	
Whole, Dried	1 Item	1	0.1	0	0	0	0	

Pink Bean (See Bean, Pink)

	Serv.	K-Cal.	Fat	Prot.	Carb.	Fib.	Sod.	FAC

Piñon (See Pine Nut)

Pinto Bean (See Bean, Pinto)

Pistachio
(1 Cup equals approximately 5 Oz)
(1 Oz equals approximately 22 nuts)

	Serv.	K-Cal.	Fat	Prot.	Carb.	Fib.	Sod.	FAC
Dried	1 Cup	739	61.9	26	32	14	8	FA
Dried	1 Oz	164	13.7	6	7	3	2	
Dry-Roasted	1 Oz	172	15	4	8	3	2	
Dry-Roasted, Salted	1 Oz	172	15	3	8	3	222	
Natural (Blue Diamond)	1 Oz	140	12	6	4	3	210	
Red (Blue Diamond)	1 Oz	140	12	6	3	3	230	
Red (Fisher)	1 Oz	97	8.6	3	3	1	29	

Pistachio Butter

	Serv.	K-Cal.	Fat	Prot.	Carb.	Fib.	Sod.	FAC
(Maranatha)	2 Tbsp	200	17	5	9	4	0	

Pita (See Bread, Pita)

Pizza, Fast Food

Bacon
Super Deli, Pan (Round

	Serv.	K-Cal.	Fat	Prot.	Carb.	Fib.	Sod.	FAC
Table)	1 Slice	260	13.5	12	26	0	380	

Cheese
(Pizza Hut):

	Serv.	K-Cal.	Fat	Prot.	Carb.	Fib.	Sod.	FAC
Big Foot	1 Slice	186	6	10	25	2	525	
Pan	1 Slice	261	11	12	28	2	501	
Thin Crust	1 Slice	205	8	11	21	2	534	
(Round Table) Thin Crust	1 Slice	160	6.2	7	16	0	240	

Pepperoni
(Pizza Hut):

	Serv.	K-Cal.	Fat	Prot.	Carb.	Fib.	Sod.	FAC
Lovers, Pan	1 Slice	332	17	15	28	2	777	
Pan	1 Slice	265	12	11	28	2	569	
Thin	1 Slice	215	10	11	21	0	627	
(Round Table) Thin	1 Slice	170	8	8	17	0	240	

Sausage

	Serv.	K-Cal.	Fat	Prot.	Carb.	Fib.	Sod.	FAC
(Pizza Hut) Pan	1 Slice	293	15	12	27	2	617	
Thin	1 Slice	236	12	11	21	2	650	

Vegetable
(Pizza Hut) Veggie

	Serv.	K-Cal.	Fat	Prot.	Carb.	Fib.	Sod.	FAC
Lovers, Thin	1 Slice	186	7	9	22	2	545	

(Round Table):

	Serv.	K-Cal.	Fat	Prot.	Carb.	Fib.	Sod.	FAC
Garden Delight, Thin	1 Slice	150	5.6	7	18	1	250	
Garden Pesto, Thin	1 Slice	170	7.7	7	18	1	220	
Gourmet Veggie, Pan	1 Slice	220	7.4	9	28	1	230	
Veggie Salute, Pan	1 Slice	190	5.1	8	28	1	190	

	Serv.	K-Cal.	Fat	Prot.	Carb.	Fib.	Sod.	FAC
Pizza Crust								
(Boboli) Cheese, 12"	⅛ Pie	178	3.2	7	25	0	311	
(Contadina)Fresh	1 Serv	170	2.5	5	31	2	430	
(Nature's Hilight)								
Brown Rice	⅛ Pie	53	0.2	1	10	0	0	
(Pillsbury)	⅛ Pie	90	1	3	17	2	195	
(Robin Hood) Mix	⅛ Pie	80	1	2	17	1	170	
Pizza, Frozen								
Canadian Bacon								
(Jeno's)	7 Oz	430	18	17	49	2	1,150	C
(Totino's)	½ Pizza	320	15	14	33	2	900	C
Cheese								
(Amy's Kitchen)	⅓ Pizza	310	11	13	39	2	490	C
(Celeste):								
	¼ Pizza	320	16	14	32	3	590	AC
Small	1 Item	540	25	23	60	4	1,090	AC
Zesty 4	¼ Pizza	330	16	14	34	3	610	AC
(Nature's Hilights) Soy								
Cheese	1 Item	560	12	30	84	NV	1,000	AC
(Red Baron) 4 Cheese	¼ Pizza	430	21	20	41	2	810	C
(Stouffer's):								
	1 Serv	320	15	14	32	2	640	
Extra Cheese	1 Serv	370	19	17	33	3	720	C
Lean Cuisine, Extra								
Cheese	1 Serv	350	12	21	39	NV	850	AC
(Tombstone) W/								
Pepperoni, 12"	¼ Pizza	425	22.5	19	36	2	937	FC
(Totino's):								
My Classic Deluxe	1 Serv	210	9	10	23	2	420	C
Three Cheese, Pan	1 Serv	290	10	15	33	2	510	FC
(Wt Watchers) Extra								
Cheese	1 Item	390	12	23	49	6	590	C
Combination								
(Digiorno)	⅙ Pizza	380	17	18	40	3	1,100	C
(Red Baron):								
Special Deluxe	¼ Pizza	340	18	13	32	2	690	C
Supreme	¼ Pizza	350	18	15	32	2	710	C
(Tony's) Supreme	¼ Pizza	340	20	13	28	2	610	C
Hamburger								
(Jeno's)	1 Serv	180	9	8	17	0	500	C
(Pappalos):								
Thin Crust	1 Serv	240	8	14	28	2	470	C
Pan	1 Serv	310	12	17	34	1	580	C
(Totino's) Party	½ Pizza	350	18	15	33	2	860	C
Pepperoni								
(Celeste) Small	1 Item	520	27	19	53	4	1,280	AC

	Serv.	K-Cal.	Fat	Prot.	Carb.	Fib.	Sod.	FAC
(Digiorno)	⅛ Pizza	370	16	18	40	3	1,080	C
(Jeno's)	1 Item	500	26	17	49	2	1,170	C
(Pappalos) Deep	¼ Pizza	425	18	21	46	2	900	FC
(Red Baron)	¼ Pizza	450	24	19	40	2	920	C
(Stouffer's)	1 Serv	350	18	15	34	0	820	C
(Tombstone):								
LT	1 Serv	272	10	15	30	2	682	C
Thin Crust	1 Serv	263	16	12	18	2	628	C
W/Sausage, LT	1 Serv	260	10	14	30	2	610	C
(Tony's)	⅓ Pizza	450	28	18	33	2	890	
(Totino's):								
My Classic Deluxe	1 Serv	260	13	12	23	2	630	C
Pan	1 Serv	330	14	16	34	2	730	C
(Wt Watchers)	1 Item	390	12	23	46	4	650	C
(Wolfgang Puck) W/								
Mushroom	½ Pizza	390	15	21	43	3	690	C
Sausage								
(Celeste) Small	1 Item	530	27	23	52	5	1,400	AC
(Fox):								
Deluxe	1 Serv	260	13	10	26	2	630	A
Deluxe W/Pepperoni	1 Serv	260	13	10	26	2	640	A
(Jeno's)	1 Item	510	27	17	49	3	1,070	FAC
(Pappalos)	¼ Pizza	370	16	18	38	2	710	C
(Stouffer's):								
	1 Serv	360	18	16	32	2	830	C
Lean Cuisine	1 Serv	350	11	23	40	NV	960	C
(Totino's):								
Pan	1 Serv	320	13	16	34	NV	630	C
Party	1 Item	760	40	30	68	4	1,740	FAC
W/Pepperoni	1 Serv	340	15	16	34	NV	720	C
(Wolfgang Puck)	½ Pizza	380	18	19	36	7	650	C
Vegetable								
(Amy's Kitchen):								
No Cheese	⅓ Pizza	270	8	6	43	3	470	A
W/Spinach	⅓ Pizza	320	111	13	40	2	490	AC
(Celeste) Suprema, Small	1 Item	480	23	20	52	5	1,270	AC
(Tombstone) LT, RF	¼ Pizza	300	9	32	39	15	625	FAC
(Totino's) Party	1 Serv	300	13	11	36	3	910	FAC
(Wolfgang Puck) Grilled								
Vegetable	½ Pizza	200	0	6	42	2	430	CA

Pizza, French Bread, Frozen
Cheese

	Serv.	K-Cal.	Fat	Prot.	Carb.	Fib.	Sod.	FAC
(Healthy Choice)	1 Item	290	1	24	47	5	480	C
(Pappalos)	1 Serv	360	15	16	40	NV	830	C
(Stouffer's) *Lean Cuisine*	1 Item	350	8	22	48	4	400	C

	Serv.	K-Cal.	Fat	Prot.	Carb.	Fib.	Sod.	FAC
(Pizza, French Bread, Frozen cont.)								
Combination								
(Healthy Choice)								
Supreme	1 Serv	300	4	20	45	5	480	C
(Pappalos)	1 Serv	430	21	19	41	NV	1,120	C
(Stouffer's):								
Deluxe...........................	1 Serv	440	22	19	42	5	980	AC
Lean Cuisine, Deluxe .	1 Item	330	6	23	45	5	560	C
Pepperoni								
(Pappalos)	1 Serv	410	20	16	41	NV	1,130	C
(Pillsbury):								
....	1 Serv	430	19	19	46	NV	940	C
W/Sausage	1 Serv	450	21	19	47	NV	950	C
(Stouffer's):								
....	1 Serv	420	20	18	42	3	930	C
Lean Cuisine...............	1 Item	330	7	20	46	4	590	C
Sausage								
(Healthy Choice)	1 Item	290	3	21	45	5	450	C
(Pappalos)	1 Serv	410	18	18	41	NV	1,000	C
(Stouffer's) *Lean Cuisine*	1 Item	350	10	22	42	NV	600	C
Vegetable								
(Stouffer's) Deluxe	1 Serv	400	17	18	43	5	830	AC

Pizza, Individual Serving, Frozen
Pocket
	Serv.	K-Cal.	Fat	Prot.	Carb.	Fib.	Sod.	FAC
(Amy's Kitchen)	1 Item	290	9	14	38	3	390	
Roll								
(Jeno's) Pepperoni.........	1 Serv	230	13	7	22	2	390	
(Totino's):								
Hamburger (.5 Oz)	1 Item	35	1.4	2	4	0	57	
Pepperoni (.5 Oz).......	1 Item	36	1.7	2	4	0	58	
Sausage (.5 Oz)	1 Item	35	1.5	1	4	0	58	
3 Cheeses (.5 Oz)......	1 Item	36	1.5	2	4	0	61	
Single								
(Tombstone):								
Pepperoni, Thin	1 Serv	306	18	14	21	2	728	C
Supreme, Thin	1 Serv	308	18	15	22	3	713	AC
(Totino's):								
Cheese........................	1 Piece	170	7	7	20	1	350	
Combination.................	1 Piece	200	10	7	20	1	630	
Pepperoni....................	1 Piece	190	9	7	20	1	530	
Sausage......................	1 Piece	200	10	7	20	1	540	

Pizza Sauce (Also See Pasta Sauce)
	Serv.	K-Cal.	Fat	Prot.	Carb.	Fib.	Sod.	FAC
(Contadina):								
....	1 Cup	100	2	4	16	4	120	A
Italian Cheese..............	1 Cup	120	4	4	16	4	1,400	A
Pepperoni....................	1 Cup	120	4	4	16	4	1,440	A
(Eden).............................	1 Cup	160	5	6	24	6	640	A

	Serv.	K-Cal.	Fat	Prot.	Carb.	Fib.	Sod.	FAC
Plantain								
Flower	1 Oz	12	0.3	1	2	0	1	
Ripe	1 Item	218	0.7	2	57	4	7	FA
Cooked	1 Cup	179	0.3	1	48	4	8	FA
Green, Fried	1 Item	375	18.6	2	57	4	12	A
Ripe, Fried	1 Item	506	27.3	3	71	5	9	A
Plum								
Fresh								
French Prune	1 Oz	20	0	0	6	1	0	
French Prune	1 Lb	319	0	0	96	9	0	A
Japanese	1 Item	36	0.4	1	9	1	0	
Purple	1 Oz	10	0	0	2	0	2	
Purple	1 Cup	160	1.8	2	38	4	0	A
Canned W/								
Extra Heavy Syrup	1 Cup	264	0.3	1	69	3	50	A
Heavy Syrup	1 Cup	230	0.3	1	60	3	49	A
Juice	1 Cup	146	0.1	1	38	3	3	A
Light Syrup	1 Cup	159	0.3	1	41	3	50	A
Water	1 Cup	102	0	1	28	2	2	A
Plum Sauce								
(Dynasty)	1 Tbsp	30	0.7	1	6	0	80	
(La Choy)	1 Tbsp	25	0.1	0	6	0	4	
Poi (Also See Taro)								
Fresh	1 Cup	269	0.3	1	65	1	29	FA
Poke								
Greens, Cooked	1 Cup	31	0.6	4	5	3	386	A
Polenta								
Mix								
Dry (Beretta)	1 Oz	100	0	3	22	2	0	
Dry (Bob's Red Mill)	¼ Cup	130	0.5	3	27	2	0	
Dry (Golden Pheasant)	1 Oz	112	0.5	2	25	1	1	
Prepared (Fantastic)	1 Cup	260	5	8	46	4	550	A
Ready-To-Serve								
(San Gennaro)	3.3 Oz	74	0	2	16	1	310	
Polish Sausage (See Sausage, Kielbasa)								
Pollack								
Atlantic, Broiled	3 Oz	100	1	21	0	0	93	
Atlantic, Raw	3 Oz	78	0.8	16	0	0	72	
Walleye, Broiled	3 Oz	96	1	20	0	0	99	
Walleye, Raw	3 Oz	69	0.7	15	0	0	84	

	Serv.	K-Cal.	Fat	Prot.	Carb.	Flb.	Sod.	FAC
Pomegranate—Chinese Apple								
Raw, 3⅜" Diameter	5.5 Oz	105	0.5	1	26	1	5	
Pomegranate Juice								
(R.W. Knudsen)	1 Cup	150	0	0	37	NV	10	A
Pomelo—Pummelo—Chinese Grapefruit								
Raw, Sections	1 Oz	13	0	0	3	0	5	A
Raw, Sections	1 Cup	72	0.1	1	18	2	2	A
Pomfret								
Raw	3 Oz	123	7	15	0	0	75	
Fried	3 Oz	204	13	20	3	0	150	
Pompano								
Raw	3 Oz	139	8.1	16	0	0	55	
Broiled	3 Oz	179	10.3	20	0	0	65	
Popcorn								
Unpopped	1 Cup	754	9.8	25	150	NV	6	
Popped	1 Cup	40	0.5	1	8	1	0	
Popped, Oil, Salted	1 Cup	55	3.1	1	6	1	97	
Unpopped (Orville)	1 Tbsp	46	0.4	2	12	3	1	
Popcorn, Frozen								
(Pillsbury):								
Butter	1 Cup	70	4.3	1	7	NV	160	
Original	1 Cup	70	4.3	1	7	4	140	
Salt-Free	1 Cup	57	2.3	1	8	NV	0	
Popcorn, Microwave, Popped								
Butter-Flavored								
(Betty Crocker):								
Pop-Secret	1 Cup	38	2.5	1	4	1	53	
Pop-Secret, LT	1 Cup	22	0.8	1	3	1	32	
Pop-Secret, No Salt	1 Cup	33	2	1	4	1	2	
(Jolly Time) American's								
Best	1 Cup	90	0	1	35	1	10	
(Newman's Own) LT	1 Cup	37	0.9	1	6	1	28	
(Orville) LT	1 Cup	20	0.5	1	3	1	30	
(Pop Qwiz)	1 Cup	33	2	1	4	1	57	
Natural								
(Bearito) Organic	1 Cup	25	0.3	1	5	1	0	
(Betty Crocker) *Pop-Secret*, LT	1 Cup	22	0.8	1	3	1	43	
(Healthy Choice)	1 Cup	15	0	1	4	1	25	
(Jolly Time) LT	1 Cup	20	1	1	4	1	25	
(Newman's Own)	1 Cup	49	3	1	5	1	50	
(Pop Qwiz)	1 Cup	33	2	1	4	1	57	

	Serv.	K-Cal.	Fat	Prot.	Carb.	Fib.	Sod.	FAC
Popcorn, Packaged								
(Auburn Farms):								
Butterscotch	1 Cup	180	0	0	42	2	210	
Caramel	1 Cup	180	0	0	42	2	210	
(Barbara's) Caramel								
Corn, No Chol	1 Cup	173	4.7	1	32	1	120	
(Bearito):								
Butter	1 Cup	60	4	1	4	1	47	
Buttery LT, Organic	1 Cup	40	1.7	1	5	1	40	
LT	1 Cup	40	1.7	1	5	1	40	
White Cheddar,								
Organic	1 Cup	73	5	1	6	1	100	
(Healthy Choice) Natural								
Flavor	1 Cup	20	0	1	5	1	35	
(Keebler):								
Honey Caramel	1 Oz	120	3	1	22	2	180	
White Cheddar	1 Cup	70	5	1	7	3	135	
(Smartfood) White								
Cheddar	1 Cup	91	5.7	2	8	1	180	
(Ultra Slim-Fast)								
Caramel	1 Oz	110	2	2	25	3	120	
(Wt Watchers) Caramel	1 Oz	100	1	1	22	1	45	
Popover								
Baked	1 Oz	64	2.6	2	7	2	62	
From Mix	1 Item	67	1.5	3	10	NV	143	
Home Recipe, 2% Milk	1 Item	88	3	3	11	0	82	
Home Recipe, Whole								
Milk	1 Item	90	3.4	3	11	NV	82	
Poppy Seed								
(McCormick)	1 Tsp	17	1.2	1	1	1	1	
Poppyseed Oil								
	1 Tbsp	120	14	0	0	0	0	A
Pop-Tarts (See Pastry, Toaster)								
Pork								
Feet								
Pickled	3 Oz	173	13.7	12	0	0	786	
Simmered	3 Oz	165	10.5	16	0	0	25	
Ground								
Cooked	3 Oz	252	17.6	22	0	0	62	
Liver								
Braised	3 Oz	141	3.7	22	3	0	42	FA
Loin, Center								
Lean/Fat, Roasted	3 Oz	246	17	22	0	0	54	
Lean, Roasted	3 Oz	193	9.9	24	0	0	54	

	Serv.	K-Cal.	Fat	Prot.	Carb.	Fib.	Sod.	FAC
(Pork cont.)								
Loin, Chop								
Lean/Fat-Roasted..........	3 Oz	255	18	22	0	0	47	
Lean, Roasted................	3 Oz	198	10.5	24	0	0	54	
Loin, Rib End								
Lean/Fat, Roasted.........	3 Oz	258	18	22	0	0	51	
Lean, Roasted................	3 Oz	210	11.7	24	0	0	62	
Loin, Whole								
Lean/Fat, Roasted.........	3 Oz	258	19	20	0	0	51	
Lean, Roasted................	3 Oz	192	10.5	23	0	0	50	
Pig's Hocks								
Cooked	3 Oz	60	4.1	5	0	0	60	
Rinds								
Barbecue Flavor.............	1 Oz	153	9	16	0	0	756	
Plain..............................	1 Oz	155	8.9	17	0	0	521	
Shoulder, Arm								
Lean/Fat, Roasted.........	3 Oz	237	16.1	21	0	0	59	
Lean, Roasted................	3 Oz	172	7.4	24	0	0	80	
Shoulder, Butt								
Lean/Fat, Roasted.........	3 Oz	250	17.5	22	0	0	57	
Lean, Roasted................	3 Oz	202	11.2	24	0	0	67	
Shoulder, Whole								
Lean/Fat, Roasted.........	3 Oz	251	17.5	22	0	0	57	
Lean, Roasted................	3 Oz	193	9.8	24	0	0	70	
Spareribs								
Lean/Fat, Raw................	3 Oz	270	23.2	14	0	0	65	
Braised	3 Oz	339	25.8	25	0	0	77	
Lean/Fat, Braised...........	3 Oz	286	21.5	22	0	0	79	
Tenderloin End								
Lean/Fat, Roasted.........	3 Oz	236	15	24	0	0	50	
Lean, Roasted................	3 Oz	193	9.1	27	0	0	66	
Pork Entree								
Canned								
(Campbell's) W/Tomato								
Sauce.........................	1 Cup	260	4	10	48	12	840	
(Hunt's)	1 Cup	260	2.4	12	55	9	1,032	
(La Choy) Chow Mein....	1 Cup	78	2.2	7	9	2	1,183	
(Luck's):								
W/Beans	1 Serv	240	6	12	35	10	530	F
W/Tomato Sauce........	1 Cup	300	2	12	56	12	1,260	
Frozen								
(Banquet) Pork Cutlet	1 Item	410	24	11	39	4	1,060	
(Hormel) Loin and Gravy	8 Oz	320	17.6	37	4	NV	1,064	
(La Choy) Sweet & Sour	1 Cup	241	6.2	5	43	4	1,733	
Pork Lard								
....	1 Tbsp	115	12.8	0	0	0	0	

	Serv.	K-Cal.	Fat	Prot.	Carb.	Fib.	Sod.	FAC
Pork Rind								
....	1 Oz	155	8.8	17	0	0	520	
Potato								
Fresh								
Whole	1 Oz	21	0	1	4	1	1	
Whole, Baked................	1 Item	220	0.2	5	51	5	16	A
Whole, Baked................	1 Cup	257	0.2	5	59	6	19	A
Whole, Raw...................	1 Cup	181	0.3	5	41	4	17	A
Whole, Boiled................	1 Cup	212	0.3	5	49	4	12	A
Flesh, Raw...................	1 Cup	190	0.2	5	43	4	14	A
Flesh, Baked	1 Cup	237	0.3	5	55	5	13	A
Flesh, Boiled	1 Cup	200	0.2	4	47	3	12	A
Skin, Baked.................	2 Oz	115	0.1	2	27	5	12	
Skin, Microwaved	1 Oz	37	0	1	8	2	5	
Skin, Raw...................	1 Oz	16	0	1	4	1	3	
Canned								
(Del Monte) Sliced	1 Cup	90	0	2	20	3	540	
(S & W) Whole, New	1 Cup	120	0	2	28	2	520	
(S & W) Piknik:								
Shoestring,.................	1 Oz	160	10.3	1	15	1	103	
Shoestring, 50% Less								
Salt...................	1 Cup	220	16	3	21	1	80	
Shoestring, Santa Fe								
BBQ	1 Cup	270	18	3	27	3	360	
Frozen								
(Flav R Pac) Redskin	1 Cup	80	0	1	21	1	47	
(Health Valley)...............	1 Cup	73	0	2	15	1	173	
Frozen, French Fries								
(Cascadian Farms).........	3 Oz	200	8	2	19	2	10	
(Inland Valley)	3 Oz	200	9	2	29	2	220	
(Lynden):								
3/8"...................	3 Oz	120	4	2	20	2	50	
Crinkle........................	3 Oz	120	4	2	20	3	45	
Shoestring...................	3 Oz	140	6	2	23	2	60	
(Ore-Ida):								
Crinkles.......................	3 Oz	140	3.5	2	23	2	20	
Fast-Fried....................	3 Oz	150	6	2	23	2	240	
Golden	3 Oz	120	4	2	20	2	25	
Frozen, Hash Browns								
(Golden Grill).................	1 Cup	236	13.6	3	26	2	288	
(Inland Valley) FF	1 Cup	91	0	3	21	3	20	
(Lynden)......................	1 Cup	225	9	3	33	3	90	
(Redi Shred)..................	1 Cup	268	13.6	4	32	3	322	
Mashed								
Home Recipe, W/Milk	1 Cup	162	1.2	4	37	4	636	A
Home Recipe, W/Milk/								
Butter	1 Cup	224	8.9	4	35	4	622	A

	Serv.	K-Cal.	Fat	Prot.	Carb.	Fib.	Sod.	FAC
Potato Chips								
Barbeque								
(Auburn Farms)								
Mesquite, FF	1 Oz	100	0	3	23	1	140	
(Barbara's)	1 Oz	128	8	2	13	1	184	
(Frito-Lay):								
Lay's	1 Chip	10	0.7	0	1	0	15	
Ruffles, Mesquite	1 Chip	10	0.6	0	1	0	8	
(Guiltless Gourmet)								
Baked	1 Oz	110	1.5	2	22	1	200	
(Keebler) *Ripplin's*	1 Chip	13	0.8	8	1	0	20	
(Louise's):								
Mesquite	1 Oz	110	1	2	24	2	180	
Mesquite, FF	1 Oz	110	0	3	23	2	180	
(Michael) W/Honey	1 Chip	7	0.3	0	1	0	13	
(Pringles):								
	1 Oz	150	10	2	15	NV	200	
Light	1 Chip	9	0.4	0	1	0	10	
LT	1 Oz	144	6.7	1	19	NV	111	
Mesquite	1 Chip	13	0.8	0	1	0	18	
Cheese								
(Auburn Farms) Cheddar, FF	1 Chip	3	0	0	1	0	6	
(Barbara's) Au Gratin	1 Oz	150	10	2	15	1	260	
(Frito-Lay) *Ruffles,* Cheddar & Sour Cream	1 Chip	12	0.8	0	1	0	18	
(Kettle)	1 Oz	141	7.7	2	16	1	225	
(O'Boisies):								
Cheddar	1 Chip	9	0.6	0	1	0	8	
Tato Skins, Cheese N' Bacon	1 Chip	8	0.5	0	1	0	9	
(Pringles):								
Cheddar & Sour Cream	1 Chip	13	0.8	0	1	0	17	
Cheeze Ums	1 Chip	11	0.7	0	1	0	14	
Original								
(Auburn Farms) FF	1 Chip	3	0	0	1	0	5	
(Frito-Lay):								
Lay's	1 Chip	8	0.6	0	1	0	7	
Ruffles	1 Oz	150	10	2	14	1	125	
(Keebler) *Ripplin's*	1 Chip	12	0.9	0	1	0	16	
(Kettle)	1 Oz	152	9.8	2	15	1	168	
(Louise's):								
	1 Oz	110	1	2	24	2	180	
FF	1 Oz	110	0	3	23	2	180	
(O'Boisies)	1 Chip	9	0.6	0	1	0	11	
(Pringles):								
	1 Chip	11	0.8	0	1	0	12	
Light	1 Oz	144	6.7	1	19	NV	111	

	Serv.	K-Cal.	Fat	Prot.	Carb.	Fib.	Sod.	FAC
Ranch								
(Frito Lay):								
Lay's, Tangy	1 Chip	9	0.5	0	1	0	13	
Ruffles	1 Chip	12	0.7	0	1	0	22	
(Keebler) Ripplin's	1 Chip	13	0.8	0	1	0	20	
(Pringles):								
	1 Chip	11	0.7	0	1	0	9	
LT	1 Chip	9	0.4	0	1	0	10	
Sour Cream and Onion								
(Auburn Farms)	1 Chip	3	0	0	1	0	5	
(Frito-Lay):								
Lay's	1 Chip	7	0.4	0	1	0	8	
Ruffles	1 Chip	12	0.8	0	1	0	13	
(Guiltless Gourmet)	1 Oz	110	1.5	2	22	1	200	
(Kettle)	1 Oz	151	9.6	2	15	1	177	
(O'Boisies):								
	1 Chip	10	0.6	0	1	0	13	
Tato Skins	1 Chip	8	0.6	0	1	0	9	
(Pringles):								
	1 Oz	144	6.7	1	19	NV	122	
	1 Chip	11	0.7	0	1	0	10	
LT	1 Chip	9	0.4	0	1	0	8	

Potato Dish, Frozen

(Serving size given in Oz to reflect weight of 1 serving)

	Serv.	K-Cal.	Fat	Prot.	Carb.	Fib.	Sod.	FAC
(Bryan) Scalloped W/								
Ham Puree	1 Oz	36	1.6	2	4	NV	61	
(Green Giant) Broccoli								
Au Gratin	5.5 Oz	130	4	4	19	2	580	A
(Healthy Choice):								
Casserole, Garden	9.2 Oz	200	4	11	30	6	520	A
Cheddar Broccoli	10.5 Oz	310	5	13	53	8	500	AC
(Hormel) Scalloped								
Potato & Ham	1 Cup	360	23	10	28	3	1,280	
(Kraft):								
Au Gratin	3.7 Oz	140	5	4	20	NV	500	
Broccoli Au Gratin	3.7 Oz	140	5	5	20	1	500	
Scalloped Potatoes	3.7 Oz	140	5	4	20	2	490	
Two Cheese	3.7 Oz	140	5	4	20	1	450	
(Stouffer's):								
Au Gratin	1 Cup	260	12	8	30	2	1,180	C
Baked, Broccoli/								
Cheese	10 Oz	320	15	15	30	4	770	AC
Scalloped	1 Cup	280	12	8	34	4	900	C
(Stouffer's) Lean Cuisine:								
Baked, Broccoli/								
Cheddar Sauce	10.2 Oz	220	6	12	30	5	580	AC
Baked/Sour Cream	10.2 Oz	230	5	9	38	NV	570	AC

	Serv.	K-Cal.	Fat	Prot.	Carb.	Fib.	Sod.	FAC
(Potato Dish, Frozen cont.)								
Cheddar, Deluxe.........	10.2 Oz	230	6	13	32	6	570	AC
(Swanson) Scalloped,								
Ham	9 Oz	290	12	16	29	4	1,020	C
(Wt Watchers):								
Baked W/Broccoli/								
Cheese	10 Oz	250	7	12	35	6	590	AC
Baked W/Veg								
Primavera..............	10 Oz	220	7	10	34	6	460	AC

Potato, Fast Food
Baked

	Serv.	K-Cal.	Fat	Prot.	Carb.	Fib.	Sod.	FAC
(Arby's):								
Broccoli 'N Cheddar ...	1 Item	571	20	14	89	9	565	A
Deluxe........................	1 Item	736	36	19	86	7	499	AC
Mushroom 'N Cheese	1 Item	515	26.7	15	58	NV	923	AC
(Carl's):								
Bacon and Cheese.....	1 Item	630	29	20	76	6	1,720	A
Broccoli and Cheese..	1 Item	530	22	11	76	8	930	A
Cheese........................	1 Item	690	36	23	70	NV	1,160	AC
Chili	1 Item	500	26	18	50	NV	630	AC
Fiesta	1 Item	720	38	31	64	NV	1,470	AC
Sour Cream & Chive ..	1 Item	430	14	8	70	6	160	A
(Wendy's):								
Bacon & Cheese	1 Item	540	18	17	78	7	1,430	AC
Broccoli & Cheese......	1 Item	470	14	9	80	9	470	AC
Cheese........................	1 Item	570	23	14	78	7	640	AC
Chili & Cheese	1 Item	620	24	20	83	9	780	AC
Plain..........................	1 Item	310	0	7	71	7	25	A
Sour Cream & Chives	1 Item	380	6	8	74	8	40	A

French Fries

	Serv.	K-Cal.	Fat	Prot.	Carb.	Fib.	Sod.	FAC
(Arby's):								
Cheddar, Curly	1 Serv	333	18	5	40	0	1,016	
Curly Fries	1 Serv	300	15	4	38	0	853	
(Burger King) Medium....	1 Serv	370	20	5	43	3	240	
(Jack In The Box):								
....	1 Serv	350	17	4	45	4	190	A
Jumbo	1 Serv	400	19	5	51	4	220	A
(McDonald's):								
Large...........................	1 Serv	450	22	6	57	5	290	FA
Medium	1 Serv	320	17	4	36	3	150	
(Wendy's):								
Biggie........................	1 Serv	460	23	6	58	6	150	
Medium	1 Serv	380	19	5	47	5	120	
Small..........................	1 Serv	260	13	3	33	3	85	

Potato Flour

	Serv.	K-Cal.	Fat	Prot.	Carb.	Fib.	Sod.	FAC
(Bob's Red Mill)	3 Tbsp	120	0.5	3	27	0	10	

	Serv.	K-Cal.	Fat	Prot.	Carb.	Fib.	Sod.	FAC
(Ener-G)	1 Cup	527	1.4	14	136	10	58	**A**
Gluten-Free	1 Cup	597	1.4	14	136	10	58	**A**

Potato, Mix
Prepared
(Prepared as indicated on package)

(Betty Crocker):

	Serv.	K-Cal.	Fat	Prot.	Carb.	Fib.	Sod.	FAC
Au Gratin	1 Cup	300	12	6	44	2	1,220	
Broccoli Au Gratin	1 Cup	300	12	6	42	2	1,180	
Buds	1 Cup	480	24	9	57	3	1,380	
Cheddar 'N Bacon	1 Cup	320	12	4	44	2	1,140	
Hash Browns	1 Cup	400	16	6	62	4	1,180	
Julienne	1 Cup	280	12	6	40	2	1,340	
Scalloped	1 Cup	320	14	6	44	2	1,340	
Smokey Cheddar	1 Cup	450	18	9	66	3	1,850	
Sour Cream/Chives	1 Cup	320	14	6	46	2	1,120	
(Fantastic):								
Broccoli & Cheese	1 Cup	190	3	8	35	3	480	
Cheddar	1 Cup	180	3	7	35	3	480	
Garlic & Herb	1 Cup	180	2	6	375	3	480	
Sour Cream/Chives	1 Cup	180	2.5	6	37	3	480	
(Pillsbury) *Hungry Jack*:								
Au Gratin	1 Cup	300	9	6	48	2	1,240	
Cheddar & Bacon	1 Cup	300	9	8	48	4	1,080	
Flakes	1 Cup	320	14	6	40	2	480	
Sour Cream & Chives	1 Cup	320	12	6	46	2	1,120	

Unprepared

	Serv.	K-Cal.	Fat	Prot.	Carb.	Fib.	Sod.	FAC
(Arrowhead Mills) Flakes	1 Cup	270	0	6	60	3	60	
(Barbara's) Mashed	1 Cup	210	0	6	51	3	30	
(General Mills):								
Au Gratin	1 Cup	200	3	4	40	2	1,100	
Cheddar	1 Cup	180	2	4	40	2	1,140	
Cheddar N Bacon	1 Cup	200	3	4	40	2	1,220	
Cheesy Scalloped	1 Cup	150	3	3	29	2	750	
Hash Browns	1 Cup	260	0	6	60	4	60	
Julienne	1 Cup	180	2	4	36	2	1,140	
Potato Buds	1 Cup	240	0	6	54	3	60	
Scalloped	1 Cup	200	2	4	42	2	1,120	
Smokey Cheddar	1 Cup	200	2	4	42	2	1,080	
Sour Cream/Chives	1 Cup	200	3	4	42	2	1,000	
Twice-Baked Cheddar/Onion	1 Cup	330	9	6	57	3	1,712	

Potato Pancake
Mix

	Serv.	K-Cal.	Fat	Prot.	Carb.	Fib.	Sod.	FAC
Hungry Jack (Pillsbury)	1 Cup	560	0	16	128	8	2,880	
(Manischewitz)	3 Tbsp	80	1	2	18	2	500	
(Panni)	3 Tbsp	150	0	3	36	2	720	

	Serv.	K-Cal.	Fat	Prot.	Carb.	Fib.	Sod.	FAC
(Potato Pancake cont.)								
Prepared								
(Casbah)	1 Oz	105	1	3	23	2	263	
Home Recipe	3 Oz	207	11.6	5	22	2	306	A

Poultry Seasoning

	Serv.	K-Cal.	Fat	Prot.	Carb.	Fib.	Sod.	FAC
	1 Tsp	5	0.1	0	1	0	0	

Preserves (Also See Fruit Spread; Jam; Jelly; Marmalade)

	Serv.	K-Cal.	Fat	Prot.	Carb.	Fib.	Sod.	FAC
(Knott's Berry Farm)	2 Tsp	36	0	0	8	NV	0	
(R.W. Knudsen)	2 Tsp	35	<1	<1	8	NV	NV	
(R.W. Knudsen) Organic	2 Tsp	25	<1	<1	7	NV	NV	
(Polaner)	2 Tsp	35	0	0	9	NV	5	
(Smucker's) Low Sugar	1 Tbsp	25	0	0	6	0	0	

Pretzel
Bavarian

	Serv.	K-Cal.	Fat	Prot.	Carb.	Fib.	Sod.	FAC
(Barbara's)	1 Item	50	0.8	3	10	2	85	
(Frito-Lay)								
Rold Gold	1 Item	37	0.7	1	7	0	147	
(Keebler)	1 Item	40	0.7	1	8	0	200	
Dutch Style								
(Mister Salty)	1 Item	60	0.5	2	13	1	290	
Minis								
(Barbara's):								
	1 Item	6	0.1	0	1	0	16	
9 Grain	1 Item	50	0.8	2	10	2	90	
NSA	1 Item	6	0.1	0	1	0	2	
(Frito-Lay) Rold Gold,								
Rods	1 Item	37	0.5	1	7	0	123	
(Keebler)	1 Item	2	0	0	0	0	10	
Mustard								
(Frito-Lay) Rold Gold, W/								
Honey	1 Item	13	0.7	0	2	0	23	
(Barbara's) W/Honey	1 Item	50	0.5	2	11	2	68	
Sourdough								
(Louise's) FF	1 Oz	90	0	1	19	1	470	
(Frito Lay) Rold Gold, FF	1 Item	80	0	2	17	1	300	
Sticks								
(Frito-Lay) Rold Gold, FF	1 Item	2	0	0	0	0	11	
Twists								
(Bearitos) WW	1 Oz	110	1	4	21	NV	350	
(Frito-Lay):								
Rold Gold	1 Item	11	0.1	0	2	0	51	
Rold Gold, Tiny, FF	1 Item	6	0	0	1	0	23	

Prickly Pear (See Cactus Pear)

	Serv.	K-Cal.	Fat	Prot.	Carb.	Fib.	Sod.	FAC
Prosciutto (See Ham, Luncheon Meat)								
Prune								
Canned W/								
Heavy Syrup..................	1 Cup	246	0.5	2	65	9	7	
Heavy Syrup, Stewed								
(S & W)	1 Piece	26	0	0	7	1	2	
Dehydrated								
Cooked	1 Cup	316	0.7	3	83	NV	6	A
Uncooked	1 Cup	447	1	5	118	NV	7	A
Dried								
Cooked, Sweetened.......	1 Cup	295	0.5	3	78	9	5	
Cooked, Unsweetened...	1 Cup	227	0.5	2	60	14	4	
Uncooked	1 Cup	339	0.7	4	89	10	6	A
Pitted (Del Monte)..........	1 Cup	480	0	4	136	12	20	
Pitted (Dole)	2 Oz	140	1	1	36	NV	10	
Prune Juice								
(Del Monte)	1 Cup	170	0	1	43	1	20	FA
(S & W)	1 Cup	178	0	2	40	1	10	
(Sunsweet)	1 Cup	180	0	0	43	2	75	
W/Pulp	1 Cup	180	0	0	43	2	75	
Prune Whip								
....	1 Cup	194	0.2	6	45	4	242	
Psyllium Seed								
Ground............................	1 Cup	67	0.7	4	108	97	47	F
Pudding, Prepared from Mix								
Banana, Prepared W/								
2% Milk............................	1 Cup	286	4.8	8	51	0	465	C
2% Milk, Instant	1 Cup	306	5	8	58	0	870	C
Whole Milk......................	1 Cup	314	8.4	8	51	0	462	C
Whole Milk, Instant	1 Cup	332	8.5	8	58	0	867	C
Chocolate, Prepared W/								
2% Milk............................	1 Cup	301	5.7	9	56	0	298	C
2% Milk, Instant	1 Cup	300	5.6	9	56	0	835	C
Whole Milk......................	1 Cup	443	11.3	10	81	0	273	C
Whole Milk, Instant	1 Cup	326	9.1	9	55	0	835	C
Coconut Cream, Prepared W/								
2% Milk............................	1 Cup	291	7	9	50	0	456	C
2% Milk, Instant	1 Cup	315	6.8	9	56	0	723	C
Whole Milk......................	1 Cup	319	10.6	8	50	0	454	C
Whole Milk, Instant	1 Cup	344	10.3	9	56	0	723	C
Lemon, Prepared W/								
2% Milk, Instant	1 Cup	309	5	8	59	0	788	C
Whole Milk, Instant	1 Cup	338	8.5	8	59	0	785	C

	Serv.	K-Cal.	Fat	Prot.	Carb.	Fib.	Sod.	FAC
(Pudding, Prepared from Mix cont.)								
Rice, Prepared W/								
2% Milk	1 Cup	323	4.6	10	61	0	317	C
Whole Milk	1 Cup	351	8.1	10	60	0	314	C
Tapioca, Prepared W/								
2% Milk	1 Cup	293	4.8	8	56	0	344	C
Whole Milk	1 Cup	321	8.2	8	55	0	341	C
Vanilla, Prepared W/								
2% Milk	1 Cup	283	4.8	8	52	0	448	C
2% Milk, Instant	1 Cup	295	4.8	8	56	0	812	C
Whole Milk	1 Cup	311	8.4	8	52	0	448	C
Whole Milk, Instant	1 Cup	324	8.2	8	56	0	812	C

Pudding, Ready-To-Serve
Chocolate

	Serv.	K-Cal.	Fat	Prot.	Carb.	Fib.	Sod.	FAC
(Diamond Crystal)	4 Oz	220	10	7	27	NV	390	
(Jell-O):								
FF	4 Oz	100	0	3	23	0	190	
Fudge	4 Oz	171	6	3	28	0	121	
Fudge, LT	4 Oz	101	1	3	22	0	113	
LT	4 Oz	104	2	3	21	0	113	
(Swiss Miss):								
	4 Oz	166	5.7	3	26	0	177	
Fudge	4 Oz	175	5.6	3	28	0	207	
Fudge, FF	4 Oz	103	0.3	2	23	0	150	
(Ultra Slim-Fast)	4 Oz	100	1	2	21	2	240	F
(Yoplait) Double	4 Oz	180	4	6	30	1	95	
Lemon								
(Hunt's)	4 Oz	162	3.3	0	33	0	100	
(Imagine Foods)	4 Oz	150	3	1	33	1	50	
Milk Chocolate								
(Hunt's) Swirl	4 Oz	164	5.6	2	26	0	175	
(Jell-O)	4 Oz	173	6	4	29	0	126	
(Yoplait)	4 Oz	180	4	6	30	NV	105	
Tapioca								
(Jell-O)	4 Oz	140	4	0	26	0	160	
(Swiss Miss) FF	4 Oz	100	0.3	2	22	0	151	
Vanilla								
(Diamond Crystal)	4 Oz	220	10	7	25	NV	400	
(Jell-O):								
	4 Oz	160	5	3	25	0	170	
FF	4 Oz	100	0	2	23	0	240	
LT	4 Oz	104	2	3	20	0	118	
(Nutra/Balance) Low								
Lactose	5 Oz	242	7.5	8	36	0	94	
(Swiss Miss):								
	4 Oz	156	5.6	2	24	0	181	
FF	4 Oz	93	0.4	2	21	0	170	
(Yoplait)	4 Oz	150	3	6	25	NV	100	

	Serv.	K-Cal.	Fat	Prot.	Carb.	Fib.	Sod.	FAC

Pudding, Ready-To-Serve, Nondairy Alternative
(Imagine Foods)

Butterscotch................	1 Cup	150	3	1	31	0	45	
(Rice Dream):								
Almond.........................	1 Cup	300	4	2	62	NV	60	
Carob	1 Cup	260	0	2	62	NV	60	
Coconut.......................	1 Cup	300	4	2	64	NV	20	

Puff Pastry (See Pastry, Puff)

Puff Pastry Shells (See Pastry, Puff)

Pummelo (See Pomelo)

Pumpkin

Raw, Cubed	1 Cup	30	0.1	1	8	1	1	A
Boiled, Mashed	1 Cup	49	0.2	2	12	3	2	A
Canned (Libby's)............	1 Cup	80	1	4	18	10	10	A

Pumpkin Pie Mix

Canned............................	1 Cup	281	0.4	3	71	22	562	A
Canned (Libby's)............	1 Cup	240	0	2	60	6	450	A

Pumpkin Pie Spice

Ground............................	1 Tsp	6	0.2	0	1	0	1	

Pumpkin Seed—Squash Seed

Fresh	1 Oz	154	15.6	7	4	0	5	
Dried...............................	1 Cup	747	63.3	34	25	5	25	FA
Kernels, Roasted............	1 Cup	1,185	95.6	75	31	9	41	FA
Whole, Roasted, Salted.	1 Cup	285	12.4	12	34	9	368	FA

Purslane

....	1 Oz	13	0.1	1	2	1	2	A

Q

	Serv.	K-Cal.	Fat	Prot.	Carb.	Fib.	Sod.	FAC
Quail								
Breast, Meat Only, Raw	3 Oz	104	2.5	19	0	0	45	
Meat/Skin, Raw	3 Oz	163	10.1	17	0	0	45	
Meat Only, Cooked	3 Oz	195	11.7	21	0	0	236	
Quiche								
(Nancy's):								
Broccoli/Cheddar	6 Oz	450	26	19	36	2	780	AC
Florentine	6 Oz	440	26	19	35	1	630	AC
Monterey	6 Oz	470	29	19	34	1	720	AC
Quince								
Raw (3 Oz)	1 Item	52	0.1	0	14	2	4	A
Quinoa								
Whole or Ground	1 Cup	636	9.9	22	117	10	36	F
Chips, *Amazing Bakes*								
(Barbara's)	1 Item	4	0	0	1	0	6	
(Arrowhead Mills):								
Flakes	1 Cup	315	3	9	69	7	15	
Flour...........................	1 Cup	528	8	16	96	9	40	F
Pasta...........................	2 Oz	180	2	5	35	3	5	
Seed............................	1 Cup	560	9	20	100	16	0	F

R

	Serv.	K-Cal.	Fat	Prot.	Carb.	Fib.	Sod.	FAC
Rabbit								
Raw	3 Oz	116	4.7	17	0	0	25	
Raw, Wild	3 Oz	97	2	19	0	0	42	
Breaded, Fried	3 Oz	189	7.4	24	5	0	270	
Stewed	3 Oz	175	7.2	26	0	0	31	
Stewed, Skinless	3 Oz	147	3	28	0	0	38	
Stewed, Wild	3 Oz	147	3	28	0	0	38	
Radicchio								
Leaf	1 Item	2	0	0	0	0	2	
Shredded	1 Cup	9	0.1	1	2	0	9	
Shredded	3 Oz	19	0.2	1	4	1	19	FA
Radish								
(Also See Daikon—Chinese Radish)								
Raw	1 Oz	5	0	0	1	0	7	
Raw	1 Item	1	0	0	0	0	1	
Raw	3 Oz	14	0.5	1	3	1	20	A
Radish Seed Sprouts								
Raw	1 Cup	16	1	1	1	NV	2	
Raisin								
Dark								
Seeded	1 Cup	488	0.9	4	129	11	46	F
Seedless	1 Oz	84	0.1	1	20	0	4	
Seedless, (Sun-Maid)	1 Cup	520	0	4	124	11	40	F
Golden								
Seedless	1 Cup	498	0.8	6	131	7	20	F
Seedless	1 Oz	86	0.1	1	23	NV	3	
Raisin Juice Concentrate								
(Sun-Maid)	3.3 Oz	287	0.5	1	70	2	37	F

Ramen (See Soup Mix, Ramen; Noodle, Japanese)

	Serv.	K-Cal.	Fat	Prot.	Carb.	Flb.	Sod.	FAC
Raspberry								
Fresh								
Raw	1 Oz	9	0	0	2	2	0	
Raw	1 Cup	60	0.7	1	14	6	0	A
Canned W/								
Heavy Syrup	1 Cup	233	0.3	2	60	8	8	A
Frozen								
Sweetened	1 Cup	258	0.4	2	65	11	3	A
(Cascadian)	1 Cup	60	0.5	1	15	7	0	A
(Flav R Pac)	1 Cup	50	0	1	11	2	0	A
W/Syrup	1 Oz	46	0	0	11	1	8	
Raspberry Juice								
(Fruitopia) W/Lemonade	1 Cup	120	0	0	29	0	27	
(R.W. Knudsen) Nectar..	1 Cup	120	0	0	30	NV	25	
W/Peach	1 Cup	120	0	0	31	NV	25	
(Snapple) Royale	1 Cup	120	0	0	29	NV	28	
Raspberry Syrup								
(R.W. Knudsen)	1 Tbsp	37	0	0	9	0	0	
Ravioli, Canned								
Beef								
(Chef Boyardee):								
Mini	1 Cup	240	6	8	37	3	1,180	
Smurfs	1 Cup	230	5	9	38	6	1,160	
(Franco-American) W/								
Meat Sauce	1 Cup	300	10	11	42	3	1,160	
(Hunt's) *Homestyle*	1 Cup	221	7.7	10	32	4	1,116	A
(Libby's)	1 Cup	230	9	11	29	7	1,040	
Cheese								
(Chef Boyardee)								
W/Beef Sauce	1 Cup	220	3	9	38	4	1,110	
Chicken								
(Chef Boyardee)	1 Cup	180	4	7	29	NV	1,100	
Ravioli Entree, Fresh								
(Contadina):								
Beef/Garlic	1 Cup	280	11.2	14	31	2	280	
Cheese	1 Cup	280	12	13	31	2	350	C
Cheese, LT	1 Cup	240	5	13	35	2	340	
Garden, LT	1 Cup	232	4.8	12	34	2	296	
(DiGiorno):								
Cheese	1 Cup	350	15	14	40	2	390	AC
Chicken/Garlic	1 Cup	270	2	17	45	1	580	
Sausage, Italian	1 Cup	453	16	21	55	3	840	

	Serv.	K-Cal.	Fat	Prot.	Carb.	Fib.	Sod.	FAC
Ravioli Entree, Frozen								
(Serving size given in Oz to reflect weight of 1 serving)								
Beef								
(Bernardi)	7.5 Oz	450	19	22	48	3	930	C
(Don Miguel)	3 Oz	190	5	9	28	4	370	
(Stouffer's)	9.5 Oz	370	14	17	43	5	680	
Cheese								
(Amy's Kitchen)	9.6 Oz	340	12	15	44	6	580	
(Bernardi)	7.5 Oz	410	15	21	48	2	570	C
(Digiorno) LT	3.5 Oz	270	2	17	45	1	580	C
(Healthy Choice)								
Parmigiana	9 Oz	250	4	11	44	6	290	
(Stouffer's):								
Lean Cuisine	8.5 Oz	240	7	11	34	4	590	
Tomato Sauce	9.6 Oz	360	14	16	42	4	720	C
(Wt Watchers)	9 Oz	280	6	17	39	5	560	AC
Chicken								
(Bernardi)	7.5 Oz	450	17	21	52	2	420	C
(Don Miguel) Lucca	3 Oz	180	4	11	26	4	450	
Florentine								
(Bernardi)	7.5 Oz	370	10	21	53	3	440	C
(Wt Watchers)	8.5 Oz	190	2	8	37	5	420	A
Refried Beans (See Beans, Refried)								
Relish								
(Claussen) Sweet	1 Tbsp	15	0	0	3	0	85	
(Heinz) Hot Dog	1 Tbsp	15	0	0	4	0	105	
Sweet	1 Tbsp	10	0	0	4	0	110	
(Vlasic):								
Curry, Sweet	1 Tbsp	15	0	0	4	0	140	
Dill	1 Tbsp	1	0	0	1	0	200	
Hamburger	1 Tbsp	20	0	0	5	NV	125	
Hot Dog	1 Tbsp	20	0	0	4	0	125	
Hot Piccalilli	1 Tbsp	17	0	0	4	0	80	
Sweet	1 Tbsp	15	0	0	4	0	110	
Rhubarb								
Raw, Diced	1 Cup	26	0.2	1	6	2	5	
Cooked, Sweetened	1 Cup	278	0.1	1	75	5	2	C
Frozen (Flav R Pac)	1 Cup	30	0.5	1	5	2	0	
Rice								
Raw								
(All values for uncooked Rice)								
Arborio								
Brown, Org (Lundberg)	¼ Cup	160	1	5	33	3	0	
White, Org (Lundberg)	¼ Cup	160	1	4	35	1	0	

	Serv.	K-Cal.	Fat	Prot.	Carb.	Flb.	Sod.	FAC
(Rice cont.)								
Basmati								
Brown (Lundberg)	¼ Cup	170	2	4	38	2	0	
White (Arrowhead Mills).	¼ Cup	150	1	3	33	2	0	
Brown								
Long Grain (S & W).......	¼ Cup	150	1	3	32	1	0	
Medium Grain.................	¼ Cup	172	1.3	4	36	2	2	
Quick (S & W)................	¼ Cup	75	0.5	2	17	1	2	
Short Grain, Org (Lundberg)	¼ Cup	170	1.5	3	40	3	0	
Glutinous								
Black................................	¼ Cup	158	1	4	32		1	
White	¼ Cup	171	0.3	3	38	2	3	
White								
Long Grain	¼ Cup	169	0.3	3	37	2	3	
Long Grain, Instant	¼ Cup	90	0	2	20	1	1	
Medium Grain.................	¼ Cup	175	0.3	3	39	1	0	
Organic (Lundberg)	¼ Cup	180	0.5	4	38	1	0	
Short Grain.....................	¼ Cup	179	0.3	3	40	1	0	
Wild								
....	¼ Cup	143	0.4	6	30	3	4	F
Cooked								
(All values for cooked rice)								
Basmati								
Brown (Fantastic)	1 Cup	204	1	6	44	NV	6	
White (Fantastic)............	1 Cup	206	0	4	46	NV	2	
Brown								
Converted (Uncle Ben's)	1 Cup	180	2	4	42	2	22	
Instant (Minute)	1 Cup	253	2.2	6	50	3	15	
Long Grain (Hinode)	1 Cup	200	2	4	40	1	13	
Medium Grain.................	1 Cup	218	1.6	5	46	4	2	
Short Grain (Lundberg)..	1 Cup	232	1.2	5	50	3	0	
Glutinous								
White	1 Cup	234	0.5	5	51	2	12	
White								
Converted (Uncle Ben's)	1 Cup	170	0	4	38	0	0	
Instant (Minute)	1 Cup	226	0	5	51	0	7	
Long Grain	1 Cup	205	0.4	4	45	1	2	
Long Grain, Instant	1 Cup	162	0.3	3	35	1	5	
Medium Grain.................	1 Cup	242	0.4	4	53	1	0	
Medium Grain (Hinode) .	1 Cup	226	0.7	4	51	0	7	
Parboiled	1 Cup	200	0.5	4	43	1	5	
Short Grain.....................	1 Cup	242	0.4	4	53	1	0	
Wild								
....	1 Cup	166	0.6	7	35	3	5	F

Rice and Beans, Prepared from Mix

(Bearitos):

Cajun............................	8.7 Oz	140	1	7	26	5	490	A

	Serv.	K-Cal.	Fat	Prot.	Carb.	Fib.	Sod.	FAC
Cuban	8.7 Oz	150	1	7	27	5	490	**A**
Mexican	8.7 Oz	160	1	7	30	4	490	**A**
(Fantastic):								
Bombay Curry	10 Oz	260	3	12	46	8	470	**A**
Cajun	10 Oz	240	1.5	10	47	6	480	**A**
Caribbean	10 Oz	230	1.5	10	44	6	480	**A**
Northern Italian	10 Oz	240	1.5	8	49	4	460	**A**
Szechuan	10 Oz	210	2	7	41	3	480	**A**
Tex-Mex	10 Oz	270	2	10	53	8	540	**A**

Rice Beverage

	Serv.	K-Cal.	Fat	Prot.	Carb.	Fib.	Sod.	FAC
(Amazake) All Flavors	1 Cup	200	4	4	36	5	20	
(Eden) Soybean Blend	1 Cup	120	3	7	16	0	80	
(Rice Dream):								
Carob	1 Cup	150	2.5	1	32	0	100	
Chocolate	1 Cup	170	3	1	36	2	115	
Chocolate, Enriched	1 Cup	170	3	1	36	0	115	**C**
Original, Enriched	1 Cup	120	2	1	25	0	90	**C**
Original Lite	1 Cup	120	2	1	28	NV	80	
Vanilla, Enriched	1 Cup	130	2	1	28	0	90	**C**
Vanilla Lite	1 Cup	120	2	1	30	NV	80	
(Westbrae):								
Concentrate	4 Fl Oz	100	3	1	18	0	70	**C**
Plain	1 Cup	100	3	1	18	0	70	**C**
Vanilla	1 Cup	120	3	1	22	0	70	**C**

Rice Bran

	Serv.	K-Cal.	Fat	Prot.	Carb.	Fib.	Sod.	FAC
Coarse	1 Oz	49	0.6	1	10	10	2	
Crude (3 Oz)	1 Cup	262	17.3	11	41	17	4	**FA**
Fine	1 Oz	107	4.5	4	13	2	7	

Rice Bran Oil

	Serv.	K-Cal.	Fat	Prot.	Carb.	Fib.	Sod.	FAC
	1 Tbsp	120	13.6	0	0	0	0	**A**

Rice Cake
Brown Rice, Flavored

	Serv.	K-Cal.	Fat	Prot.	Carb.	Fib.	Sod.	FAC
(Hain):								
Apple Cinnamon, Mini	1 Item	10	0	0	2	0	0	
Barbecue, Mini	1 Item	14	0.6	0	2	NV	10	
Honey Nut, Mini	1 Item	12	0.2	0	2	NV	11	
Ranch, Mini	1 Item	13	0.6	0	2	0	32	
(Lundberg):								
Popcorn	1 Item	60	0.5	1	12	NV	140	
Popcorn, Unsalted	1 Item	60	0.5	1	12	NV	3	
Sesame, Mini	1 Item	10	0	0	3	NV	1	
Unsalted	1 Item	60	0	1	14	2	0	

Flavored

	Serv.	K-Cal.	Fat	Prot.	Carb.	Fib.	Sod.	FAC
(Hain):								
Apple Cinnamon	1 Item	50	0	1	11	0	10	

	Serv.	K-Cal.	Fat	Prot.	Carb.	Fib.	Sod.	FAC
(Rice Cake cont.)								
Cheese, Mini	1 Item	14	0.5	0	2	0	27	
Honey Nut	1 Item	50	0	1	11	0	25	
W/Popcorn, Butter	1 Item	40	0	1	9	3	60	
W/Popcorn, Caramel	1 Item	50	0	1	11	0	20	
(Lundberg):								
Buckwheat	1 Item	60	0	1	14	2	120	
Creamy Dill, Mini	1 Item	12	0.2	0	3	0	11	
Rye, Caraway	1 Item	60	0	1	14	2	120	
(Quaker):								
Apple Cinnamon	1 Item	50	0	1	11	0	0	
Caramel Corn, Mini	1 Item	10	0	0	2	0	5	
Cheddar, White, Mini	1 Item	8	0	0	2	0	20	
Cinnamon Crunch	1 Item	50	0	1	11	0	25	
Honey Nut, Mini	1 Item	10	0	0	2	0	5	

Rice Dish, Frozen

	Serv.	K-Cal.	Fat	Prot.	Carb.	Fib.	Sod.	FAC
(Budget Gourmet):								
Stir Fry W/Veg	8 Oz	350	16	7	44	3	670	
Wild Rice W/Veg	8.5 Oz	400	16	8	56	2	780	A
(Cascadian) Teriyaki	9 Oz	270	7	9	44	2	630	A
(Green Giant):								
Medley	10 Oz	240	3	6	46	3	880	
W/Broccoli	10 Oz	320	12	8	44	2	1,000	A
W/Broccoli W/Cheese Sauce	5.5 Oz	160	5	5	26	2	490	A
White & Wild	10 Oz	250	5	6	45	3	1,000	
(Wt Watchers):								
Risotto/Cheese/ Mushrooms	10 Oz	290	8	11	44	4	540	AC
Sante Fe W/Beans	10 Oz	290	9	12	41	10	670	C

Rice Dish, Mix (Also See Pilaf, Prepared)

(Prepared from mix)

Beef

	Serv.	K-Cal.	Fat	Prot.	Carb.	Fib.	Sod.	FAC
(Farmhouse)	1 Cup	200	1	5	45	2	690	
(Rice-A-Roni)	1 Cup	300	8	8	48	NV	1,060	
W/Mushroom	1 Cup	290	6	7	51	2	1,265	

Broccoli Au Gratin

(Farmhouse)	1 Cup	210	2	5	44	2	620	
(Rice-A-Roni)	1 Cup	370	17	7	47	2	885	

Chicken

(Farmhouse)	1 Cup	180	1.5	4	42	4	670	
(Rice-A-Roni):								
	1 Cup	320	9.5	7	51	1	1,095	
Fast Cook	1 Cup	250	6.5	6	41	1	920	
W/Broccoli	1 Cup	290	7.5	7	51	2	1,405	

	Serv.	K-Cal.	Fat	Prot.	Carb.	Fib.	Sod.	FAC
W/Mushroom	1 Cup	360	14	8	52	2	1,480	
W/Vegetables	1 Cup	290	7	6	52	2	1,470	
Herb, Spiced								
(Farmhouse):								
Saffron	1 Cup	190	0.5	4	42	4	1,080	
Wild Herb	1 Cup	200	2	5	43	2	730	
(Knorr) Risotto, Onions/								
Herb	1 Cup	300	1.5	6	66	1	1,390	
(Lundberg):								
One Step Chili	1 Cup	180	1	6	42	5	420	
One Step Curry	1 Cup	160	1.5	5	38	5	400	
One Step Garlic	1 Cup	160	1	6	37	5	480	
(Rice-A-Roni) W/Herb								
Butter	1 Cup	310	9	6	53	1	1,160	
Oriental								
(Farmhouse) Fried	1 Cup	200	2	6	48	2	860	
(La Choy) Fried	1 Cup	236	1.1	5	53	2	1,024	
(Rice-A-Roni):								
	1 Cup	290	10	6	43	1	930	
Fried	1 Cup	320	11	6	51	2	1,595	
Stir Fry	1 Cup	290	5.5	6	53	1	1,080	
Spanish								
(Fantastic) W/Beans	1 Cup	210	1.5	9	49	8	140	A
(Farmhouse)	1 Cup	180	1.5	5	42	4	840	
(Rice-A-Roni):								
	1 Cup	270	8	6	46	3	1,210	
Fast Cook	1 Cup	250	5.5	6	44	2	1,005	

Rice Flour

Brown (Bob's Red Mill)	1 Cup	560	4	12	124	5	20	
White (Bob's Red Mill)	1 Cup	583	2.7	11	127	5	0	
White Rice, Coarse								
(Ener-G)	1 Cup	366	1	6	80	2	3	

Rice Pudding (See Pudding, Prepared From Mix, Rice)

Rice Syrup

Brown, Org (Lundberg)	¼ Cup	170	0	0	42	0	5	

Roast Beef Hash (See Hash, Roast Beef)

Roast Beef, Luncheon Meat (See Beef, Roast, Luncheon Meat)

Rockfish

Raw	3 Oz	82	1.4	116	0	0	53	
Broiled	3 Oz	103	1.7	20	0	0	66	

Rocket (See Arugula)

	Serv.	K-Cal.	Fat	Prot.	Carb.	Fib.	Sod.	FAC
Roe								
Fresh	3 Oz	123	4.8	19	1	0	126	
Broiled	3 Oz	174	7	25	2	0	24	
Roll								
Brown and Serve								
(Pepperidge Farm):								
Club	1 Item	100	1	3	19	1	190	
French	½ Item	120	1	4	24	1	250	
Hearth	1 Item	50	1	2	10	0	100	
Plain, Brown & Serve	1 Item	85	2.1	2	14	1	148	
Dinner								
(Awrey's) Sesame Seed	1 Item	60	1	2	12	1	140	
(Ener-G) Tapioca,								
Gluten-Free	1 Item	151	5.7	2	24	1	6	
(Home Pride) Wheat	1 Item	160	4	5	26	2	270	
White	1 Item	65	2	2	11	1	115	
(Pepperidge Farm):								
Butter Crescent	1 Item	110	6	2	13	0	150	
Finger Poppyseed	1 Item	50	2	2	8	0	80	
Golden Twist	1 Item	110	5	2	14	0	150	
Old-Fashioned	1 Item	50	2	2	7	NV	85	
Parker House	1 Item	60	1	2	9	0	80	
Potato	1 Item	90	3	2	14	1	125	
(Pillsbury) Butterflake	1 Item	130	5	3	19	1	530	
Crescents	1 Item	100	5.5	2	11	0	215	
(Wonder)	1 Item	80	1	2	14	1	140	
Hard								
French	1 Item	105	1.6	3	19	1	231	
Kaiser	1 Item	167	2.5	6	30	1	310	
Submarine Hoagie	1 Item	400	8	11	72	4	683	
(Pepperidge Farm)								
French	1 Item	100	1	4	20	1	230	
Sourdough	1 Item	100	1	4	19	1	240	
Sweet								
(Hostess) Cinnamon	1 Item	220	6	4	39	1	260	
(Mrs. Smith's) Cinnamon	1 Item	320	15	5	41	0	300	
(Pepperidge Farm)								
Cinnamon	1 Item	250	12	4	33	2	220	
(Pillsbury):								
Caramel W/Icing	1 Item	170	7	2	25	1	330	
Cinnamon Raisin W/								
Icing	1 Item	180	7	2	26	1	310	
Cinnamon W/Icing	1 Item	140	5	2	21	0	330	
Raisins/Nuts Home								
Recipe	1 Item	196	7.3	4	30	NV	185	

	Serv.	K-Cal.	Fat	Prot.	Carb.	Fib.	Sod.	FAC
(Wt Watchers)								
Cinnamon...................	1 Item	180	5	4	31	NV	170	
Roselle								
Raw	1 Cup	28	0.4	1	6	0	3	
Rosemary								
Fresh	1 Oz	28	1.3	0	4	NV	4	
Ground (McCormick)......	1 Tsp	6	0	0	1	1	0	
Roughy, Orange								
Raw	3 Oz	60	0.6	12	0	0	54	
Broiled	3 Oz	76	0.8	16	0	0	69	
Rugola (See Arugula)								
Rum (See Alcoholic Beverages, Liqueur)								
Rutabaga								
Raw	1 Cup	50	0.3	2	11	4	28	**A**
Raw	1 Lb	163	0.9	5	37	11	90	**FAC**
Boiled, Mashed	1 Cup	94	0.5	3	21	4	48	**A**
Rye								
Whole	1 Cup	566	4.2	25	118	25	10	**FA**
Flakes, Rolled (Arrow-								
head Mills)	1 Cup	330	1.5	12	72	12	0	**FA**
Rye Flour								
(Arrowhead Mills) Whole								
Grain	1 Cup	400	4	20	80	16	0	**FA**
(Bob's Red Mill) Dark	1 Cup	440	4	16	88	4	0	**FA**
Light	1 Cup	400	2	8	84	4	0	
(Ener-G) Dark,								
Breadmaker	1 Cup	445	3.9	18	86	36	1	**FA**
Medium, *Breadmaker* .	1 Cup	355	2	10	75	9	1	
(Pillsbury)......................	1 Cup	400	2	12	83	NV	0	
(Robin Hood) Stone								
Ground.........................	1 Cup	360	2	13	86	13	10	

S

	Serv.	K-Cal.	Fat	Prot.	Carb.	Fib.	Sod.	FAC
Sablefish								
Raw	3 Oz	165	13	11	0	0	30	
Broiled	3 Oz	213	16.7	14	0	0	63	
Smoked	3 Oz	216	16.9	15	0	0	618	
Saccharin (See Sweetener, Alternative)								
Safflower Oil								
....	1 Cup	1,927	218	0	0	0	0	A
(Saffola)	1 Tbsp	120	14	0	0	0	0	A
(Spectrum)	1 Tbsp	120	14	0	0	0	0	A
Saffron								
Dried	1 Tbsp	7	0.1	0	1	0	3	
Sage								
Fresh	1 Oz	34	1.3	1	4	NV	1	
Ground (McCormick)	1 Tsp	4	0	0	0	0	0	
Salad Dressing, Bottled								
Balsamic								
(Cook's) *Triple H* FF	1 Tbsp	10	0	0	3	NV	23	
(Newman's Own)	1 Tbsp	45	5	0	2	0	175	
(S & W) LT	1 Tbsp	18	0	0	4	0	230	
Blue Cheese								
(Hidden Valley) LF	1 Tbsp	10	0	0	2	0	135	
(Kraft) Free, FF	1 Tbsp	25	0	0	6	1	170	
(Spectrum) LF	1 Tbsp	17	1	0	2	0	110	
(Walden Farms) FF	1 Tbsp	13	0	0	2	0	120	
(Wish-Bone)	1 Tbsp	85	8	1	1	0	140	
Buttermilk								
(Hains) Old-Fashioned	1 Tbsp	65	7	0	1	0	95	
(Kraft):								
Ranch	1 Tbsp	75	8	0	1	0	115	
Seven Seas	1 Tbsp	80	8	0	1	NV	130	

	Serv.	K-Cal.	Fat	Prot.	Carb.	Fib.	Sod.	FAC
Caesar								
(Cook's) *Triple H*..............	1 Tbsp	50	5	1	1	0	30	
(Kraft) Golden..................	1 Tbsp	70	7	0	1	NV	180	
(Newman's Own).............	1 Tbsp	75	8	1	1	0	225	
(Spectrum) South- western, LF..................	1 Tbsp	20	1	1	2	0	115	
(Wt Watchers) FF	1 Tbsp	5	0	0	1	0	195	
(Wish-Bone) Creamy......	1 Tbsp	90	9	1	1	0	145	
Coleslaw								
(Best Foods) *Step 1*	1 Tbsp	80	8	0	2	0	90	
(Hidden Valley) LF	1 Tbsp	17	0	0	5	0	100	
(Kraft) *Miracle Whip*.......	1 Tbsp	70	6	0	3	0	105	
Cucumber								
(Kraft).............................	1 Tbsp	75	7.5	0	1	0	110	
Dijon								
(Cook's) *Triple H*, Oil- Free.............................	1 Tbsp	8	0	0	2	0	100	
(Hain).............................	1 Tbsp	65	6.5	0	2	0	140	
Dill								
(Spectrum) Creamy, Org, FF	1 Tbsp	12	0	1	2	0	95	
French								
(Cook's) *Triple H*, FF	1 Tbsp	10	0	0	3	0	80	
(Kraft):								
FF..............................	1 Tbsp	25	0	0	6	0	150	
Seven Seas, Creamy .	1 Tbsp	60	6	0	2	NV	240	
(Walden Farms) FF........	1 Tbsp	15	0	0	3	0	145	
(Wt Watchers) FF	1 Tbsp	20	0	0	4	0	100	
Garlic								
(Cook's):								
Triple H, Garlic Lovers	1 Tbsp	50	5	0	1	0	95	
Triple H, Gusto, FF	1 Tbsp	6	0	0	1	0	90	
(Kraft) Creamy..................	1 Tbsp	55	5.5	0	1	0	175	
(Spectrum) Creamy, Org, FF	1 Tbsp	10	0	0	2	0	90	
Honey Mustard								
(Cook's) *Triple H*............	1 Tbsp	50	6	0	2	0	80	
(Kraft) Free, Dijon, FF ...	1 Tbsp	25	0	0	6	1	165	
(Spectrum) LF	1 Tbsp	17	1	0	2	0	100	
(Walden Farms) FF........	1 Tbsp	13	0	0	3	0	120	
(Wt Watchers) FF	1 Tbsp	22	0	0	5	0	75	
Italian								
(Hidden Valley) Lo Cal ..	1 Tbsp	25	3	0	1	0	120	
(Kraft):								
FF..............................	1 Tbsp	5	0	0	1	0	145	
Seven Seas, Creamy .	1 Tbsp	55	6	0	1	0	255	
Seven Seas, Free, FF	1 Tbsp	5	0	0	1	0	240	
Sour Cream	1 Tbsp	50	5	0	1	0	120	

	Serv.	K-Cal.	Fat	Prot.	Carb.	Fib.	Sod.	FAC
(Salad Dressing, Bottled cont.)								
(Spectrum) Zesty, LF.....	1 Tbsp	15	1	0	1	0	110	
(Walden Farms):								
FF................................	1 Tbsp	5	0	0	1	0	145	
FF, LS.........................	1 Tbsp	5	0	0	1	0	0	
Parmesan, FF............	1 Tbsp	13	0	0	2	0	180	
(Wt Watchers) FF..........	1 Tbsp	15	0	0	3	0	180	
(Wish-Bone)...................	1 Tbsp	40	4	0	1	0	245	
Peppercorn								
(Cook's) *Triple H*, Ranch								
FF................................	1 Tbsp	5	0	0	2	NV	155	
(Kraft) FF.....................	1 Tbsp	25	0	0	6	1	180	
(Wt Watchers) FF..........	1 Tbsp	8	0	0	2	0	85	
Ranch								
(Hidden Valley):								
....	1 Tbsp	40	3	0	1	0	135	
LT................................	1 Tbsp	30	3	0	1	0	130	
(Kraft):								
FF................................	1 Tbsp	25	0	0	6	0	155	
Seven Seas, FF.........	1 Tbsp	25	0	0	6	1	165	
Seven Seas, Viva.......	1 Tbsp	80	8	0	1	NV	135	
(Newman's Own)............	1 Tbsp	90	9	1	1	0	170	
(Walden Farms) FF........	1 Tbsp	13	0	0	2	0	145	
(Wt Watchers) FF..........	1 Tbsp	17	0	0	3	0	135	
Russian								
(Kraft) Creamy................	1 Tbsp	60	5	0	2	NV	150	
(Walden Farms) FF........	1 Tbsp	15	0	0	3	0	145	
(Wish-Bone)..................	1 Tbsp	55	3	0	8	0	175	
Thousand Island								
(Kraft) Free, FF.............	1 Tbsp	23	0	0	6	1	150	
(Walden Farms) FF........	1 Tbsp	10	0	0	4	0	120	
(Wish-Bone):								
....	1 Tbsp	70	6	0	4	0	170	
FF................................	1 Tbsp	17	0	0	5	0	145	
Soy								
(Nasoya):								
Creamy Dill.................	1 Tbsp	30	2.5	0	2	0	68	
Sesame Garlic............	1 Tbsp	30	2.5	0	2	0	63	
(Newman's Own) LT......	1 Tbsp	10	0.3	0	2	0	190	
Salad Dressing, Mix								
(Prepared as directed)								
(Good Seasons):								
Caesar	1 Tbsp	75	8	0	2	0	150	
Cheese Garlic.............	1 Tbsp	70	8	0	1	0	165	
Garlic/Herb.................	1 Tbsp	70	8	0	1	0	170	
Italian	1 Tbsp	70	7.5	0	1	0	110	
Italian, FF....................	1 Tbsp	5	0	0	2	0	145	
Italian, Zesty LT..........	1 Tbsp	25	3	0	1	0	135	

	Serv.	K-Cal.	Fat	Prot.	Carb.	Flb.	Sod.	FAC
(Hain) Caesar, FF	1 Tbsp	5	0	0	1	0	165	
(Hidden Valley):								
Bacon......................	1 Tbsp	60	6	1	1	0	110	
Blue Cheese..............	1 Tbsp	60	6	1	1	0	100	
Buttermilk	1 Tbsp	55	6	0	1	0	120	
Original, LF	1 Tbsp	15	0.5	0	1	0	120	
Original, Milk.............	1 Tbsp	60	6	0	1	0	105	

Salad Mix
Greens Only
(Dole):

	Serv.	K-Cal.	Fat	Prot.	Carb.	Flb.	Sod.	FAC
Classic Coleslaw	3 Oz	25	0	1	5	2	25	A
Classic Iceberg..........	3 Oz	15	0	1	4	1	15	A
French Blend	3 Oz	20	0	1	4	2	20	A
Italian	3 Oz	15	0	1	2	2	10	A
Romaine......................	3 Oz	15	0	1	2	2	10	A

Complete W/Dressing
(Dole):

	Serv.	K-Cal.	Fat	Prot.	Carb.	Flb.	Sod.	FAC
Oriental	3.5 Oz	120	6	2	13	2	240	A
Romano	3.5 Oz	150	12	3	9	2	570	A
Spinach Bacon	3.5 Oz	160	9	3	18	2	630	A
(Wt Watchers):								
Caesar, FF..................	3.5 Oz	60	0	2	11	1	600	
European, FF..............	3.5 Oz	60	0	2	13	2	530	
Garden, FF	3.5 Oz	60	0	2	12	1	270	

Salad, Fast Food
Arby's

	Serv.	K-Cal.	Fat	Prot.	Carb.	Flb.	Sod.	FAC
Chef	14.5 Oz	205	9.5	19	13	NV	796	
Roast Chicken	14.5 Oz	149	2	20	12	5	418	A
Burger King								
Chicken	10.7 Oz	200	10	21	7	3	110	A
Garden, W/O Dressing	7.5 Oz	100	5	6	7	3	110	A
Side, W/O Dressing....	4.7 Oz	60	3	3	4	2	55	
Carl's Jr								
Taco To Go	14.7 Oz	310	19	30	5	NV	920	AC
Del Taco								
Chicken	7 Oz	254	19	12	8	NV	476	
Chicken Deluxe	9 Oz	716	47	26	55	NV	1,419	
Taco	10.5 Oz	235	19	9	9	NV	268	
Taco Deluxe	9.2 Oz	741	49	26	57	NV	1,280	
Hardee's								
Chicken N Pasta	14.5 Oz	230	3	27	23	NV	380	
Jack In The Box								
Side W/O Dressing.....	4 Oz	70	4	4	3	2	80	A
Long John Silver's								
Garden........................	8.7 Oz	170	9	9	13	2	380	
Mixed Vegetables.......	4 Oz	60	2	2	9	6	330	
Ocean Chef Salad......	8.2 Oz	110	1	12	13	NV	730	

	Serv.	K-Cal.	Fat	Prot.	Carb.	Fib.	Sod.	FAC
(Salad, Fast Food cont.)								
Mighty Taco								
Beef Taco	14.2 Oz	438	18.5	24	45	5	858	
Chicken Taco..............	13.7 Oz	381	12	29	39	3	793	
Subway								
Roasted Chicken								
Breast.......................	10.5 Oz	143	3	20	9	1	845	A
Seafood & Crab.........	10.2 Oz	238	17	13	9	2	573	
Subway Club	10.2 Oz	123	3	14	10	1	1,041	A
Tuna...........................	10.2 Oz	345	31	9	9	1	604	A
Turkey	10 Oz	99	2	10	10	NV	1,083	A
Taco Bell								
Taco LT, W/Chips	19 Oz	680	25	35	81	10	1,620	AC
Taco Lt, W/O Chips ...	16.5 Oz	330	9	30	35	10	1,610	A
Taco Time								
Chicken Taco..............	11 Oz	571	31	32	41	NV	821	
Taco	9.2 Oz	447	20	24	44	NV	1,186	
Wendy's								
Caesar, W/O Dressing	3 Oz	110	5	8	8	2	660	
Chicken, W/O								
Dressing......................	12 Oz	200	8	25	10	4	690	AC
Garden Deluxe W/O								
Dressing......................	9.5 Oz	110	6	7	10	4	320	A
Side, W/O Dressing....	5.5 Oz	60	3	4	5	2	160	A
Taco	18 Oz	590	30	29	53	10	1,230	AC
Tuna...........................	2 Oz	100	6	7	4	0	270	
Salami								
(Serving size given in Oz to reflect weight of 1 slice)								
(Buon Gusto)..................	1 Oz	100	8	7	1	0	290	
(Gallo)..............................	1 Oz	110	8	7	1	0	580	
(Marco Polo)....................	1 Oz	110	8	7	1	0	580	
(Oscar Mayer):								
....	0.8 Oz	45	3.5	3	1	0	295	
Genoa	0.3 Oz	33	3	2	0	0	163	
Mixed Meat...................	0.8 Oz	55	4.5	3	0	0	250	
Thin Slice.....................	0.3 Oz	33	2.8	2	0	0	155	
(Louis Rich) Turkey........	1 Oz	40	2.5	4	0	0	280	
Salami, Alternative								
Meatless (Worthington)..	1 Slice	43	2.7	4	1	1	310	
Salmon								
Atlantic								
Raw, Farmed..................	3 Oz	120	5.4	17	0	0	37	
Broiled, Farmed..............	3 Oz	180	10.5	19	0	0	51	
Broiled, Wild	3 Oz	152	6.9	22	0	0	48	
Chinook								
Raw	3 Oz	153	9	17	0	0	49	

	Serv.	K-Cal.	Fat	Prot.	Carb.	Fib.	Sod.	FAC
Broiled	3 Oz	210	12	22	0	0	54	
Chum								
Raw	3 Oz	102	3.2	17	0	0	43	
Raw, Frozen	3 Oz	106	3	20	0	0	77	
Broiled	3 Oz	130	3.9	21	0	0	49	
Poached (9 Oz)	1 Cup	294	6.8	58	0	0	206	
Coho								
Raw, Farmed	3 Oz	136	6.5	18	0	0	40	
Raw, Frozen	3 Oz	102	3.9	17	0	0	63	
Raw, Wild	3 Oz	123	4.8	18	0	0	40	
Broiled, Farmed	3 Oz	151	7	21	0	0	44	
Broiled, Wild	3 Oz	120	3.6	20	0	0	48	
Poached, Farmed (9 Oz)	1 Cup	327	9.1	61	0	0	153	
Poached, Wild	3 Oz	156	6.4	23	0	0	45	
King, Alaska								
Raw	3 Oz	191	11.8	20	0	0	41	
Broiled	3 Oz	189	11.5	21	0	0	56	
Pink								
Raw	3 Oz	99	2.9	17	0	0	57	
Poached (9 Oz)	1 Cup	374	13.8	63	0	0	149	
Sockeye								
Raw	3 Oz	143	7.3	18	0	0	40	
Broiled	3 Oz	184	9.3	23	0	0	56	

Salmon, Canned
Pink

	Serv.	K-Cal.	Fat	Prot.	Carb.	Fib.	Sod.	FAC
(Bumble Bee)	2 Oz	70	2	14	0	0	220	
(Chicken of the Sea)	2 Oz	60	2	10	0	0	280	
(Chicken of the Sea)	1 Cup	360	20	48	0	0	1,080	
Red								
(Bumble Bee)	2 Oz	110	7	13	0	0	270	
Sockeye								
(Bumble Bee)	3.5 Oz	180	10	20	0	NV	500	
(S & W)	3 Oz	150	9	17	0	0	368	

Salmon, Smoked—Lox

	Serv.	K-Cal.	Fat	Prot.	Carb.	Fib.	Sod.	FAC
(Lasco)	2 Oz	60	1	10	3	0	960	
(Vita) Nova	3 Oz	80	1.5	11	1	NV	960	

Salsa
(Del Monte):

	Serv.	K-Cal.	Fat	Prot.	Carb.	Fib.	Sod.	FAC
Fire Roasted	1 Tbsp	5	0	0	1	0	105	
Garlic	1 Tbsp	5	0	0	1	0	105	
Thick & Chunky	1 Tbsp	5	0	0	1	0	105	
Traditional	1 Tbsp	5	0	0	1	0	105	
(Frito-Lay):								
Con Queso, *Tostitos*	1 Tbsp	20	1	1	3	0	325	
Doritos	1 Tbsp	8	0	0	2	1	100	

	Serv.	K-Cal.	Fat	Prot.	Carb.	Flb.	Sod.	FAC
(Salsa cont.)								
(Guiltless Gourmet):								
Red Pepper, Roasted.	1 Tbsp	5	0	0	1	0	60	
Southwestern Grill	1 Tbsp	5	0	0	1	0	75	
Tomatillo	1 Tbsp	5	0	0	1	1	80	
Tomato, Medium.........	1 Tbsp	5	0	0	1	0	70	
(Hunt's) Alfresco,								
Homestyle	1 Tbsp	5	0	0	1	0	910	
(Old El Paso):								
Cheese........................	1 Tbsp	20	1.5	0	2	0	150	
Chunky.......................	1 Tbsp	8	0	1	2	1	115	
Green Chili.................	1 Tbsp	5	0	0	1	0	55	
Picante, Mild..............	1 Tbsp	5	0	0	1	0	115	
(Rosarita):								
Chile, Green	1 Tbsp	4	0.1	0	1	0	84	
Extra Chunky	1 Tbsp	3	0.1	0	1	0	114	
Green Tomatillo	1 Tbsp	4	0.1	0	1	0	94	
Jalapeño Picante	1 Tbsp	4	0	0	1	0	120	
Roasted, Mild..............	1 Tbsp	5	0.2	0	1	0	116	
Traditional	1 Tbsp	4	0.1	0	1	0	117	
(S & W) *Sun Vista*	1 Tbsp	3	0	0	1	0	85	
Salsify—Oyster Plant								
Cooked	1 Cup	91	0.2	4	21	4	334	
Salt								
Idodized (Morton)	1 Tsp	0	0	0	0	0	2,300	
Kosher (Morton)	1 Tsp	0	0	0	0	0	1,800	
Non-Iodized (Morton)	1 Tsp	0	0	0	0	0	2,300	
Sea (Hain)	1 Tsp	0	0	0	0	0	2,255	
Salt Substitute, Seasoned								
(Dolph's)	1 Tsp	0	0	0	0	0	0	
(Health Valley) Instead								
of Salt	1 Tsp	11	0.5	1	2	0	3	
(Lawry's) Salt-Free.........	1 Tsp	3	0	0	1	0	7	
(Morton)	1 Tsp	2	0	1	0	0	0	
Sandwich, Fast Food								
Chicken								
(Arby's):								
BBQ	7 Oz	388	13	23	47	2	1,002	
Breast Fillet................	7.2 Oz	445	22.5	22	52	NV	958	
Deluxe Grilled.............	8 Oz	430	20	23	41	3	848	
Roast Deluxe, LT	7 Oz	276	6	20	33	4	848	
(Burger King):								
....	8 Oz	710	43	26	54	2	1,400	
Broiler...........................	8.7 Oz	550	29	30	41	2	480	A

	Serv.	K-Cal.	Fat	Prot.	Carb.	Flb.	Sod.	FAC
(Carl's Jr):								
BBQ	6.7 Oz	310	6	31	34	3	830	
Club	8.7 Oz	550	29	35	37	3	1,160	C
Santa Fe	8 Oz	530	30	30	36	3	1,230	
(Hardee's) Grilled	6.5 Oz	290	9	23	30	2	880	A
(Jack In The Box):								
	5.5 Oz	400	18	20	38	0	1,290	
Caesar	8.2 Oz	520	26	27	44	4	1,050	C
Ched/Bacon	7.7 Oz	540	30	30	37	0	1,520	C
Grilled	7.5 Oz	430	19	29	36	0	1,070	
Sourdough Ranch	8 Oz	490	21	29	45	1	1,060	
Spicy Crispy	8 Oz	560	27	24	55	0	1,020	A
Supreme	8.5 Oz	620	36	25	48	0	1,520	A
(KFC)	6 Oz	482	27	21	39	NV	1,060	A
(Subway):								
Breast	8.5 Oz	321	5	26	42	3	1,055	A
Chicken	8.2 Oz	317	5	26	43	2	1,065	A
(Wendy's):								
Breaded	7.2 Oz	440	18	28	44	2	840	
Club	7.7 Oz	500	23	32	44	2	1,090	
Grilled	6.2 Oz	290	7	24	35	2	720	
Fish								
(Arby's) Filet	7.7 Oz	529	27	23	50	2	864	
(Carl's Jr) *Catch Fish*	7.5 Oz	560	30	17	54	5	1,220	
(Jack In The Box)								
Supreme	8.7 Oz	590	32	22	51	0	1,170	
(Long John Silver's):								
	5.5 Oz	320	13	17	40	NV	800	
Platter	13.2 Oz	870	38	26	108	NV	1,110	AC
Ham								
(Arby's) W/Cheese	6 Oz	359	14	24	34	2	1,283	
(Subway)	7.5 Oz	270	4	17	42	2	1,291	A
Roast Beef								
(Arby's):								
Deluxe, LT	6.5 Oz	296	10	18	33	6	826	
Giant	8 Oz	555	28	35	43	5	1,561	
Jr	4.5 Oz	324	14	17	35	NV	779	
Regular	5.5 Oz	388	19	23	33	3	1,009	
Sub	10.7 Oz	700	42	38	44	4	2,034	C
(Carl's Jr) Deluxe	9.2 Oz	540	26	28	46	NV	1,340	AC
(Hardee's)	5.6 Oz	410	23	24	28	1	1,140	
Tuna								
(Arby's) Sub	10 Oz	663	37	74	50	NV	1,342	C
(Subway) Wheat, LT								
Mayo	8.2 Oz	372	15	15	43	3	866	A
Turkey								
(Arby's):								
Deluxe	8.2 Oz	510	24	28	46	NV	1,220	

	Serv.	K-Cal.	Fat	Prot.	Carb.	Flb.	Sod.	FAC
(Sandwich, Fast Food cont.)								
Deluxe, LT Roast	7 Oz	260	7	20	33	4	1,262	
Sub..............................	9.7 Oz	550	27	31	47	2	2,084	AC
(Carl's Jr) Club..............	9.2 Oz	530	23	30	50	NV	2,890	C
(Subway):								
Jumbo Del	8.2 Oz	290	6	22	37	1	1,926	
White............................	7.5 Oz	273	4	16	44	2	1,303	A
Vegetable								
(Subway) *Veggie*								
Delite........................	5.5 Oz	219	2	8	42	2	526	A

Sandwich, Frozen

(Serving size given in Oz to reflect weight of 1 serving)

	Serv.	K-Cal.	Fat	Prot.	Carb.	Flb.	Sod.	FAC
(Amy's Kitchen) *Pocketful:*								
Cheese Pizza	4.5 Oz	290	9	14	38	3	390	C
Spinach Feta	4.5 Oz	200	7	9	27	2	420	C
Vegetable Pot Pie	4.5 Oz	230	6	7	37	2	420	A
(Hot Pockets):								
Beef and Cheddar......	4.5 Oz	360	18	14	36	1	830	C
Ham & Cheese...........	4.5 Oz	340	15	14	37	4	840	C
Pepperoni....................	4.5 Oz	350	17	13	38	2	780	C
Turkey & Ham W/ Cheese..........................	4.5 Oz	320	13	14	35	1	680	C
(Red Baron) *Pizza Pouches:*								
Ham & Cheese...........	1 Item	320	15	14	33	1	980	
Pepperoni....................	1 Item	340	17	15	32	2	740	C
Steak & Cheese	1 Item	280	12	12	32	1	840	
(Wt Watchers):								
Bagel/Ham/Cheese.....	3 Oz	200	5	12	27	1	470	
Chicken Broc Ched	5 Oz	250	6	13	40	1	310	
Classic Omelet	3.7 Oz	220	5	15	26	2	410	C
Dijon Turkey Pretzel...	4 Oz	230	4	16	36	3	500	
English Muffin	4 Oz	210	5	13	28	2	420	
Garden Omelet	3.5 Oz	220	6	10	31	2	440	
Grilled Chicken	4 Oz	210	5	18	24	2	420	
Ham & Cheddar Pretzel	4 Oz	260	8	15	33	3	580	
Ham & Cheese Pocket	5 Oz	240	7	14	32	5	480	
Pizza Pocket...............	5 Oz	300	7	17	46	4	490	
Reuben Pocket...........	5 Oz	250	6	12	42	5	400	

Sandwich Seasoning Mix

	Serv.	K-Cal.	Fat	Prot.	Carb.	Flb.	Sod.	FAC
(Hunt's) *Manwich:*								
Barbeque	4 Tbsp	60	0.2	1	14	1	888	
Bold.............................	4 Tbsp	65	1	1	13	NV	802	
Burrito	4 Tbsp	25	0.2	1	5	NV	560	
Mexican.......................	4 Tbsp	26	0.2	1	4	1	560	
Original.......................	4 Tbsp	32	0.4	1	6	1	365	

	Serv.	K-Cal.	Fat	Prot.	Carb.	Fib.	Sod.	FAC
Taco	4 Tbsp	32	0.1	1	8	1	590	
Thick & Chunky	4 Tbsp	44	0.5	1	9	1	740	

Sandwich Spreads (See Luncheon Meat, Canned)

Sapodilla
Raw (6 Oz)	1 Item	141	1.9	1	34	9	20	A
Raw	1 Cup	200	2.7	1	48	13	30	A

Sapote
Raw (8 Oz)	1 Item	302	1.4	5	76	6	23	A

Sardine, Canned
Packed In Water
(Chicken of the Sea)	3 Oz	150	10	14	0	0	75	C

Packed in Oil
(Chicken of the Sea)
Smoked	3 Oz	220	16	18	0	0	400	C
(King Oscar)	3 Oz	240	16	18	0	0	350	C
(S & W) Norwegian								
Brisling	2 Oz	160	13	10	0	0	190	
Skinless/Boneless	2 Oz	100	6	12	0	0	250	
(Spirit of Norway)	3 Oz	240	16	18	0	0	350	C

Sauce (See individual listings)

Sauerkraut
(Claussen)	½ Cup	10	0	0	2	2	420	
(Del Monte)	½ Cup	25	0	1	6	NV	775	
(Eden) Organic	½ Cup	25	0	2	4	3	580	
(S & W)	½ Cup	20	0	0	2	0	720	

Sausage
Beef
(Eckrich)	1 Oz	100	9	3	<1	0	275	
(Hillshire Farm):								
Cheddar, Smoked	1 Oz	95	7.5	4	1	0	250	
Hot Links	1 Oz	95	8.5	4	1	0	280	
Smoked	1 Oz	90	8	4	1	0	245	
Smoked, Bun Size	1 Oz	90	8	4	1	0	285	
Summer, Semi-Dry	1 Oz	95	8.5	5	1	0	306	
(Jones Dairy Farm)								
Golden	1 Item	75	6.1	4	0	0	159	
(Oscar Mayer) Smokies	1.5 Oz	120	11	5	1	0	420	
(Swift) Premium	1 Item	120	12	4	1	0	250	

Bratwurst
(Eckrich)	1 Item	310	30	11	1	0	820	

	Serv.	K-Cal.	Fat	Prot.	Carb.	Flb.	Sod.	FAC
(Sausage cont.)								
(Hillshire Farm):								
Fresh..........................	1 Oz	95	8.5	4	1	0	205	
Fresh, Spicy................	1 Oz	90	8.5	4	1	0	245	
Link, Fully Cooked......	1 Oz	85	8	4	1	0	190	
Breakfast								
(Healthy Choice):								
Links...........................	1 Item	25	0.8	4	2	0	150	
Patty...........................	1 Item	25	0.8	4	2	0	150	
(Louis Rich) Turkey........	1 Oz	60	4	6	1	0	220	
(Mr. Turkey)..................	1 Oz	76	5.4	7	0	0	266	
(Shelton) Turkey Link.....	1 Item	140	14	6	0	0	260	
(Swift Premium)								
Brown & Serve...........	2 Oz	210	19	7	2	0	410	
(Turkey Store) Link	1 Oz	70	5.5	4	1	0	180	
Cheese								
(Hillshire Farm):								
Cheddarwurst..............	1 Oz	95	8.5	4	1	0	240	
Summer,, Semi-Dry	1 Oz	100	9	5	1	0	302	
(Oscar Mayer):								
Cheese Smokies	1 Item	130	12	6	1	0	450	
Lil' Cheese Smokies...	1 Item	30	2.7	1	0	0	100	
Chicken								
(Brooks Farm) Lemon....	3 Oz	120	5	15	2	0	510	
Italian								
(Hillshire Farm):								
Hot, Fresh...................	1 Oz	90	8.5	4	1	0	250	
Mild, Fresh..................	1 Oz	95	8.5	4	1	0	245	
NY Style Pork	1 Item	170	19	14	1	0	780	
Kielbasa								
(Armour)	1 Item	230	19	9	5	0	820	
(Healthy Choice) LF........	1 Item	100	3	11	7	0	480	
(Hillshire Farm):								
Beef.............................	1 Oz	95	8.5	4	1	0	275	
LT................................	1 Oz	65	5.5	4	1	0	256	
Mild.............................	1 Oz	95	8.5	4	1	0	265	
(John Morrel).................	1 Item	270	23	10	4	0	1,100	
Knockwurst								
(Hillshire Farm)...............	1 Oz	90	8	4	1	0	230	
Pork								
(Hormel):								
Brown & Serve	1 Item	77	7	3	0	0	222	
Little Sizzlers	1 Item	77	7	3	0	0	200	
(Jimmy Dean).................	1 Item	97	9	3	0	0	166	
(Jimmy Dean).................	2 Oz	250	24	10	0	0	540	
(Jones Dairy Farm)								
Brown & Serve	1 Item	95	9	3	1	0	140	
(Oscar Mayer)	1 Item	90	8	5	1	0	225	

	Serv.	K-Cal.	Fat	Prot.	Carb.	Fib.	Sod.	FAC
Smoked								
(Armour) *Hot & Spicy*	1 Item	230	19	9	5	NV	820	
(Healthy Choice):								
....	1 Oz	35	0.8	5	3	0	240	
LF.................................	1 Item	100	3	12	7	0	480	
(Hillshire Farm):								
....	1 Oz	95	9	4	1	0	260	
Country Recipe...........	1 Oz	90	8	4	1	0	245	
Flavorseal, LT.............	1 Oz	65	5.5	4	1	0	256	
(John Morrel)	1 Item	270	23	10	4	0	1,100	
(Old Smokehouse)								
Summer	1 Oz	110	10	4	1	0	400	
(Oscar Mayer) Smokie....	1 Item	130	12	5	1	0	430	
Turkey								
(Butterball) Sweet								
Italian	1 Item	170	10	19	0	0	640	
(Louis Rich):								
....	1 Item	45	3	6	0	0	235	
Hot/Original	1 Oz	48	3.2	5	0	0	172	
(Mr. Turkey):								
Polish	1 Item	47	2.7	4	1	0	259	
Smoked........................	1 Oz	46	2.6	4	1	0	309	
(Shelton's):								
Italian	1 Item	160	16	7	0	0	310	
Patty.............................	1 Item	140	11	10	0	0	370	
(Turkey Store) Italian,								
Hot	1 Oz	47	3	5	1	0	227	
Sausage, Alternative								
(Ivy Food) *Meat of*								
Wheat..........................	3.5 Oz	199	0.9	34	13	NV	330	
(Morningstar):								
Breakfast Links...........	1 Item	32	1.2	4	1	1	169	
Breakfast Patty	1 Item	68	2.8	8	2	2	264	
Breakfast Strip............	1 Item	28	2.2	1	1	0	110	
Garden Vege Patty.....	1 Item	104	2.6	11	9	4	382	
Grillers........................	1 Item	140	6.9	14	5	3	256	
(Natural Touch) Pattie,								
Garden Grain..............	1 Item	160	8	7	15	NV	200	
Savory								
(McCormick)	1 Tsp	7	0	0	2	1	0	
Scallion (See Onion, Green)								
Scallop								
Raw	1 Item	26	0.2	5	1	0	48	
Raw	3 Oz	74	0.7	16	2	0	155	
Raw	1 Cup	119	1	23	3	0	217	

	Serv.	K-Cal.	Fat	Prot.	Carb.	Fib.	Sod.	FAC
(Scallop cont.)								
Fried, Breaded	1 Item	33	1.7	3	2	0	72	
Steamed	3 Oz	93	1.2	19	2	0	225	

Scallop Alternative (See Surimi)

Scallop Entree, Frozen

	Serv.	K-Cal.	Fat	Prot.	Carb.	Fib.	Sod.	FAC
(Mrs. Paul's) Fried	1 Piece	17	0.7	1	2	0	30	
(Stouffer's) Lean Cuisine, W/Vegeta-								
bles/Rice	1 Item	220	3	17	32	NV	1,200	
(Stouffer's) W/Shrimp								
Mariner.......................	1 Item	400	16	23	40	NV	1,120	

Scone

	Serv.	K-Cal.	Fat	Prot.	Carb.	Fib.	Sod.	FAC
Gluten-Free (Ener-G)	1 Item	429	23.2	5	37	1	566	
Plain..............................	1 Item	150	6.6	4	19	1	246	
Whole Wheat.................	1 Item	145	6.7	5	18	3	174	

Sea Bass

	Serv.	K-Cal.	Fat	Prot.	Carb.	Fib.	Sod.	FAC
Raw, All Varieties...........	3 Oz	83	1.7	16	0	0	58	
Broiled	3 Oz	105	2.2	20	0	0	74	

Seafood Entree, Frozen

	Serv.	K-Cal.	Fat	Prot.	Carb.	Fib.	Sod.	FAC
Creole/Rice (Swanson) ..	8 Oz	214	5.4	6	36	1	720	A
Gumbo (Hormel)	8 Oz	80	1	10	6	NV	1,168	
Newburg (Budget								
Gourmet).....................	10 Oz	350	12	17	43	0	660	FA
Newburg (Healthy								
Choice)........................	8 Oz	200	3	13	30	1	440	

Seasoning and Coating Mix
Chicken
(Kraft):

	Serv.	K-Cal.	Fat	Prot.	Carb.	Fib.	Sod.	FAC
Shake 'N Bake	1 Pkg	320	8	8	56	0	1,840	F
Shake 'N Bake, BBQ .	1 Pkg	360	8	0	72	0	3,280	A
Shake 'N Bake, Italian								
Herb......................	1 Pkg	320	4	8	56	0	2,400	
Oven Fried, Extra								
Crispy	1 Pkg	480	8	16	80	0	3,360	F
Oven Fried, Home								
Style	1 Pkg	320	8	8	56	0	3,760	

Fish

	Serv.	K-Cal.	Fat	Prot.	Carb.	Fib.	Sod.	FAC
(Kraft) Shake 'N Bake....	1 Pkg	280	6	4	56	4	1,680	

Pork

	Serv.	K-Cal.	Fat	Prot.	Carb.	Fib.	Sod.	FAC
Oven Fried, Extra Crispy	1 Pkg	480	12	16	88	0	2,720	F
(Kraft) Shake 'N Bake,								
BBQ	1 Pkg	280	0	0	64	0	2,000	A

	Serv.	K-Cal.	Fat	Prot.	Carb.	Fib.	Sod.	FAC
Seasoning, Dry Mix								
(Bag 'N Season):								
Beef Stew	1 Tsp	15	0	1	2	NV	670	
Chicken	1 Tbsp	20	0	1	4	0	460	
Meatloaf	1 Tsp	8	0	1	1	0	195	
Pork Chop	1 Tsp	8	0	0	2	NV	295	
Pot Roast	1 Tsp	10	0	1	1	NV	390	
Spareribs	1 Tbsp	30	0	1	6	1	590	
Swiss Steak	1 Tsp	15	0	0	3	NV	430	
(Kikkoman):								
Chinese Chicken	1 Tbsp	25	0	1	4	0	1,980	
Chow Mein	1 Tbsp	20	0	1	3	0	0	
Sichuan Shrimp	1 Tbsp	23	0	0	4	0	480	
Stir Fry, Broc/Beef	1 Tbsp	23	0	1	5	0	720	
Thai Noodles	1 Tbsp	30	0	0	6	0	645	
(McCormick):								
Beef Stew	1 Tsp	8	0	0	2	0	205	
Chili	1 Tbsp	23	0.4	1	4	1	233	
Fried Rice	1 Tbsp	20	0	1	4	0	600	
Sloppy Joes	1 Tsp	15	0	0	3	0	350	
Stir Fry	1 Tsp	10	0	0	2	0	260	
Taco, Mild	1 Tsp	10	0	0	2	0	230	
(Old El Paso):								
Burrito	1 Tsp	10	0	0	2	1	145	
Taco	1 Tsp	10	0	0	3	0	275	
Seaweed								
Raw								
Irish Moss	1 Oz	14	0	0	3	0	19	F
Kelp, Kombu	1 Oz	12	0.2	0	3	0	66	F
Laver, Nori	1 Oz	10	0.1	2	1	0	14	F
Wakame	1 Oz	13	0.2	1	3	0	247	F
Dried								
Agar	1 Oz	87	0.1	2	23	2	29	F
Alaria, Maine	1 Cup	54	0	3	9	9	904	AC
Black, Alaska	1 Cup	40	0.3	4	6	NV	150	F
Dulse	1 Cup	45	0.6	5	8	1	86	F
Hai-Tai	1 Oz	71	0.3	0	17	2	574	F
Kelp, Maine	1 Cup	51	0	3	9	9	937	F
Laver, Nori, Maine	1 Cup	66	0	6	9	9	339	FA
Ribbon, Alaska	1 Cup	42	0.1	3	8	4	162	F
Spirulina	1 Oz	82	2.2	16	7	1	297	F
(Eden):								
Agar Agar Bar	1 Tbsp	10	0	0	2	2	10	
Arame	1 Cup	60	0	2	15	14	240	F
Hiziki	1 Cup	60	0	0	12	12	320	FC
Kombu (4" Piece)	1 Item	10	0	0	2	1	90	
Nori	1 Piece	10	0	1	1	1	5	
Wakame	1 Cup	50	0	4	8	8	1,320	F

	Serv.	K-Cal.	Fat	Prot.	Carb.	Flb.	Sod.	FAC
(*Seaweed cont.*)								
Wakame Flakes, Instant	1 Cup	50	0	4	8	8	1,440	F

Seitan
(Arrowhead Mills) Quick Mix	1 Cup	450	3	63	42	6	60	
(Grand Life)	2 Oz	74	1	14	2	0	242	
(Light Life) BBQ	4 Oz	160	2	24	12	0	360	
Teriyaki	4 Oz	160	2	26	10	0	320	
(White Wave) Philly Steak	1 Slice	20	0	5	1	0	35	
Traditional	1 Piece	140	0	31	4	1	240	

Seltzer (See Soft Drink, Unflavored)

Semolina
Flour	1 Oz	102	0.3	4	21	1	0	
Flour	1 Cup	601	1.8	21	122	7	2	F

Sesame Butter (Also See Tahini)
(Bearitos)	2 Tbsp	220	19	6	6	NV	35	
(Maranatha)	2 Tbsp	200	17	6	8	2	0	C
(Roaster Fresh)	2 Tbsp	168	15	5	6	0	3	

Sesame Flour
LF	1 Cup	333	1.8	50	36	NV	39	
Meal, Partially Defatted	1 Oz	160	13.6	5	7	NV	11	

Sesame Oil
(Eden) Toasted	1 Tbsp	130	14	0	0	0	0	A
(Spectrum)	1 Tbsp	120	14	0	0	0	0	A

Sesame Seed
Decorticated	1 Tsp	16	1.5	1	0	0	1	
Whole, Roasted	1 Oz	160	13.6	5	7	4	3	C
(Arrowhead Mills) Kernel	1 Cup	840	80	28	20	20	0	FAC
Whole Brown (5 Oz)	1 Cup	800	80	28	32	20	40	FAC
(McCormick) Whole, Raw	1 Tsp	21	1.6	1	0	0	7	

Sesame Seed Seasoning
(Eden):								
Garlic, Organic	1 Tsp	20	1	0	0	0	70	
Plain, Organic	1 Tsp	20	1	0	0	0	80	
Seaweed, Organic	1 Tsp	20	1	0	0	0	70	

	Serv.	K-Cal.	Fat	Prot.	Carb.	Fib.	Sod.	FAC
Sesame Stick								
(Barbara's)	1 Oz	103	2.3	5	20	0	400	
(Flavor Tree)	½ Cup	270	18.2	6	21	0	700	
Shad, American								
Raw	3 Oz	172	12	15	0	0	45	
Broiled	3 Oz	214	15	19	0	0	55	
Shallot								
Raw	1 Tbsp	1	0	0	0	NV	0	
Freeze-Dried	1 Tbsp	3	0	0	1	NV	1	
Shark								
Raw	3 Oz	110	3.8	18	0	0	67	
Fin	1 Oz	108	0	27	0	0	8	
Fried W/Batter	3 Oz	194	11.7	16	5	0	104	
Sheanut Oil								
	1 Tbsp	120	14	0	0	0	0	
Sheephead								
Raw	3 Oz	92	2	17	0	0	60	
Cooked	3 Oz	107	1.4	22	0	0	62	
Sherbet (See Sorbet)								
Shortbread (See Cookie, Shortbread)								
Shortening								
(Crisco)	1 Tbsp	110	12	0	0	0	0	A
(Crisco) Butter Flavor	1 Tbsp	110	12	0	0	0	0	A
(Wesson)	1 Tbsp	100	12	0	0	0	0	A
Shoyu (See Soy Sauce)								
Shrimp								
Fresh								
Raw	3 Oz	90	1.5	16	1	0	125	
Boiled	1 Cup	127	1.4	27	0	0	287	
Boiled, Bay	1 Cup	90	0	22	0	0	800	
Fried	3 Oz	206	10.4	18	10	0	292	
Canned								
(Crown Prince)	2 Oz	60	0.5	13	<1	0	360	
(Orleans)	2 Oz	44	0	10	0	0	650	
(Pacific Pearl)	2 Oz	70	0.5	15	1	0	310	
Frozen								
(Contessa) Cooked	3 Oz	60	0	13	0	0	480	
Uncooked	4 Oz	80	0	2	1	0	470	

	Serv.		K-Cal.	Fat	Prot.	Carb.	Fib.	Sod.	FAC

Shrimp Alternative (See Surimi)

Shrimp Entree, Frozen

	Serv.		K-Cal.	Fat	Prot.	Carb.	Fib.	Sod.	FAC
Creole (Light and Elegant)	10	Oz	200	2	11	31	2	1,045	A
Creole (Ultra Slim-Fast)	12	Oz	240	4	12	45	3	430	A
Marinara (Healthy Choice)	10.5	Oz	220	0.5	10	44	5	220	A
Marinara (Ultra Slim-Fast)	12	Oz	290	3	17	53	5	280	A
Marinara (Wt Watchers)	9	Oz	200	2	8	37	4	590	A
Primavera (Right Course)	10	Oz	240	7	12	32	NV	590	
W/Chicken Cantonese, *Lean Cuisine*, (Stouffer's)	10	Oz	270	9	22	25	NV	920	
W/Clams, Linguini, LT (Mrs. Paul's)	10	Oz	240	5	12	36	4	750	
W/Vegetable Marinara (Healthy Choice)	12.5	Oz	270	3	15	46	5	540	A
W/Vegetable, Stir Fry (Chef Choice)	5	Oz	118	1	10	17	1	470	A

Shrimp Paste

	Serv.		K-Cal.	Fat	Prot.	Carb.	Fib.	Sod.	FAC
Canned	1	Cup	608	31.8	70	5	0	473	FC
Canned	1	Oz	46	0.6	8	2	0	405	

Shrimp, Prepared, Frozen

	Serv.		K-Cal.	Fat	Prot.	Carb.	Fib.	Sod.	FAC
(Gorton's):									
Beer Batter	3.3	Oz	250	15	9	19	0	630	
Breaded	3.2	Oz	230	13	10	18	0	550	
Popcorn	3	Oz	240	13	9	22	0	780	
Scampi	3.2	Oz	250	16	9	18	0	410	
(Van De Kamp's)									
Breaded	4	Oz	280	14	12	28	2	58	

Smelt

	Serv.		K-Cal.	Fat	Prot.	Carb.	Fib.	Sod.	FAC
Raw	3	Oz	83	2.1	15	0	0	51	
Broiled	3	Oz	105	2.6	19	0	0	66	
Canned	1	Item	40	2.7	4	0	0	NV	
Dried, Alaska	3.3	Oz	361	11.9	59	0	0	NV	
Fried, Breaded	1	Cup	652	32.5	56	32	9	1,393	

Smoothie

	Serv.		K-Cal.	Fat	Prot.	Carb.	Fib.	Sod.	FAC
(Odwalla):									
Boyzenberry Mango	1	Cup	140	0	1	34	2	20	A
Raspberry	1	Cup	140	0	4	20	4	26	A

	Serv.	K-Cal.	Fat	Prot.	Carb.	Fib.	Sod.	FAC
Strawberry Banana.....	1 Cup	100	0	1	28	4	10	**A**

Snack Bar (Also See Breakfast Bar; Diet Bar; Sport Bar)
Chocolate
(Fi-Bar) W/Almonds........	1 Item	140	4.5	3	23	2	25	
(Health Valley) W/								
Cherry, FF	1 Item	110	0	3	26	4	30	

Fruit
(Barbara's):								
Apple, FF	1 Item	50	0	1	13	0	10	
Apricot, FF..................	1 Item	50	0	1	11	0	10	
Raspberry, FF.............	1 Item	50	0	1	13	0	10	
(Fi-Bar) Cranberry, LF ...	1 Item	120	2.5	1	27	3	25	
Yogurt Coated, Berry .	1 Item	120	2	2	23	4	15	
(Health Valley):								
Apple FF	1 Item	140	0	3	35	3	0	
Apricot Bake	1 Item	100	3	2	16	2	15	
Date Bakes, FF	1 Item	70	0	2	18	2	30	
Fruit & Fitness.............	1 Item	100	2.5	2	18	2	13	
Oat Bran/Nuts.............	1 Item	150	4	4	28	3	5	
Raisin, FF	1 Item	140	0	2	35	3	5	

Granola
(Barbara's):								
Apple Filling, FF	1 Item	110	0	2	27	2	90	
Blueberry, FF..............	1 Item	110	0	2	27	2	90	
Choc Chip....................	1 Item	80	2	1	15	1	5	
Oat/Honey...................	1 Item	80	2	2	15	2	85	
Peanut Butter..............	1 Item	80	3	2	14	2	5	
(Ener-G) Almond	1 Item	150	7.7	6	14	2	23	
(Health Valley):								
Blueberry, FF..............	1 Item	140	0	2	35	3	5	
Date Almond, FF........	1 Item	140	0	2	35	3	5	
Raisin, FF	1 Item	140	0	2	35	3	5	
Strawberry, FF	1 Item	140	0	2	35	3	5	
(Kellogg's) Nutri-Grain:								
Almond, LF	1 Item	80	1.5	2	16	1	60	
Apple Cinnamon	1 Item	140	3	2	27	1	60	
Cinn Raisin, LF...........	1 Item	80	1.5	2	16	1	60	
Strawberry...................	1 Item	140	3	2	27	1	60	
(Nature Valley):								
Cinnamon.....................	1 Item	105	4	2	17	1	70	
Clusters.......................	1 Item	150	3	2	28	2	115	
Oat Bran	1 Item	105	4	3	16	2	85	
Oats 'N Honey.............	1 Item	100	3	2	18	2	85	
Peanut Butter..............	1 Item	110	5	3	15	1	75	

Snack Mix
(Fisher) Nut 'N Crunchies:								
Fiesta	1 Cup	560	28	16	64	4	1,320	

	Serv.	K-Cal.	Fat	Prot.	Carb.	Fib.	Sod.	FAC
(Snack Mix cont.)								
Golden Crisp	1 Cup	560	28	16	60	4	1,280	
Honey	1 Cup	560	24	16	68	4	840	
(General Mills) *Chex*:								
BBQ	1 Cup	260	10	6	42	4	800	F
Cheddar	1 Cup	260	8	6	40	2	620	F
Traditional	1 Cup	225	7.5	5	35	3	615	F
(Pepperidge Farm):								
Classic	1 Oz	140	8	4	14	NV	360	
Smoked	1 Oz	150	9	4	13	NV	350	
Spicy	1 Oz	140	8	4	14	NV	340	

Snail—Escargot

	Serv.	K-Cal.	Fat	Prot.	Carb.	Fib.	Sod.	FAC
Raw	3 Oz	75	1.2	14	2	0	60	A
Raw, Giant African	3 Oz	63	1.2	8	4	0	60	A
Broiled	3 Oz	111	3.7	15	2	0	95	A
Steamed	3 Oz	150	2.4	27	3	0	100	A

Snap Bean (See Green Bean)

Snap Pea (See Pea, Fresh)

Snapper

	Serv.	K-Cal.	Fat	Prot.	Carb.	Fib.	Sod.	FAC
Raw, Golden Striped	3 Oz	90	1.5	18	0	0	66	
Raw, Red	3 Oz	90	1.9	18	0	0	75	
Broiled	3 Oz	109	1.5	22	0	0	48	

Snow Pea (See Pea, Frozen)

Soba (See Noodle, Soba)

Soda (See Soft Drink)

Soft Drink (Also See Water)
Cherry

	Serv.	K-Cal.	Fat	Prot.	Carb.	Fib.	Sod.	FAC
(Coca-Cola) Cherry								
Cola	1 Cup	104	0	0	28	0	4	
(Dr Pepper)	1 Cup	101	0.3	0	26	0	25	
Diet	1 Cup	2	0	0	0	0	12	
(Minute Maid) Black								
Cherry	1 Cup	110	0	0	29	0	11	
(Pepsi) Wild	1 Cup	112	0	0	29	0	0	
(R.W. Knudsen) Spritzer	1 Cup	113	0	0	28	0	13	
(Shasta) Cherry Cola	1 Cup	92	0	0	25	0	15	
(Snapple) Cherry Lime								
Rickey	1 Cup	110	0	0	27	0	0	
French Cherry	1 Cup	120	0	0	29	0	0	

	Serv.	K-Cal.	Fat	Prot.	Carb.	Flb.	Sod.	FAC
Citrus								
(Coca-Cola):								
Fresca	1 Cup	3	0	0	0	0	1	
Mello Yello	1 Cup	120	0	0	32	0	9	
Mello Yello, Diet	1 Cup	3	0	0	0	0	0	
(Mountain Dew)	1 Cup	118	0	0	1	0	0	
Cola								
(Coca-Cola):								
	1 Cup	105	0	0	29	0	4	
Classic	1 Cup	96	0	0	27	0	10	
Diet	1 Cup	1	0	0	0	0	4	
Mr. Pibb	1 Cup	96	0	0	28	0	7	
Mr. Pibb, Diet	1 Cup	1	0	0	0	0	4	
Tab	1 Cup	1	0	0	0	0	4	
(Hansen's) Diet	1 Cup	8	0	0	2	0	0	
(Pepsi)	1 Cup	104	0	0	26	0	0	
Diet	1 Cup	0	0	0	0	0	1	
(Shasta)	1 Cup	97	0	0	26	0	0	
(Spree)	1 Cup	97	0	0	26	0	0	
Creme								
(A & W)	1 Cup	112	0	1	29	0	16	
(Hire)	1 Cup	117	0	1	31	0	52	
(Snapple)	1 Cup	130	0	0	33	0	0	
Fruit								
(Hansen) Peach Mango	1 Cup	88	0	0	24	0	0	
(Health Valley) Wild Berry	1 Cup	95	0.6	1	22	0	18	
(Minute Maid):								
Peach	1 Cup	110	0	0	29	0	9	
Pineapple	1 Cup	110	0	0	30	0	9	
Raspberry	1 Cup	111	0	0	30	0	9	
Strawberry	1 Cup	122	0	0	33	0	9	
(R.W. Knudsen) Mango Fandango	1 Cup	127	0	1	30	0	20	
(Snapple):								
Kiwi Strawberry	1 Cup	130	0	0	33	0	6	
Passion Supreme	1 Cup	120	0	0	29	0	0	
Peach Melba	1 Cup	120	0	0	31	0	4	
Ginger Ale								
(Canada Dry)	1 Cup	90	0	0	21	0	7	
(Coca-Cola) Fanta	1 Cup	86	0	0	23	0	4	
(Health Valley)	1 Cup	102	0.6	1	24	0	20	
(R.W. Knudsen) Spritzer	1 Cup	107	0	1	27	0	17	
(Schweppes)	1 Cup	86	0	0	21	0	13	
(Shasta)	1 Cup	80	0	0	22	0	8	
(Spree)	1 Cup	80	0	0	22	0	0	
Grape								
(Canada Dry)	1 Cup	130	0	0	32	0	21	
(Coca-Cola) Fanta	1 Cup	117	0	0	31	0	9	

	Serv.	K-Cal.	Fat	Prot.	Carb.	Fib.	Sod.	FAC
(Soft Drinks cont.)								
(Minute Maid)	1 Cup	121	0	0	32	0	9	
(R.W. Knudsen) Spritzer	1 Cup	113	0	1	27	0	20	
(Schweppes)....................	1 Cup	124	0	0	31	0	20	
Lemon								
(Minute Maid) Lemonade	1 Cup	106	0	0	28	0	0	
(Schweppes) Bitter								
Lemon	1 Cup	107	0	0	27	0	17	
Sour Lemon	1 Cup	103	0	0	25	0	16	
Lemon-Lime								
(Coca-Cola) *Fresca*........	1 Cup	3	0	0	0	0	1	
(Hansen's)	1 Cup	88	0	0	24	0	0	
(R.W. Knudsen) Spritzer	1 Cup	113	0	1	28	0	17	
(Schweppes)....................	1 Cup	96	0	0	24	0	40	
(7-Up)	1 Cup	98	0	0	26	0	17	
(Slice)	1 Cup	99	0	0	25	0	45	
(Spree).............................	1 Cup	102	0	0	28	0	0	
(Sprite).............................	1 Cup	96	0	0	26	0	22	
Diet..............................	1 Cup	3	0	0	0	0	0	
Orange								
(Coca-Cola) *Fanta*..........	1 Cup	118	0	0	32	0	9	
(Minute Maid)	1 Cup	118	0	0	32	0	0	
Diet..............................	1 Cup	2	0	0	0	0	0	
(Orangina)	1 Cup	94	0	0	23	0	90	
Root Beer								
(Coca-Cola)	1 Cup	120	0	0	34	0	4	
Fanta............................	1 Cup	111	0	0	29	0	4	
(Hansen's) Creamy	1 Cup	104	0	0	29	0	0	
(Health Valley) Old-								
Fashioned	1 Cup	80	0.6	1	17	0	8	
Sarsaparilla	1 Cup	102	0.6	1	23	0	18	
(Snapple)	1 Cup	110	0	0	29	0	0	
Unflavored								
Club, Carbonated............	1 Cup	0	0	0	0	0	50	
Tonic Water/Quinine,								
Carbonated	1 Cup	83	0	0	21	0	10	
(Schweppes) Seltzer	1 Cup	0	0	0	0	0	8	

Sorbet—Sherbet (Also See Fruit Bar, Frozen)

	Serv.	K-Cal.	Fat	Prot.	Carb.	Fib.	Sod.	FAC
(Baskin Robbins):								
Pink Raspberry								
Lemonade, FF.........	1 Cup	220	0	0	58	0	20	
Raspberry, FF..............	1 Cup	240	0	0	60	0	20	
Raspberry Cranberry,								
FF	1 Cup	220	0	0	58	0	20	
(Ben & Jerry's):								
Cranberry Orange, FF	1 Cup	260	0	0	64	0	20	A
Devil's Food.................	1 Cup	320	4	4	72	4	120	
Mango Lime, FF	1 Cup	260	0	0	64	0	20	A

	Serv.	K-Cal.	Fat	Prot.	Carb.	Fib.	Sod.	FAC
Strawberry Kiwi, FF....	1 Cup	260	0	0	66	0	40	A
(Häagen-Dazs):								
Orange W/Cream	1 Cup	401	18	5	54	0	93	A
Raspberry W/Cream...	1 Cup	373	18.2	5	47	1	91	
(Healthy Choice):								
Orange W/Cream	1 Cup	180	4	4	34	2	100	C
Raspberry Sorbet	1 Cup	180	4	4	34	2	100	C
Strawberry...................	1 Cup	180	4	4	34	2	100	C

Sorghum

Dry, Whole	1 Cup	651	6.3	22	143	NV	12	C
Syrup	1 Cup	565	0	0	150	0	22	C
Syrup	1 Tbsp	61	0	0	16	0	2	

Sorrel

Fresh	1 Cup	30	1	3	4	1	6	A

Soup, Bouillon

Beef

(Bovril)	2 Tsp	15	0	2	1	0	1,840	
(Hormel) *Herb-Ox*...........	1 Cube	10	0	0	1	0	700	
(Knorr)	½ Cube	20	1.5	1	1	0	1,200	
(Maggi)	1 Cube	5	0	0	0	0	1,120	
(Steero):								
....	1 Cube	5	0	0	1	0	600	
Granular.....................	1 Tsp	5	0	0	1	0	900	
Reduced Sodium........	1 Tsp	5	0	0	1	0	600	
(Wt Watchers)	1 Pkg	10	0	0	2	0	800	

Chicken

(Bovril)	2 Tsp	5	0	0	0	0	740	
(Hormel) *Herb-Ox*...........	1 Cube	10	0	0	1	0	1,040	
(Knorr)	½ Cube	20	1.5	1	1	0	1,200	
(Maggi)	1 Cube	5	0	0	0	0	1,060	
(Wt Watchers)	1 Pkg	10	0	0	2	0	830	

Fish

(Knorr)	½ Cube	10	1	1	0	0	960	

Vegetable

(Knorr)	½ Cube	15	1	1	1	0	980	
(Maggi)	1 Cube	5	0	0	1	0	820	

Soup, Canned

(All soups ready to serve unless indicated condensed [cond])

Asparagus, Cream of

(Campbell's) PFC...........	1 Cup	80	4	2	10	NV	820	
(Soup Supreme)..............	1 Cup	160	9	4	17	1	920	

	Serv.	K-Cal.	Fat	Prot.	Carb.	Flb.	Sod.	FAC
(Soup, Canned cont.)								
Bean								
(Campbell's):								
Ham, Chunky..............	1 Cup	190	2	13	29	9	880	**FA**
Rice Creole, Chunky ..	1 Cup	210	8	10	27	6	720	**FA**
W/Bacon, PFC............	1 Cup	140	4	6	21	NV	840	**FA**
Healthy Request, W/								
Bacon, PFC............	1 Cup	140	4	6	21	NV	470	**FA**
(Hain) Black Bean..........	1 Cup	130	0.5	8	26	8	480	**FA**
(Health Valley):								
Black Bean Vegetable,								
FF................................	1 Cup	110	0	11	24	12	280	**FA**
Bean Vegetable, FF ...	1 Cup	140	0	10	32	13	250	**FA**
(Healthy Choice) Ham ...	1 Cup	170	1.5	9	31	7	480	**FA**
(Soup Supreme):								
Black Bean	1 Cup	150	3	9	23	7	1,450	**FA**
Red Beans W/Rice.....	1 Cup	130	1.5	5	26	5	770	**FA**
Royal Navy Bean	1 Cup	140	2	7	24	5	1,110	**FA**
SW White Bean..........	1 Cup	120	1.5	6	22	5	780	**FA**
Beef								
(Campbell's):								
Beef Noodle, PFC	1 Cup	70	3	4	7	NV	830	
Beef W/Veg & Barley,								
Cond................................	1 Cup	160	4	10	22	4	1,840	**A**
Beefy Mushroom, PFC	1 Cup	60	3	4	5	NV	960	
Broth Dbl Rich, Cond,								
FF..............................	1 Cup	30	0	6	2	0	1,800	
Country Vegetable,								
Chunky	1 Cup	160	4	13	18	3	900	**A**
(Health Valley) Broth, FF	1 Cup	20	0	5	0	0	160	
(Swanson) Broth, Clear .	1 Cup	20	1	2	1	0	820	
Broccoli								
(Campbell's) W/Cheese,								
Cond	1 Cup	220	14	6	18	4	1,720	**A**
(Health Valley) FF..........	1 Cup	70	0	6	16	7	240	**A**
Broccoli, Cream of								
(Campbell's) *Healthy*								
Request, Cond............	1 Cup	140	4	4	18	2	960	**A**
(Soup Supreme) W/								
Cheese..........................	1 Cup	190	12	6	16	1	890	**A**
(Soup Supreme) W/								
Mushroom	1 Cup	180	11	6	16	2	760	**A**
Celery, Cream of								
(Campbell's) PFC............	1 Cup	100	7	2	8	NV	820	
(Campbell's) *Healthy*								
Request, Cond.............	1 Cup	140	4	4	22	2	960	**C**
Chicken								
(Campbell's):								
Alphabet, PFC	1 Cup	80	3	3	10	NV	800	**A**

	Serv.	K-Cal.	Fat	Prot.	Carb.	Fib.	Sod.	FAC
Cream, PFC...............	1 Cup	110	7	2	9	NV	810	
Dumplings, PFC	1 Cup	80	3	4	9	NV	960	
Healthy Request,								
Cream, PFC............	1 Cup	110	7	3	9	0	490	A
(Health Valley) Natural								
Broth	1 Cup	42	2	5	1	0	0	
(Healthy Choice) Hearty	1 Cup	130	2.5	8	20	1	460	A
(Progresso) Hearty W/								
Rotini............................	1 Cup	90	2	10	8	0	860	A
(Soup Supreme) Cream.	1 Cup	160	8	8	14	2	910	A
Chicken Broth								
(Campbell's) PFC...........	1 Cup	30	2	1	2	0	710	
(Hain)................................	1 Cup	40	2.7	3	2	NV	92	
(Health Valley) FF..........	1 Cup	30	0	6	0	0	170	
(Shelton's):								
....	1 Cup	35	2.5	2	0	0	580	
FF...............................	1 Cup	10	0	2	0	0	60	
(Swanson) Clear	1 Cup	30	2	2	1	0	1,000	
Chicken Gumbo								
(Campbell's) PFC...........	1 Cup	60	2	2	8	NV	900	
W/Sausage	1 Oz	13	0.4	1	1	0	101	A
(Soup Supreme).............	1 Cup	90	2.5	5	11	1	1,300	
Chicken Mushroom								
(Campbell's) PFC,								
Creamy	1 Cup	120	8	3	8	NV	920	
(Campbell's) Chunky......	1 Cup	210	17	9	12	1	1,020	A
Chicken Noodle								
(Campbell's):								
Chunky.........................	1 Cup	130	3	9	16	2	1,050	A
PFC.............................	1 Cup	60	2	3	8	NV	900	
Creamy, Cond	1 Cup	260	14	10	24	4	1,760	A
Healthy Request.........	1 Cup	160	3	9	25	2	480	A
Healthy Request, PFC	1 Cup	60	2	3	8	0	440	
Homestyle	1 Cup	100	3.5	7	11	1	980	A
Homestyle, PFC	1 Cup	70	3	3	8	NV	880	
(Hain) No Salt	1 Cup	100	4	7	9	NV	75	A
(Healthy Choice)	1 Cup	140	3	9	20	1	400	A
(Progresso).....................	1 Cup	80	2	9	8	1	730	A
(Soup Supreme).............	1 Cup	100	2.5	3	16	1	1,120	A
Chicken W/Rice								
(Campbell's):								
Chunky.........................	1 Cup	140	3	9	18	2	840	A
Healthy Request.........	1 Cup	120	5	4	20	1	960	A
W/Rice, PFC..............	1 Cup	60	2	3	7	NV	870	
(Healthy Choice)	1 Cup	110	3	7	15	1	430	A
(Progresso) W/Veg.........	1 Cup	110	3	7	12	1	790	A
(Soup Supreme) W/Wild								
Rice................................	1 Cup	210	12	8	17	0	1,230	A

	Serv.	K-Cal.	Fat	Prot.	Carb.	Fib.	Sod.	FAC
(Soup, Canned cont.)								
Chicken W/Vegetables								
(Campbell's):								
....	1 Cup	90	1	7	13	3	870	A
Healthy Request.........	1 Cup	160	4	6	24	2	960	A
PFC............................	1 Cup	70	3	3	8	NV	850	
(Hain)........................	1 Cup	100	3	7	12	NV	85	A
Clam Chowder, Manhattan								
(Campbell's) PFC............	1 Cup	70	2	2	10	NV	820	
Clam Chowder, New England								
(Campbell's):								
....	1 Cup	240	15	7	21	2	980	
PFC............................	1 Cup	80	3	3	12	NV	870	
Chunky......................	1 Cup	130	4	6	20	3	900	
(Health Valley)...............	1 Cup	13	0.3	1	2	0	19	
(Healthy Choice)	1 Cup	120	1.5	6	23	2	480	
(Jake's) Cond................	1 Cup	300	16.5	6	30	5	930	
(Progresso)....................	1 Cup	110	2	12	11	3	710	
(Snows):								
Cond	1 Cup	160	3	6	26	0	1,520	
Healthy Value	1 Cup	120	1.5	8	20	3	480	
(Soup Supreme).............	1 Cup	180	6	9	22	1	730	
Corn								
(Campbell's):								
Chowder, Chunky.......	1 Cup	250	15	10	18	3	870	A
LS..............................	1 Cup	191	5	3	31	NV	33	
(Health Valley) Country								
Corn & Vegetable,								
FF.............................	1 Cup	70	0	5	17	7	135	FA
(Soup Supreme) Green								
Chili Cheese	1 Cup	170	5	6	28	2	1,220	A
Lentil								
(Campbell's) Hearty,								
Homecook..................	1 Cup	130	0.5	7	24	5	860	A
(Hain)........................	1 Cup	170	0.5	12	30	11	480	A
(Health Valley):								
LS..............................	1 Cup	193	2.3	9	31	19	28	
W/Carrots, FF.............	1 Cup	90	0	10	25	14	220	A
(Healthy Choice)	1 Cup	150	1	9	29	5	420	A
(Progresso)....................	1 Cup	140	2	9	22	7	750	
Minestrone								
(Campbell's):								
Chunky......................	1 Cup	140	5	5	22	2	800	A
PFC............................	1 Cup	80	2	3	13	NV	900	A
Healthy Request.........	1 Cup	120	2	4	24	3	480	A
(Fantastic) Prepared	1 Cup	150	1	6	29	4	480	A
(Hain) LS......................	1 Cup	135	3.4	6	22	NV	63	A
(Health Valley) FF...........	1 Cup	80	0	8	21	11	210	FA

	Serv.	K-Cal.	Fat	Prot.	Carb.	Flb.	Sod.	FAC
(Healthy Choice):								
....	1 Cup	110	1	6	23	3	390	A
Cond	1 Cup	180	2	8	34	4	960	A
(Progresso)......................	1 Cup	130	2.5	6	22	5	960	A
(Soup Supreme).............	1 Cup	70	2.5	3	11	2	1,030	A
Mushroom, Cream of								
(Campbell's):								
PFC..............................	1 Cup	100	7	2	8	NV	820	A
Healthy Request,								
Cond......................	1 Cup	140	5	2	20	0	960	C
LS..................................	1 Cup	200	14	3	18	3	65	
RF	1 Cup	140	7	2	20	2	1,880	
(Soup Supreme).............	1 Cup	200	15	4	13	1	940	
Onion								
(Campbell's):								
Cond	1 Cup	140	5	4	20	6	1,960	
Creamy, PFC...............	1 Cup	100	5	2	12	NV	830	
(Soup Supreme) French								
Onion	1 Cup	80	4	2	11	1	1,110	
Potato, Cream of								
(Campbell's) Cream,								
PFC..............................	1 Cup	80	3	1	12	NV	870	
(Soup Supreme).............	1 Cup	190	9	5	22	1	750	A
Split Pea								
(Anderson) FF................	1 Cup	130	0	10	24	<1	740	A
W/Bacon	1 Cup	140	1	10	22	<1	760	A
(Campbell's):								
Ham/Bacon, PFC........	1 Cup	160	4	9	24	NV	780	
Ham, Chunky..............	1 Cup	190	3	14	27	3	1,120	A
LS..............................	1 Cup	240	4	12	38	5	50	A
(Hain) LS..........................	1 Cup	150	1	13	27	4	70	A
W/Vegetables...............	1 Cup	110	0.5	7	20	7	480	A
(Health Valley)..............	1 Cup	102	1.1	10	13	14	28	A
W/Carrot, FF..............	1 Cup	110	0	8	17	4	230	A
(Healthy Choice) W/Ham	1 Cup	160	2	11	25	2	400	A
(Progresso) W/Ham	1 Cup	160	4	9	20	5	830	AC
(Soup Supreme)								
W/Ham..........................	1 Cup	120	1.5	9	18	6	1,030	A
Tomato								
(Anderson)......................	1 Cup	130	3	2	24	2	880	A
(Campbell's):								
PFC..............................	1 Cup	90	2	1	17	NV	680	A
Cream, PFC................	1 Cup	110	3	1	20	NV	810	A
Fiesta, Cond, FF	1 Cup	140	0	2	32	2	1,720	AC
Healthy Request,								
Cond......................	1 Cup	180	4	4	36	2	920	A
Italian, Cond	1 Cup	200	1	4	46	4	1,640	A
LS..................................	1 Cup	170	6	4	28	2	60	A

	Serv.	K-Cal.	Fat	Prot.	Carb.	Fib.	Sod.	FAC
(Soup, Canned cont.)								
(Health Valley):								
....	1 Cup	147	3.4	3	24	1	45	A
Vegetable, FF.............	1 Cup	80	0	6	17	5	240	FA
(Healthy Choice)	1 Cup	110	1.5	5	21	3	420	A
(Muir Glen) Org............	1 Cup	60	0	3	12	3	660	A
(Progresso) Tortellini......	1 Cup	120	5	5	13	2	910	A
(Soup Supreme)								
Florentine.....................	1 Cup	90	1.5	3	16	2	1,000	A
Turkey								
(Campbell's) Noodle,								
PFC..............................	1 Cup	70	2	3	9	NV	880	
Vegetable, PFC..........	1 Cup	70	3	2	8	NV	710	A
(Hain) Rice	1 Cup	80	3	7	8	NV	820	A
Rice, LS	1 Cup	100	3	6	11	NV	65	A
(Healthy Choice) Rice....	1 Cup	90	2.5	6	13	1	360	
Vegetable.....................	1 Cup	120	2.5	7	18	2	490	
Vegetable								
(Campbell's):								
California, Cond..........	1 Cup	120	2	6	20	4	1,700	A
Chunky.......................	1 Cup	130	3	3	22	4	870	A
Country.......................	1 Cup	110	1	3	19	2	760	A
Healthy Request..........	1 Cup	100	1	3	20	2	470	A
Healthy Request,								
Cond.........................	1 Cup	180	2	6	32	4	960	A
Mediterranean,								
Chunky	1 Cup	140	5	4	21	1	850	A
Vegetarian, PFC.........	1 Cup	80	2	3	13	NV	790	A
W/Pasta, Cond	1 Cup	180	2	4	36	4	1,660	A
(Bearitos) Southwest,								
FF..............................	1 Cup	70	0	4	15	2	500	A
(Fantastic) Tomato Rice								
Parmesano...................	1 Serv	200	2	6	41	2	550	A
(Hain):								
Broth	1 Serv	40	0	1	9	NV	95	A
Vegetarian, LS.............	1 Serv	150	5	5	23	NV	80	A
(Health Valley):								
Barley, FF...................	1 Cup	90	0	6	19	4	210	FA
14 Garden..................	1 Cup	80	0	6	17	4	250	A
Natural	1 Oz	15	0.1	1	3	1	5	A
Power Carotene..........	1 Cup	70	0	5	17	6	240	A
(Healthy Choice):								
Country	1 Cup	100	0.5	4	23	2	430	A
Garden	1 Cup	120	1	5	26	3	400	A
(Soup Supreme):								
Beef/Barley	1 Cup	90	2	5	14	2	830	A
Creole	1 Cup	110	3	4	20	2	1,660	A
Garden	1 Cup	70	1.5	3	13	3	560	A
Harvest.......................	1 Cup	90	1.5	3	17	3	960	A

	Serv.	K-Cal.	Fat	Prot.	Carb.	Fib.	Sod.	FAC
Zesty Italian	1 Cup	70	1	3	14	2	720	A

Soup, Fast Food
(Arby's):
Boston Clam Chowder	1 Cup	190	9	9	18	1	968	
Cream of Broccoli.......	1 Cup	160	8	7	15	4	1,008	
French Onion..............	1 Cup	67	3	2	7	1	1,248	
Lumberjack Mixed Vegetable	1 Cup	90	4	2	10	1	1,152	
Old-Fashioned Chicken Noodle.......	1 Cup	80	4	6	11	1	848	
Pilgrim Clam Chowder	1 Cup	193	11	10	18	2	1,157	
Roast Beef and Vegetable	1 Cup	96	3	5	14	0	996	
Split Pea and Ham....	1 Cup	200	10	8	21	4	1,029	
Tomato Florentine	1 Cup	84	2	3	15	0	910	
Wisconsin Cheese......	1 Cup	280	18	10	20	4	1,064	

Soup Mix
(Prepared as indicated on package, unless specified as mix)
Bean
(Fantastic):
Black Bean Salsa.......	10 Oz	240	1.5	11	46	8	450	A
5 Bean	10 Oz	230	1	12	43	10	480	A
Jumpin' Black Bean....	10 Oz	210	1	12	39	8	470	A
W/Spanish Rice...........	10 Oz	210	1.5	9	49	8	140	
(Health Valley) W/Rice...	1 Cup	100	0	5	22	4	190	
(Nile Spice):								
Black Bean	10 Oz	170	1.5	11	35	11	600	
Black Bean Salsa, Org	10 Oz	190	1	9	34	6	630	
Red Beans W/Rice.....	10 Oz	170	1	10	36	10	650	

Chicken Noodle
(Health Valley) W/
Vegetable....................	1 Cup	110	0	5	24	3	190	
(Hormel)..........................	1 Cup	110	2.5	8	13	0	790	
(Knorr)	1 Cup	90	1.5	5	16	0	770	
(Lipton)	1 Cup	80	2	3	12	0	650	
(Wyler's)	⅛ Pkg	80	0.5	2	17	1	960	A

Chicken Rice
(Campbell's)	1 Cup	120	2.5	5	20	2	1,130	
(Hormel)..........................	1 Cup	110	3	5	17	1	950	

Corn
(Fantastic).......................	10 Oz	180	1	7	36	8	510	A
(Health Valley).................	1 Cup	100	0	5	21	3	190	
(Nile Spice)......................	10 Oz	110	2	3	22	3	400	

	Serv.	K-Cal.	Fat	Prot.	Carb.	Fib.	Sod.	FAC
(Soup Mix cont.)								
Couscous								
(Fantastic):								
Creole Vegetable........	10 Oz	220	1.5	10	41	6	590	A
Lentil	10 Oz	230	1	12	44	7	480	A
Nacho Cheddar	10 Oz	200	3	8	36	6	590	A
(Nile Spice):								
Almondine	10 Oz	200	2.5	7	37	2	490	
Garbanzo	10 Oz	220	2.5	9	39	2	500	
Lentil Curry	10 Oz	200	1.5	10	36	4	730	
Minestrone	10 Oz	180	1.5	8	34	2	590	A
Parmesan.....................	10 Oz	200	3	8	34	2	570	A
Lentil								
(Fantastic) Hearty...........	10 Oz	230	1	15	41	12	480	A
(Health Valley)................	1 Cup	130	0	7	28	5	190	
(Nile Spice):								
....	10 Oz	180	1.5	12	31	3	500	A
Curry W/Rice, Org......	10 Oz	180	1	10	33	3	570	A
Minestrone								
(Fantastic).....................	10 Oz	150	1	6	29	4	480	A
(Nile Spice)...................	10 Oz	140	1	8	30	8	590	
Miso, Dry Mix								
(Kikkoman):								
Red	1 Pkg	35	1	2	4	0	790	
Tofu............................	1 Pkg	35	1	3	4	0	740	
Tofu Spinach	1 Pkg	35	1	3	4	0	790	
White...........................	1 Pkg	35	1	3	4	0	820	
(Westbrae):								
Red	1 Pkg	35	1.5	2	3	0	750	
White...........................	1 Pkg	35	1.5	2	3	0	780	
Mushroom								
(Fantastic) Creamy.........	10 Oz	120	0	6	24	2	570	
(Nile Spice)...................	10 Oz	140	2.5	4	26	1	610	
Noodle								
(Fantastic):								
W/Vegetable Miso	1 Serv	130	1	5	25	2	540	
W/Vegetable Tomato..	1 Serv	150	1	5	31	3	490	
Onion								
(Campbell's)..................	1 Tbsp	25	0	1	5	0	660	
(Knorr)	1 Cup	45	1	1	8	0	790	
(Mrs. Grass)	1 Cup	35	0.5	1	6	0	980	
Ramen								
(Also See Noodle, Japanese)								
(Campbell's):								
Beef.............................	1 Cup	190	8	5	26	NV	1,010	
Chicken	1 Cup	190	8	5	26	NV	970	
Oriental	1 Cup	190	8	2	26	NV	930	
Pork.............................	1 Cup	190	6	5	26	NV	860	

	Serv.	K-Cal.	Fat	Prot.	Carb.	Fib.	Sod.	FAC
(Fantastic):								
Chicken-Free	1 Cup	140	0.5	8	26	4	540	
Vegetable Curry	1 Cup	140	1	6	28	3	490	A
Vegetable Tomato	1 Cup	150	1	5	31	3	490	
(Maruchan):								
Beef	1 Cup	190	8	5	26	1	770	
Chicken	1 Cup	190	8	5	26	1	780	
Chili	1 Cup	190	8	5	26	1	710	
Oriental	1 Cup	190	8	4	26	1	900	
(Top Ramen):								
Beef	1 Cup	190	7	4	28	1	700	
Cajun Chicken	1 Cup	180	7	4	26	1	890	
Chicken	1 Cup	190	7	4	27	1	910	
Oriental	1 Cup	190	7	4	28	1	830	
Pork	1 Cup	190	7	4	27	1	860	
Spinach								
(Knorr) Cream	1 Cup	70	2.5	2	9	0	600	
Split Pea								
(Fantastic)	10 Oz	190	1	12	35	8	470	
(Nile Spice)	10 Oz	200	1	13	35	8	600	
Tomato								
(Fantastic) W/Rice	10 Oz	200	2	6	41	2	550	A
(Knorr)	1 Cup	80	2	2	13	0	890	A
(Nile Spice):								
Org	10 Oz	120	3	4	19	3	420	A
W/Rice	10 Oz	130	3	5	23	1	550	A
Vegetable								
(Campbell's):								
	1 Cup	100	2	3	17	2	850	
Beef	1 Cup	90	2	5	13	2	780	
(Fantastic):								
Broccoli & Cheddar	10 Oz	130	1.5	6	23	2	480	A
Creole	10 Oz	220	1.5	10	41	6	590	A
W/Barley	10 Oz	150	0.5	6	29	6	470	
W/Noodle, Curry	10 Oz	140	1	6	28	3	490	A
(Hormel) Beef	1 Cup	90	1	6	15	1	790	
(Knorr)	1 Cup	30	0.5	1	6	1	730	A
(Nile Spice):								
Org	10 Oz	110	1.5	3	21	1	600	A
W/Barley, Org	10 Oz	130	1.5	5	29	5	460	A

Sour Cream (See Cream, Sour)

Sourdock

Young Leaves	1 Cup	28	0.6	2	5	NV	NV	A

Soursop

Raw, Pulp	1 Cup	148	0.7	2	38	7	32	A

	Serv.	K-Cal.	Fat	Prot.	Carb.	Fib.	Sod.	FAC
Soybean								
Boiled, W/O Salt	1 Cup	298	15.4	29	17	10	2	**FAC**
Dried................................	1 Cup	774	37.1	68	56	17	4	**FAC**
Edamame	1 Cup	240	12	20	16	18	0	**FAC**
Green, Boiled	1 Cup	254	11.5	22	20	8	25	**FAC**
Green, Raw.....................	1 Cup	376	17.4	33	28	11	38	**FAC**
Soybean Cakes (See Tofu)								
Soybean Curd (See Tofu)								
Soybean, Fermented								
(Natto).............................	1 Cup	370	19	31	25	9	12	**C**
Soybean Kernel								
Dry-Roasted	1 Cup	774	37.2	68	56	14	3	**FAC**
Roasted	1 Cup	810	43.7	61	58	30	200	**FAC**
Soybean Oil								
(Springfield)	1 Tbsp	120	13.6	0	0	0	0	**A**
Soybean, Sprouted								
Raw	1 Cup	85	4.7	9	7	1	10	**F**
Steamed	1 Cup	76	4.2	8	6	1	9	**F**
Stir-Fried.........................	3.3 Oz	125	7.1	13	9	1	14	**FA**
Soy Beverage								
Malt								
(Westsoy):								
Almond......................	1 Cup	333	14.7	9	41	NV	187	**A**
Almond, LT	1 Cup	213	5.3	7	35	NV	187	
Banana, LT	1 Cup	213	4	7	37	NV	187	
Carob	1 Cup	360	14.7	8	49	NV	187	**A**
Cocoa, LT	1 Cup	140	2	3	27	NV	95	
Cocoa Mint, LT...........	1 Cup	213	4	7	35	NV	187	
Cocoa Mint	1 Cup	360	14.7	8	49	NV	187	**A**
Java	1 Cup	360	14.7	9	49	NV	187	**A**
Vanilla	1 Cup	150	5	6	20	NV	120	**A**
Vanilla, LT..................	1 Cup	110	2	3	20	NV	80	
Soy Milk								
(Eden):								
Eden Blend, W/Rice ...	1 Cup	120	3	7	16	0	80	
Edensoy Extra,								
Original....................	1 Cup	135	4	10	14	0	110	**FAC**
Edensoy Extra, Vanilla	1 Cup	150	3	6	23	0	90	**FAC**
(Health Valley) Moo	1 Cup	110	0	6	22	1	60	**C**
(Pacific):								
Original......................	1 Cup	100	5	7	5	3	40	**C**
Plain, FF	1 Cup	70	0	3	14	0	75	**C**

	Serv.	K-Cal.	Fat	Prot.	Carb.	Fib.	Sod.	FAC
(Silk) Plain, LT	1 Cup	80	2.5	4	11	0	130	
(Vitasoy):								
Carob	1 Cup	210	2	4	15	1	95	
Carob Supreme	1 Cup	210	6	8	32	NV	160	
Cocoa, LT	1 Cup	130	2	4	25	NV	130	
Original	1 Cup	160	7	9	14	1	180	
Plain, LT	1 Cup	80	0.2	4	15	1	95	
Rich Cocoa	1 Cup	210	6	8	32	NV	180	
Vanilla, Lite	1 Cup	110	2	4	20	1	95	
(Westsoy):								
Carob Plus	1 Cup	160	5	6	21	0	80	C
Original	1 Cup	150	5	7	18	NV	115	
Plain	1 Cup	150	5	6	18	NV	140	C
Plain, Lite	1 Cup	100	2	4	16	0	100	
Unsweetened	1 Cup	100	5	7	5	NV	40	
Vanilla Plus	1 Cup	150	5	6	21	0	120	C

Soy Flour

Full Fat, Raw	1 Cup	371	17.6	29	30	8	11	F
Defatted	1 Cup	329	1.2	47	38	18	20	FC
Full Fat, Roasted	1 Cup	375	18.6	30	29	8	10	F
LF	1 Cup	287	5.9	41	33	9	16	F

Soy, Grits

(Arrowhead Mills)	1 Cup	560	24	48	48	24	0	FC

Soy Meal

Defatted	1 Cup	414	2.9	55	49	NV	4	FC

Soy Protein Concentrate

	1 Oz	93	0.1	16	9	2	1	F

Soy Protein Isolate

	1 Oz	95	1	23	2	2	281	F

Soy Sauce—Shoyu—Tamari

(Eden):								
Organic	1 Tbsp	15	0	2	2	0	1,040	
Reduced Sodium	1 Tbsp	10	0	2	2	0	500	
(Kikkoman):								
LT	1 Tbsp	10	0	1	1	0	605	
Naturally Brewed	1 Tbsp	110	0	2	0	0	920	
(La Choy):								
	1 Tbsp	11	0	2	1	0	1,227	
LT	1 Tbsp	15	0	2	2	0	542	
(Sanj) Tamari Lite	1 Tbsp	16	0	2	1	0	607	
(Westbrae):								
Mild, LS	1 Tbsp	10	0	1	2	NV	430	
Wheat-Free	1 Tbsp	10	0	2	1	NV	760	

	Serv.	K-Cal.	Fat	Prot.	Carb.	Fib.	Sod.	FAC
Spaghetti (See Pasta, Spaghetti)								
Spaghetti, Canned								
(Chef Boyardee):								
Beef/Sauce	1 Cup	240	9	7	30	4	1,120	A
Meatball	1 Cup	210	8	8	27	3	960	
(Franco-American):								
Franks, *Spaghettios*	1 Cup	250	11	10	32	4	1,210	
Meatballs, *Spaghettios*	1 Cup	260	11	11	31	5	1,150	
Meatballs, Tomato								
Sauce	1 Cup	270	10	11	35	4	1,060	
Tomato & Cheese								
Sauce	1 Cup	210	2	7	41	3	1,020	
Spaghetti Entree, Frozen								
(Serving size given in Oz to reflect weight of 1 serving)								
(Healthy Choice):								
	10 Oz	310	6	16	48	4	440	
Bolognese	10 Oz	260	3	14	43	5	470	
(Light and Elegant)	10.2 Oz	290	8	16	40	NV	700	
(Stouffer's):								
	13 Oz	370	11	18	49	NV	1,510	
Lean Cuisine	11.5 Oz	290	6	14	45	4	550	
Meatballs	13.5 Oz	420	15	19	51	5	680	
(Ultra Slim-Fast)								
Beef/Mushroom	12 Oz	370	9	19	59	5	740	
(Wt Watchers)	12 Oz	290	6	14	45	5	560	
Spaghetti Sauce (See Pasta Sauce)								
Spam (See Luncheon Meat, Canned)								
Spearmint								
Dried (McCormick)	1 Tsp	2	0	0	0	0	2	
Spelt								
(Arrowhead Mills)	1 Oz	83	0.6	4	20	4	1	
Spelt Flour								
(Arrowhead Mills)	1 Cup	400	2	16	96	20	0	
Spinach								
Fresh								
Raw	1 Cup	12	0.2	2	2	2	44	FA
Raw	1 Oz	3	0.1	1	0	2	34	FA
Boiled	1 Cup	41	0.5	5	7	4	126	FA
New Zealand	1 Cup	22	0.3	2	4	NV	193	FA
Canned								
LS	1 Cup	45	0.9	5	7	5	176	FA

	Serv.	K-Cal.	Fat	Prot.	Carb.	Fib.	Sod.	FAC
Chopped (Del Monte)	1 Cup	60	0	4	8	4	720	**FA**
Whole Leaf (Del Monte)	1 Cup	60	0	4	8	4	720	**FA**
Frozen								
(Green Giant)	1 Cup	50	0	6	6	4	480	**FA**
(Health Valley)...............	1 Cup	50	2	6	10	4	164	**FA**

Spinach Dish, Frozen

Creamed (Green Giant) .	1 Cup	160	6	8	20	4	1,040	**FA**
Creamed (Stouffer's)......	1 Cup	320	24	8	16	4	760	**FAC**
Souffle (Stouffer's)	1 Cup	300	20	12	18	0	960	**FAC**
W/Butter (Green Giant)..	1 Cup	80	3	4	10	4	560	**FA**

Spirulina (See Seaweed, Dried)

Split Pea

Dried...............................	1 Oz	98	0.3	7	17	7	4	**F**
Dried...............................	1 Cup	672	2.3	48	119	50	30	**F**
Boiled..............................	1 Cup	231	0.8	16	41	16	4	**F**

Sport Bar

(Balance) Almond								
Brownie	1 Bar	190	6	14	22	2	170	**FAC**
Chocolate..................	1 Bar	190	6	14	22	1	210	**FAC**
(Clif) Berry	1 Bar	250	2	4	52	2	100	
Peanut Butter..............	1 Bar	250	4	10	45	8	150	
(Edge) Peanut Butter	1 Bar	212	3	8	40	2	80	**FAC**
(Power Bar) Mocha........	1 Bar	230	2.5	10	45	3	90	**AC**
Oatmeal Raisin	1 Bar	230	2.5	10	45	3	120	**AC**
(Shaklee) Carbo								
Crunch	1 Bar	180	4	9	27	0	85	**FA**
(Tiger's Milk) Peanut								
Butter	1 Bar	140	5	6	18	1	75	**C**
Protein Rich................	1 Bar	145	5	7	18	1	70	**C**

Sport Beverage (Also See Diet Drink; Nutritional Drink)

Bottled								
(Gatorade) Thirst-								
Quenching Drink.........	1 Cup	60	0	0	16	0	96	
(Powerade)	1 Cup	72	0	0	19	0	28	
(R.W. Knudsen)								
Recharge	1 Cup	70	0	0	18	NV	25	
Prepared From Mix								
Instant Protein								
(Shaklee)	1 Cup	220	2	32	16	0	280	**C**
Fitness	1 Cup	360	1	24	66	0	180	**FAC**
Mix								
Fiber Plan (Shaklee)	1 Tbsp	45	0	0	11	3	3	
Performance	1 Tbsp	33	0	0	8	0	38	

	Serv.	K-Cal.	Fat	Prot.	Carb.	Fib.	Sod.	FAC
Squab								
Breast Meat, Raw	3 Oz	115	3.9	15	0	0	0	
Meat/Skin, Raw	3 Oz	250	20.1	16	0	0	0	
Squash Seed (See Pumpkin Seed)								
Squash, Summer								
Crookneck								
Raw	1 Cup	24	0.4	1	5	NV	0	A
Boiled...............................	1 Cup	36	0.6	2	8	NV	0	A
Zucchini								
Raw, Sliced	1 Cup	18	0.2	2	4	2	4	A
Baby, Raw, 2 5/8"...........	1 Item	2	0	0	0	0	0	
Boiled...............................	1 Cup	29	0.1	1	7	3	5	A
Canned, Italian	1 Cup	66	0.3	2	16	NV	849	A
Frozen, Boiled.................	1 Cup	38	0.3	3	8	3	4	A
Frozen (Flav R Pac)	1 Cup	23	0	2	3	2	23	A
Squash, Winter								
Raw	1 Cup	43	0.3	2	10	2	5	FA
Acorn, Baked..................	1 Cup	115	0.3	2	30	9	8	FA
Butternut, Baked	1 Cup	82	0.2	2	22	7	8	FA
Hubbard, Baked	1 Cup	71	0.9	3	15	7	12	FA
Spaghetti, Baked............	1 Cup	46	0.4	1	10	2	25	FA
Squid—Calamari								
Raw	3 Oz	78	1.2	13	3	0	37	
Boiled...............................	3 Oz	90	1.3	15	3	0	270	
Fried	3 Oz	149	6.4	15	7	0	260	
Star Fruit (See Carambola)								
Steak Sauce								
(A-1) Original..................	1 Tbsp	15	0	0	0	0	250	
(A-1) Sweet & Tangy.....	1 Tbsp	30	0	0	8	0	200	
(Crosse & Blackwell)......	1 Tbsp	30	0	0	7	0	95	
(Heinz) *57*......................	1 Tbsp	15	0	0	4	0	220	
(Hunt's)	1 Tbsp	10	0.1	0	2	0	256	
(Kikkoman)	1 Tbsp	20	0	0	5	0	290	
Stir-Fry Sauce								
(Kikkoman)	1 Tbsp	15	0	1	3	0	530	
(La Choy):								
Mandarin Soy	1 Cup	141	0.4	5	31	3	1,704	
Sweet/Sour	1 Cup	274	0	3	71	6	1,508	
Szechwan	1 Cup	168	0.4	5	36	0	1,248	

	Serv.	K-Cal.	Fat	Prot.	Carb.	Fib.	Sod.	FAC
Strawberry								
Fresh								
Raw	1 Item	5	0	0	1	1	0	
Raw	1 Cup	45	0.6	1	11	3	1	A
Raw	1 Oz	9	0.1	0	2	1	0	
Frozen								
Sweetened, Sliced	1 Cup	245	0.3	1	66	5	8	A
Sweetened, Whole	1 Cup	199	0.4	1	54	5	3	A
Unsweetened, Whole	1 Cup	52	0.2	1	14	3	3	A
Canned W/								
Heavy Syrup	1 Cup	234	0.7	1	60	4	10	A
Strawberry Juice								
(Kern) Nectar W/Banana	1 Cup	150	0	0	36	0	6	A
(Odwalla) *"C" Monster...*	1 Cup	130	0	2	31	1	34	A
Go Man Go	1 Cup	100	1	1	26	2	25	A
(R.W. Knudsen):								
Nectar	1 Cup	120	0	0	30	NV	25	
W/Banana	1 Cup	120	0	0	30	NV	25	
W/Lemonade	1 Cup	120	0	0	29	NV	35	
(Snapple)	1 Cup	128	0	0	31	NV	36	A
Strawberry Topping, Syrup								
(Baskin Robbins)	1 Oz	60	0	0	14	0	5	
(Hershey's)	1 Tbsp	56	0	0	14	0	3	
(Nestlé) Quik	1 Tbsp	55	0	0	14	0	0	
(S & W) Lo-Cal	1 Tbsp	15	0	0	4	0	26	

String Bean (See Green Bean)

Strudel (See Pastry, Toaster Strudel)

Stuffing								
(General Foods) Chicken	1 Cup	214	2.1	7	41	0	976	
(General Mills):								
Chicken	1 Cup	220	2	8	42	NV	1,060	
Herb	1 Cup	220	2	8	44	NV	1,100	
(Kellogg's) Croutettes	1 Cup	120	0	5	25	0	460	
(Kraft) *Stove Top:*								
Chicken Flavor	1 Cup	220	2	4	20	1	878	
Chicken, Flexible	1 Cup	240	6	6	38	1	920	
Cornbread	1 Cup	220	2	6	42	2	1,018	
Cornbread, Flexible	1 Cup	220	5	6	38	2	1,000	
Rice, Wild	1 Cup	206	1.9	8	41	1	917	
(Pepperidge Farm):								
Apple & Raisin	1 Cup	280	3	8	54	4	1,040	
Chicken, Classic	1 Cup	260	3	10	48	6	980	
Cornbread	1 Cup	227	2.7	5	44	3	640	

	Serv.	K-Cal.	Fat	Prot.	Carb.	Fib.	Sod.	FAC
(Stuffing cont.)								
Country Style	1 Cup	187	2	7	36	3	507	
Cube	1 Cup	187	2	5	37	3	707	
Garden & Herb	1 Cup	300	10	8	44	4	720	
Herb Seasoned	1 Cup	227	2	7	44	4	800	
Rice, Wild & Mushroom	1 Cup	255	9	8	33	3	615	
Veg & Almond	1 Cup	280	6	10	46	4	600	A

Sturgeon

	Serv.	K-Cal.	Fat	Prot.	Carb.	Fib.	Sod.	FAC
Raw	3 Oz	100	3.4	14	0	0.	46	
Cooked	3 Oz	115	4.4	18	0	0	59	
Smoked	3 Oz	147	3.7	27	0	0	628	

Succotash

	Serv.	K-Cal.	Fat	Prot.	Carb.	Fib.	Sod.	FAC
Boiled	1 Cup	221	1.5	10	47	9	33	FA
Canned (S & W)	1 Cup	200	2	6	38	4	680	FA
Frozen (Flav R Pac)	1 Cup	150	1.5	6	33	3	75	FA

Sugar

	Serv.	K-Cal.	Fat	Prot.	Carb.	Fib.	Sod.	FAC
Brown Rice (Devansoy)	1 Tsp	18	0	0	4	0	0	
Brown, Golden (C & H)	1 Tsp	16	0	0	4	0	0	
Brown, Old-Fashioned (Domino)	1 Tsp	16	0	0	4	0	0	
Cubes (Domino)	1 Cube	8	0	2	0	0	0	
Date Sugar	1 Tsp	17	0	0	3	0	2	
Granulated	1 Cup	774	0	0	200	0	2	
Granulated	1 Tsp	15	0	0	4	0	0	
Powdered	1 Cup	405	0	0	105	0	1	
Powdered	1 Tsp	10	0	0	2	0	0	
Turbonado	1 Tsp	17	0	0	4	0	0	

Sugar Alternative (See Sweetener, Alternative)

Sunchoke (See Jerusalem Artichoke)

Sunflower Butter

	Serv.	K-Cal.	Fat	Prot.	Carb.	Fib.	Sod.	FAC
Roasted (Maranatha)	2 Tbsp	200	16	9	7	5	0	FA

Sunflower Oil

	Serv.	K-Cal.	Fat	Prot.	Carb.	Fib.	Sod.	FAC
(Spectrum)	1 Tbsp	120	14	0	0	0	0	A

Sunflower Seed Flour

	Serv.	K-Cal.	Fat	Prot.	Carb.	Fib.	Sod.	FAC
Partially Defatted	1 Cup	260	1.3	38	29	4	2	FA

Sunflower Seed, Kernel

	Serv.	K-Cal.	Fat	Prot.	Carb.	Fib.	Sod.	FAC
Dry-Roasted, Salted	1 Cup	745	63.7	25	31	9	998	FA
Oil-Roasted, Salted	1 Cup	830	77.5	29	20	9	814	FA

	Serv.	K-Cal.	Fat	Prot.	Carb.	Fib.	Sod.	FAC
Surimi								
Crab, Imitation	3 Oz	84	0.4	11	9	0	676	
Crab, Imitation (Louis Kemp)	3 Oz	80	0	9	10	0	500	
Scallops, Imitation (Louis Kemp)	3 Oz	80	0	9	11	0	560	
Shrimp, Imitation	3 Oz	86	1.3	11	8	0	599	
Sushi								
Egg, No Veg, No Fish	1 Item	32	1.3	1	4	0	86	A
Vegetables, No Fish	1 Item	38	0.1	1	9	0	58	A
Vegetables, W/Fish	1 Item	37	0.1	1	8	0	54	A
Vegetables, W/Seaweed	1 Item	30	0.1	1	7	0	24	A
Sushi Rice, Prepared								
W/Vinegar, Sugar	1 Tbsp	10	0	0	2	0	23	
W/Vinegar, Sugar	1 Cup	156	0.2	3	36	1	368	
Sweet and Sour, Entree								
Chicken (La Choy)	9 Oz	161	2.4	8	29	1	658	A
Chicken Dinner (Budget Gourmet)	10 Oz	330	5	18	55	4	700	A
Chicken Dinner (Le Menu)	11 Oz	400	18	19	41	NV	1,020	A
Noodles W/Chicken (La Choy)	9.5 Oz	256	3.1	7	49	9	697	A
Sweet and Sour Sauce								
(Contadina)	1 Tbsp	20	0.5	0	4	0	55	
(Hickory Farms)	1 Tbsp	51	0	0	12	NV	0	
(Kikkoman)	1 Tbsp	18	0	0	5	0	95	
(La Choy)	1 Tbsp	29	0.1	0	7	0	52	
Sweetener, Alternative								
(Equal)	1 Pkg	4	0	1	0	0	0	
(Fruitsource)	1 Tsp	15	0	0	4	0	0	
(Nutrasweet)	1 Tsp	0	2	0	0	0	0	
(Splenda)	1 Tsp	2	0	0	1	0	0	
(Sugar Twin)	1 Pkg	4	0	0	0	0	0	
(Sweet 'N Low)	1 Pkg	0	0	0	1	0	0	
(Wt Watchers)	1 Pkg	4	0	1	0	0	30	
Sweet Potato								
Baked, Peeled	4 Oz	117	0.1	2	28	3	11	A
Boiled, Mashed	1 Cup	344	1	5	80	6	43	A
Candied	4 Oz	144	3.4	1	29	3	74	A
Canned In Syrup, Drained	1 Cup	212	0.6	3	50	6	76	A

	Serv.	K-Cal.	Fat	Prot.	Carb.	Fib.	Sod.	FAC
(Sweet Potato cont.)								
Canned, Mashed............	1 Cup	258	0.5	5	59	4	191	**A**
Frozen, Baked................	1 Cup	176	0.2	3	41	3	14	**A**

Swiss Chard (See Chard)

Swordfish

Raw	3 Oz	103	3.4	17	0	0	76	
Broiled	3 Oz	132	4.4	22	0	0	98	

Syrup (See individual listings)

T

	Serv.	K-Cal.	Fat	Prot.	Carb.	Fib.	Sod.	FAC
Tabasco Sauce (See Pepper Sauce, Hot)								
Tabbouleh—Tabouli (Also See Bulgur)								
Dry (Casbah)	1 Oz	96	0.4	2	19	1	328	
Prepared (Fantastic)	1 Cup	240	1	8	52	12	900	A
Taco, Fast Food								
(Del Taco):								
Beef, Deluxe Double	1 Item	205	13	9	13	NV	159	
Beef, Double	1 Item	172	10	8	12	NV	150	
Chicken	1 Item	186	13	8	10	NV	276	
(Mighty Taco):								
Beans & Cheese	1 Item	179	7.5	5	22	5	386	
Beans, Cheese & Beef	1 Item	199	10	9	18	3	411	
Hard Shell	1 Item	223	12.5	13	14	2	436	
Vegetarian	1 Item	228	15	10	12	0	558	
(Taco Bell):								
Chicken, LT	1 Item	178	5.8	12	20	2	522	
Chicken Meximelt	1 Item	257	15	14	19	2	779	C
Combo Burrito	1 Item	407	16	18	46	3	1,136	C
Supreme	1 Item	228	13.5	11	13	2	295	
(Taco Time) Chicken,								
Soft	1 Item	390	12	31	34	NV	322	
Taco Sauce (Also See Salsa)								
(La Victoria) Green	1 Tbsp	0	0	0	0	0	95	
(Old El Paso)	1 Tbsp	5	0	0	1	0	80	
(Santiago)	1 Tbsp	7	0.1	0	2	0	82	
(Tico Pica)	1 Tbsp	0	0	0	0	0	255	
Taco Shell								
(Bearitos):								
Blue Corn	1 Item	70	3.5	1	9	1	3	
Yellow Corn	1 Item	70	3.5	1	9	1	3	
(Gebhardt)	1 Item	52	2.8	1	6	1	2	

	Serv.	K-Cal.	Fat	Prot.	Carb.	Flb.	Sod.	FAC
(Taco Shell cont.)								
(Old El Paso):								
....	1 Item	57	3.3	1	6	1	43	
Super	1 Item	95	6	2	11	1	75	
(Rosarita).......................	1 Item	52	2.8	1	6	1	2	

Tahini (Also See Sesame Butter)
(Arrowhead Mills)	1 Tbsp	95	9.5	3	3	2	3	
(Bearitos):								
Mideastern	1 Tbsp	110	10	5	2	NV	0	
Raw, Hulled	1 Tbsp	105	9.5	4	1	NV	0	
Toasted, Hulled	1 Tbsp	110	9.5	4	2	NV	0	
W/Salt	1 Tbsp	110	9.5	3	3	NV	18	
(Casbah).........................	1 Cup	640	52	16	40	2	640	FA
(Joyva)...........................	1 Tbsp	100	9	3	3	1	37	
(Maranatha) Roasted	1 Tbsp	105	8	3	5	1	3	

Tamale
Canned
Beef (Gebhardt)	1 Item	134	10.3	2	9	1	385	
Beef (Hormel)...............	1 Item	93	7	2	7	1	333	
Chicken (Hormel)	1 Item	70	3.6	2	7	1	340	
Derby (Hunt's)...............	1 Item	84	5.8	2	7	1	345	
(Van Camp's)	1 Item	90	5	3	11	3	540	
Frozen								
Beef (Garibaldi)	5 Oz	225	14	8	19	3	345	
Beef (Gebhardt)	3 Oz	134	10.3	2	9	1	385	
Beef (Golden West)	5 Oz	170	10	7	18	3	600	A
Chicken (Golden								
West)...........................	5 Oz	170	10	7	17	3	560	
Turkey (Garibaldi)	5 Oz	185	9	10	17	2	305	

Tamari (See Soy Sauce)

Tamarind
Leaves, Fresh	1 Oz	33	0.6	2	5	NV	NV	
Paste	1 Oz	68	0.1	1	16	2	1,199	
Pods	1 Oz	89	0.3	1	21	0	3	
Pulp	1 Cup	290	0.7	3	75	NV	30	

Tangerine
Fresh
Raw, Peeled...................	1 Item	37	0.2	1	9	2	1	A
Sections........................	1 Cup	90	0.4	1	22	NV	4	A
Canned W/								
Juice	1 Cup	92	0.1	2	24	2	12	A
Light Syrup.....................	1 Cup	154	0.3	1	41	2	15	A

	Serv.	K-Cal.	Fat	Prot.	Carb.	Flb.	Sod.	FAC
Tangerine Juice								
Fresh	1 Cup	106	0.5	1	25	0	2	A
Canned, Sweetened	1 Cup	124	0.5	1	30	1	2	A
Frozen, Diluted	1 Cup	111	0.3	1	27	NV	2	A
Tapioca Pearls (Also See Pudding, Ready-To-Serve, Tapioca)								
Dry	1 Oz	910	0	0	25	0	0	
Dry	1 Cup	544	0	0	135	1	2	
Dry, Quick-Cooking	1.5 Tsp	20	0	0	5	0	0	
Taro (Also See Poi)								
Raw	1 Oz	35	0.1	0	8	0	3	
Raw	1 Cup	111	0.2	2	28	4	11	A
Cooked, Sliced	1 Cup	187	0.1	1	46	7	20	A
Fried	1 Cup	305	10.7	1	52	8	369	A
Taro Chips								
Salted (Ray's)	1 Cup	120	6	1	20	4	40	
Unsalted (Ray's)	1 Oz	139	6	2	20	2	15	
Tarragon								
Fresh	1 Oz	14	0.3	1	2	NV	3	
Dried (McCormick)	1 Tsp	2	0	0	0	0	0	
Ground	1 Tsp	5	0.1	0	1	0	1	
Tartar Sauce								
(Best Foods)	1 Tbsp	70	8	0	0	NV	130	
(Bright Day)	1 Tbsp	50	5	0	2	0	40	
(Hellmann's) LF	1 Tbsp	20	0.8	0	4	NV	180	
(Kraft) FF	1 Tbsp	12	0	0	3	0	100	
(Kraft)	1 Tbsp	75	8	0	0	0	85	
(Wt Watchers)	1 Tbsp	35	3	0	3	NV	80	
Tea								
Brewed	1 Cup	3	0	0	0	0	7	
Herbal, Chamomile	1 Cup	2	0	0	0	0	3	
Herbal, Brewed	1 Cup	2	0	0	0	0	2	
Instant, Prepared, Sweetened	1 Cup	88	0	0	22	0	8	
Instant, Prepared, Unsweetened	1 Cup	2	0	0	0	0	7	
Tea, Iced								
Bottled/Canned								
(Fruitopia):								
Lemon Berry Intuition	1 Cup	83	0	0	22	0	0	
Mango	1 Cup	83	0	0	22	0	0	
Peachable Peach	1 Cup	80	0	0	22	0	0	

	Serv.	K-Cal.	Fat	Prot.	Carb.	Fib.	Sod.	FAC
(Tea, Iced cont.)								
(Nestea):								
Cool	1 Cup	82	0	0	22	0	32	
Cool Diet	1 Cup	1	0	0	0	0	25	
Earl Grey	1 Cup	65	0	0	18	0	4	
Lemon, Sweetened	1 Cup	80	0	0	22	0	0	
Sweetened	1 Cup	65	0	0	18	0	0	
(R.W. Knudsen):								
Cherry Spice	1 Cup	73	0	0	17	0	13	
Ginger Peach	1 Cup	73	0	0	17	0	13	
Hibiscus	1 Cup	73	0	0	17	0	13	
Hibiscus Cooler	1 Cup	90	0	0	23	0	40	
Lemon Cooler	1 Cup	90	0	0	23	0	40	
Mango Cooler	1 Cup	90	0	0	23	0	40	
Mango Van	1 Cup	73	0	0	17	0	13	
Orange Cooler	1 Cup	90	0	0	23	0	40	
Raspberry Cooler	1 Cup	90	0	0	23	0	40	
Raspberry	1 Cup	73	0	0	17	0	13	
(Snapple):								
Decaffeinated	1 Cup	100	0	0	24	NV	10	
Diet, Decaffeinated	1 Cup	0	0	0	1	NV	5	
Lemon	1 Cup	100	0	0	25	0	10	
Lemon, Decaffeinated	1 Cup	100	0	0	24	0	10	
Lemon, Diet	1 Cup	0	0	0	1	0	10	
Mango	1 Cup	111	0	0	27	0	10	
Mint	1 Cup	120	0	0	29	0	10	
Orange	1 Cup	110	0	0	27	NV	10	
Peach	1 Cup	100	0	0	26	0	10	
Plain	1 Cup	70	0	0	18	0	10	
Raspberry	1 Cup	100	0	0	26	0	10	
Strawberry	1 Cup	100	0	0	26	0	10	
Prepared From Mix								
(Crystal Light) Sugar-Free	1 Cup	4	0	0	0	0	0	
(Lipton) Lemon	1 Cup	71	0	0	19	0	0	
Sugar-Free	1 Cup	1	0	0	1	0	6	
(Nestea) Lemon	1 Cup	6	0	0	10	0	0	
Sugar-Free	1 Cup	6	0	0	1	0	5	
Teff								
Flour (Bob's Red Mill)	1 Cup	452	4	16	88	16	20	
Seed (Arrowhead Mills)	1 Cup	640	4	20	128	24	20	
Whole Grain (Arrowhead Mills)	2 Oz	200	1	7	41	8	10	
Tempeh								
(Light Life) Soy	8 Oz	364	12	48	18	2	24	F
3 Grain	8 Oz	380	8	24	50	12	34	F

	Serv.	K-Cal.	Fat	Prot.	Carb.	Fib.	Sod.	FAC
(White Wave):								
Five Grain	8 Oz	420	12	36	45	12	0	F
Original	8 Oz	450	18	48	30	18	0	F
Sea Veggie	8 Oz	360	9	36	33	24	75	FC
Soy Rice	8 Oz	420	15	36	39	15	0	F
Wild Rice	8 Oz	420	12	39	36	18	30	F
Teriyaki Sauce								
(Chun King)	1 Tbsp	17	0.4	2	3	0	994	
(Kikkoman):								
	1 Tbsp	30	0	0	8	0	960	
Glaze	1 Tbsp	25	0	1	6	0	405	
Glaze, Honey	1 Tbsp	40	0	1	9	0	385	
Marinade	1 Tbsp	15	0	1	2	0	610	
Marinade, LT	1 Tbsp	15	0	1	3	0	320	
(La Choy)	1 Tbsp	17	0.1	1	3	1	917	
(La Choy) LT	1 Tbsp	18	0	1	4	0	439	
Thyme								
Fresh	1 Oz	27	0.7	1	4	NV	5	
Dried (McCormick)	1 Tsp	17	0	0	1	0	0	
Tofu								
Firm								
(Azumaya):								
	3 Oz	60	2.5	6	3	0	0	
Extra Firm	3 Oz	80	3.5	10	2	0	0	
(Kikkoman)	3 Oz	50	2.5	6	2	0	30	
(Nasoya) Extra Firm	1 Lb	450	25	55	5	0	50	C
Flavored								
(Nasoya):								
Five Spice	3 Oz	66	3.8	8	1	0	66	
French Country	3 Oz	66	3.8	8	1	0	123	
(White Wave):								
Mexican	2 Oz	120	6	13	3	1	240	
Oriental	2 Oz	120	6	13	3	1	240	
(Wildwood) Teriyaki	3.5 Oz	150	3	16	15	NV	790	
Prepared								
(Azumaya):								
Fried, Nama, Aged	3 Oz	130	5	15	7	0	0	
Puff, Aged	3 Oz	240	9	24	12	0	0	
Silken								
(Azumaya) Soft	3 Oz	45	2	3	4	0	0	
(Morinaga Nutrition):								
Extra Firm	3 Oz	55	2	7	2	1	60	
Firm	3 Oz	50	2.5	6	2	1	30	
LT	3 Oz	35	1	5	1	1	70	
Soft	3 Oz	45	2.5	4	2	1	5	
Soft								
(Kikkoman)	3 Oz	45	2.5	4	2	0	5	

	Serv.	K-Cal.	Fat	Prot.	Carb.	Fib.	Sod.	FAC
(Tofu cont.)								
(Nasoya)	3 Oz	19	1	2	1	0	2	
(Nasoya)	1 Lb	300	15	35	10	0	25	C
Tofu Entree								
(Fantastic):								
Classic, Curry	10 Oz	440	6	28	72	8	940	A
Scrambler	10 Oz	234	10	18	18	5	526	
Scrambler W/Butter	10 Oz	342	22	18	18	5	666	
(Health Valley) Fast								
Menu, Black Beans	10 Oz	140	0	18	18	19	230	FAC
Tomatillo								
Raw	1 Cup	42	1.4	1	8	3	1	A
Raw	1 Item	11	0.4	0	2	1	0	
Tomato, Fresh								
Raw	1 Oz	6	0.1	0	1	0	1	
Raw (5 Oz)	1 Med	26	0.4	1	6	1	11	A
Boiled	1 Cup	65	1	3	14	2	26	A
Cherry, Raw	1 Med	4	0.1	0	1	0	2	
Diced	1 Cup	38	0.6	2	8	2	16	A
Green, Raw (5 Oz)	1 Med	30	0.3	1	6	1	16	A
Tomato, Canned								
Chunky								
(Del Monte)	1 Cup	90	0	0	22	4	1,120	A
Crushed								
(Angela Mia)	1 Cup	55	0.3	3	13	4	760	A
(Contadina)	1 Cup	80	0	4	16	4	600	A
(Hunt's)	1 Cup	57	0.5	2	14	3	572	A
(S & W)	1 Cup	80	0	4	16	4	380	A
Diced								
(Del Monte)	1 Cup	50	0	0	12	4	320	A
(Muir Glen) Organic	1 Cup	50	0	2	8	2	580	A
Paste								
(Contadina):								
	1 Tbsp	20	0.5	1	4	1	160	
LS	1 Tbsp	15	0	1	3	1	10	
(Del Monte)	1 Tbsp	15	0	1	4	1	12	
(Hunt's):								
	1 Tbsp	15	0.3	1	3	1	44	
LS	1 Tbsp	15	0.3	1	3	1	3	
(Muir Glen) Organic	1 Tbsp	15	0	1	3	1	10	
(S & W)	1 Tbsp	15	0	1	3	1	10	
Puree								
(Contadina) LS	1 Cup	80	0	4	16	4	60	A
(Hunt's)	1 Cup	96	1.3	4	20	6	393	A
(Muir Glen) Organic	1 Cup	80	0	4	20	4	80	A

	Serv.	K-Cal.	Fat	Prot.	Carb.	Fib.	Sod.	FAC
Stewed								
(Contadina):								
....	1 Cup	80	0	2	18	2	500	**A**
Italian	1 Cup	80	0	2	16	2	520	**A**
Mexican......................	1 Cup	80	0	2	18	2	440	**A**
(Del Monte)	1 Cup	70	0	0	12	4	320	**A**
(Hunt's):								
....	1 Cup	66	0.6	2	15	3	714	**A**
LS................................	1 Cup	66	0.6	2	15	3	62	**A**
(S & W):								
....	1 Cup	70	0	2	14	4	540	**A**
Italian	1 Cup	70	0	2	14	4	540	**A**
LS................................	1 Cup	70	0	2	14	4	30	**A**
Whole, Peeled								
(Contadina).....................	1 Cup	50	0	2	8	2	440	**A**
(Del Monte)	1 Cup	50	0	0	12	4	320	**A**
(Hunt's):								
....	1 Item	11	0.1	1	2	0	202	
LS................................	1 Item	11	0.3	1	2	1	2	
(Muir Glen) Organic	1 Cup	60	0	2	10	2	520	**A**
(S & W):								
....	1 Cup	50	0	2	8	2	440	**A**
LS................................	1 Cup	40	0	4	8	2	180	**A**
Tomato Juice								
(Campbell's)	1 Cup	50	0	2	9	1	860	**A**
(Del Monte)	1 Cup	40	0	3	7	0	550	**A**
(Hunt's)...........................	1 Cup	34	0.3	2	8	2	688	**A**
(Muir Glen) Organic	1 Cup	40	0	3	7	1	550	**A**
(R.W. Knudsen)..............	1 Cup	60	0	2	14	NV	390	**A**
(Snap E Tom)	1 Cup	46	0	2	9	2	1,298	**A**
Tomato Sauce, Canned								
(Contadina):								
....	1 Cup	80	0	4	16	4	1,120	**A**
Italian	1 Cup	60	0	4	16	4	1,280	**A**
Thick, Zesty	1 Cup	80	0	4	12	4	1,360	**A**
(Del Monte):								
....	1 Cup	80	0	NV	16	4	1,360	**A**
LS................................	1 Cup	80	0	0	16	4	80	**A**
(Health Valley)................	1 Cup	70	0.4	2	13	NV	35	**A**
(Hunt's):								
....	1 Cup	63	0.8	4	12	4	1,464	**A**
LS................................	1 Cup	63	0.8	4	12	4	49	**A**
(Muir Glen) Organic	1 Cup	80	0	4	20	4	760	**A**
(S & W):								
....	1 Cup	80	0	4	16	4	1,200	**A**

	Serv.	K-Cal.	Fat	Prot.	Carb.	Fib.	Sod.	FAC
(Tomato Sauce, Canned cont.)								
Garden	1 Cup	80	0	0	16	4	800	A
Italian Herb	1 Cup	70	0	4	18	4	940	A
LS	1 Cup	90	0	4	18	3	65	A
Mild Mexican	1 Cup	80	0	4	16	4	760	A

Tomato, Sun-Dried

	Serv.	K-Cal.	Fat	Prot.	Carb.	Fib.	Sod.	FAC
	1 Oz	77	0.1	3	19	2	34	A
	1 Cup	139	1.6	8	30	7	1,131	A
Packed in Oil, Drained	1 Cup	234	15.5	6	26	6	293	A

Topping (See individual listings)

Tortellini
Fresh

(Contadina):	Serv.	K-Cal.	Fat	Prot.	Carb.	Fib.	Sod.	FAC
Cheese	1 Cup	347	8	17	52	4	440	C
Cheese/Basil	1 Cup	360	11	16	49	3	380	C
Cheese/Garlic	1 Cup	280	5	15	50	3	390	C
Chicken/Prosciutto	1 Cup	360	13	15	46	3	440	C
Chicken/Veg	1 Cup	347	9.3	13	52	3	293	
Sausage	1 Cup	330	10	13	47	3	290	C

Frozen

(Bernardi):	Serv.	K-Cal.	Fat	Prot.	Carb.	Fib.	Sod.	FAC
Cheese	1 Cup	260	6	13	40	4	400	
Meat	1 Cup	250	6	11	38	2	490	
Spinach, Cheese	1 Cup	280	8	13	40	2	320	A
(DiGiorno):								
Cheese	1 Cup	310	9	16	41	3	310	
Mozzarella Garlic	1 Cup	300	9	15	40	1	440	C
Mushroom	1 Cup	290	7	14	42	2	510	C
(Green Giant)								
Provençale	9.6 Oz	260	6	10	44	3	840	AC

Tortellini Entree, Frozen, Cheese

(Bernardi):	Serv.	K-Cal.	Fat	Prot.	Carb.	Fib.	Sod.	FAC
Meat Sauce	1 Oz	60	2	2	7	0	90	
Red Sauce	1 Oz	50	1	2	8	NV	45	
Tomato Sauce	1 Oz	60	2	3	9	0	70	
(Le Menu) *Lightstyle*								
Dinner	1 Item	230	6	10	35	NV	460	A
(Stouffer's):								
Alfredo	1 Item	550	33	25	38	5	720	C
Tomato Sauce	1 Item	290	6	19	40	4	740	C
(Wt Watchers) Tomato Sauce	1 Item	290	4	12	51	3	510	AC

	Serv.	K-Cal.	Fat	Prot.	Carb.	Fib.	Sod.	FAC
Tortilla								
Corn								
(La Tortilla) White	1 Item	60	0.5	1	13	1	5	
(La Tortilla) Yellow	1 Item	53	0.5	1	11	1	1	
(Mission)	1 Item	40	0.5	1	7	1	10	
Flour								
(Mission):								
....	1 Item	160	4	4	25	1	360	
RF	1 Item	80	0.5	3	17	2	220	
(Gordita)	1 Item	180	5	5	28	1	410	
(La Tortilla):								
FF	1 Item	60	0	2	13	6	180	
Gorditas, LF.................	1 Item	150	2.5	4	29	2	175	
Whole Wheat, FF	1 Item	60	0	2	12	9	180	
Tortilla Chips (Also See Corn Chips)								
(Frito-Lay) *Doritos*,								
Original.........................	1 Oz	140	7	2	18	1	135	
(Guiltless Gourmet)								
Originals......................	1 Chip	6	0.1	0	1	0	1	
(Keebler) *Chacho's*	1 Chip	10	0.5	0	1	0	14	
(Louise's) FF	1 Oz	120	1.5	2	23	1	170	
(Westbrae) NS	1 Chip	9	0.5	0	1	0	0	
Baked								
(Frito-Lay):								
Tostitos, Cool Ranch..	1 Chip	11	0.3	0	2	0	16	
Tostitos, NS.................	1 Chip	8	0.1	0	2	0	0	
(Guiltless Gourmet):								
Nacho..........................	1 Chip	6	0.1	0	1	0	10	
Originals......................	1 Chip	6	0.1	0	1	0	8	
Blue Corn								
(Bearitos) (1 Oz)	15 Chip	140	7	2	18	2	120	
(Guiltless Gourmet)........	1 Chip	6	0.1	0	1	0	7	
Flavored								
(Bearitos) Nacho,								
FF (1 Oz)......................	10 Chips	110	1	3	21	1	95	
(Frito-Lay):								
Doritos, Nacho								
Cheesier..................	1 Oz	140	7	2	18	1	170	
Doritos, Ranch............	1 Oz	140	7	2	18	1	160	
Tostitos, Lime N Chili.	1 Chip	25	1.2	0	3	0	30	
(Guiltless Gourmet):								
Chili/Lime	1 Chip	6	0.1	0	1	0	10	
Ranch	1 Chip	6	0.1	0	1	0	10	
(Keebler) *Chacho's*,								
Cheesy.........................	1 Chip	11	0.6	0	1	0	19	
White Corn								
(Bearitos)........................	15 Chips	140	7	2	18	2	120	
(Frito-Lay) *Tostitos*.........	1 Chip	12	0.6	0	1	0	7	

	Serv.	K-Cal.	Fat	Prot.	Carb.	Fib.	Sod.	FAC
(Tortilla Chips cont.)								
(Guiltless Gourmet)	1 Chip	6	0.1	0	1	0	7	
(Old El Paso)	1 Chip	13	0.7	0	1	0	5	
(Santitas)	1 Chip	23	1	0	3	0	13	
Yellow Corn								
(Barbara's Bakery)	1 Chip	9	0.4	0	1	0	6	
(Bearitos) (1 Oz)	21 Chips	140	7	2	18	2	120	
Tostada, Fast Food								
(Del Taco)	1 Item	140	8	6	12	NV	333	
(Taco Bell)	1 Item	292	14.4	11	31	11	696	
(Taco Time) Meat	1 Item	409	22	24	31	NV	1,006	
Tostada Shell								
(Bearitos)	1 Item	140	7	2	17	2	0	
(Old El Paso)	1 Item	53	3.3	1	6	1	73	
(Ortega)	1 Item	50	2	0	8	0	5	
(Rosarita)	1 Item	63	2.4	1	9	0	10	
Trail Mix (4 Oz equal approximately 1 cup)								
(Dole):								
California Style	1 Oz	110	2	4	19	2	0	F
Hawaiian Style	1 Oz	125	3	2	22	2	17	F
(Fisher):								
California Style	1 Oz	140	8	2	16	2	20	F
Classic Mix	1 Oz	150	11	5	11	2	70	F
Piña Colada	1 Oz	150	10	4	13	NV	50	F
Tropical	1 Oz	140	8	4	14	2	90	F
Triticale Flour								
Flakes	1 Cup	448	2.4	17	94	22	1	FA
Grain (Bob's Red Mill)	1 Cup	440	2	16	92	20	2	FA
Whole Grain	1 Oz	95	0.4	4	20	4	1	
Tropical Fruit Juice								
(Libby's) Juicy	1 Cup	130	0	1	31	0	10	
(Kerns) Nectar	1 Cup	146	0	2	32	0	7	
(R.W. Knudsen):								
Lime Cooler	1 Cup	110	0	0	27	0	35	
Punch	1 Cup	120	0	0	29	0	20	
Rain Forest	1 Cup	120	0	0	29	0	20	
Trout								
Mixed Species								
Raw	3 Oz	126	5.6	18	0	0	44	
Broiled	3 Oz	162	7.2	23	0	0	57	
Rainbow								
Raw	3 Oz	100	3	18	0	0	25	
Raw, Farmed	3 Oz	117	4.6	18	0	0	30	

	Serv.	K-Cal.	Fat	Prot.	Carb.	Fib.	Sod.	FAC
Raw, Wild	3 Oz	105	3.1	18	0	0	27	
Broiled, Farmed	3 Oz	144	6.1	21	0	0	36	
Broiled, Wild	3 Oz	128	5	20	0	0	48	

Turmeric

Dried (McCormick)	1 Tsp	8	0	0	2	0	0	

Tuna

Bluefin, Raw	3 Oz	122	4.2	20	0	0	33	
Bluefin, Cooked	3 Oz	156	5.3	25	0	0	43	
Skipjack, Raw	3 Oz	88	1	18	0	0	32	
Skipjack, Broiled	3 Oz	111	1	24	0	0	40	
Yellowfin, Raw	3 Oz	92	1	20	0	0	32	
Yellowfin, Broiled	3 Oz	120	1	25	0	0	40	

Tuna, Alternative

Tuno (Worthington)	1 Cup	166	10.9	13	4	3	575	

Tuna, Canned
Chunk Light

(Bumble Bee) Oil	3 Oz	165	9	21	0	0	275	
Water	3 Oz	90	0.8	21	0	0	375	
(S & W) Oil	3 Oz	165	9	21	0	0	345	
Water	3 Oz	105	0.8	23	0	0	345	
(Star-Kist):								
Oil	3 Oz	165	9	20	0	0	375	
Water	3 Oz	90	0.8	20	0	0	375	
Water, LS/LF	3 Oz	90	0.8	21	0	0	150	

Chunk White

(Bumble Bee) Water	3 Oz	90	1.5	21	0	0	375	
(Star-Kist) Water	3 Oz	90	1.5	21	0	0	375	
Water, LS/LF	3 Oz	90	0.8	21	0	0	53	

Solid White

(Bumble Bee) Water	3 Oz	90	0.8	21	0	0	375	
(S & W) Oil	3 Oz	120	2.3	26	0	0	345	
(Star-Kist) Oil	3 Oz	135	4.5	23	0	0	375	
Water	3 Oz	105	1.5	23	0	0	375	

Tuna Entree, Mix
(Prepared as directed)
(Betty Crocker):

Au Gratin	1 Cup	310	12	14	36	1	930	
Cheesy Pasta	1 Cup	280	11	14	32	1	890	
Creamy Pasta	1 Cup	300	13	14	31	1	910	
Fettucine Alfredo	1 Cup	310	13	14	32	1	940	
Romanoff	1 Cup	280	8	15	38	1	800	
Tetrazzini	1 Cup	310	12	17	33	1	1,010	

	Serv.	K-Cal.	Fat	Prot.	Carb.	Fib.	Sod.	FAC
Turbot, European								
Raw	3 Oz	81	2.5	14	0	0	127	
Broiled	3 Oz	102	3	17	0	0	150	
Turkey								
Breast								
(Louis Rich) BBQ W/O								
Skin	3 Oz	90	0	18	1	0	900	
(Mr. Turkey) Roasted	3 Oz	100	3	17	1	0	800	
Dark Meat								
W/Skin, Roasted	3 Oz	188	10	23	0	0	65	
W/O Skin, Roasted	3 Oz	164	6.2	25	0	0	70	
W/O Skin, Roasted	1 Cup	262	10.1	40	0	0	111	
Ground								
Raw	1 Lb	676	37.5	79	0	0	426	
Raw	3 Oz	126	7	15	0	0	80	
Broiled	3 Oz	200	11.2	23	0	0	90	
(Louis Rich), Raw	3 Oz	142	9	15	0	0	105	
(Mr. Turkey), Raw 91%								
FF	3 Oz	129	7.9	14	1	0	70	
Leg								
Roasted W/Skin	3 Oz	175	8.2	23	0	0	64	
Light Meat								
Roasted, W/Skin	3 Oz	165	7	24	0	0	53	
Roasted, W/O Skin	1 Cup	220	4.5	42	0	0	90	
Roasted, W/O Skin	3 Oz	140	0.6	26	0	0	56	
Liver								
Simmered	1 Cup	237	8.3	34	5	0	90	**FA**
Thigh								
Roasted, W/Skin	3 Oz	133	7.2	16	0	0	370	
Turkey, Canned								
Chunk (Hormel)	2 Oz	70	3	11	0	0	340	
Chunk White (Hormel)	2 Oz	60	1	13	0	0	320	
White W/Water (Swanson)	1 Cup	360	8	64	16	4	880	
Turkey Entree, Frozen								
(Healthy Choice):								
Breast, Traditional	10.5 Oz	280	3	22	40	7	460	**A**
Country Inn	10 Oz	250	4	26	29	6	530	**A**
Fettuccine/Crema	12.5 Oz	350	4	28	50	5	370	**A**
Homestyle W/Vegs	9.5 Oz	260	2	26	34	3	490	
Medallions/Veg	12.5 Oz	350	6	29	45	NV	480	
Tetrazzini	12.5 Oz	340	6	23	49	NV	490	**A**
W/Mushroom	8.5 Oz	220	4	19	28	3	440	
(Le Menu):								
Breast, W/Gravy,								
Dinner	10.5 Oz	300	7	22	38	NV	1,020	**A**

	Serv.	K-Cal.	Fat	Prot.	Carb.	Flb.	Sod.	FAC
Lightstyle, Divan	10 Oz	260	7	25	23	NV	420	A
Lightstyle, Glazed	8.3 Oz	260	6	18	34	NV	720	
Lightstyle, Traditional ...	8 Oz	200	5	19	19	NV	610	A
(Right Course) W/Curry								
Sauce	8.7 Oz	320	8	23	40	NV	570	A
(Stouffer's):								
Homestyle....................	8 Oz	280	11	19	25	1	950	
Pie	10.5 Oz	530	33	21	36	3	1,040	A
Tetrazzini Dinner..........	10 Oz	360	17	19	33	1	1,060	
(Stouffer's) *Lean Cuisine*:								
Breast, Roast..............	10 Oz	290	4	16	48	3	530	
Breast, W/Mushroom...	8 Oz	240	7	23	20	2	790	A
Breast, W/Stuffing.......	10 Oz	290	4	16	48	3	530	
Dijon	9.5 Oz	270	10	24	22	NV	900	
Homestyle....................	9.5 Oz	230	6	18	26	3	590	A
Pie	9.5 Oz	300	9	20	34	3	590	A
(Swanson):								
Dinner..........................	11.7 Oz	300	6	20	42	4	1,130	
Hungry Man.................	17 Oz	510	15	35	59	9	1,660	
W/Dressing/Potato	9 Oz	230	5	15	30	3	1,040	
(Wt Watchers):								
Breast, Stuffed.............	9 Oz	230	5	17	28	6	680	A
Medallions....................	8.5 Oz	190	2	10	34	4	530	

Turkey Fat

....	1 Tbsp	115	12.8	0	0	0	0	

Turkey, Luncheon Meat
Breast

(Healthy Choice).............	⅓ Oz	10	0.3	2	0	0	78	
(Hillshire Farm)................	⅓ Oz	10	0.1	2	1	0	105	
(Louis Rich):								
....	1 Oz	30	1	5	0	0	280	
FF...............................	1 Oz	25	0	4	1	0	330	
(Oscar Meyer)	1 Oz	30	1	4	1	0	330	
Honey								
(Healthy Choice).............	1 Oz	35	1	5	1	0	200	
(Louis Rich)...................	1 Oz	30	0.5	5	1	0	320	
(Mr. Turkey)	⅓ Oz	10	0.2	2	1	0	103	
Roll								
Light	1 Oz	42	2.1	5	0	0	139	
Light/Dark Meat..............	1 Oz	42	2	5	1	0	166	
Smoked								
(Healthy Choice).............	⅓ Oz	10	0.3	2	0	0	70	
(Hillshire Farm)................	⅓ Oz	10	0.1	2	1	0	100	
(Louis Rich):								
....	¾ Oz	20	0.3	5	0	0	270	

	Serv.	K-Cal.	Fat	Prot.	Carb.	Fib.	Sod.	FAC
(Turkey, Luncheon Meat cont.)								
FF	1 Oz	25	0	4	1	0	300	
Hickory	1 Oz	30	0.5	5	1	0	260	
(Mr. Turkey)	⅓ Oz	8	0.1	1	1	0	188	
(Oscar Mayer)	½ Oz	10	0	2	1	0	138	

Turkey, Luncheon Meat, Alternative

	Serv.	K-Cal.	Fat	Prot.	Carb.	Fib.	Sod.	FAC
(Light Life)	3 Slices	40	0	9	1	0	290	
(White Wave)	1 Slice	40	0	7	4	1	200	
(Worthington):								
Smoked	1 Slice	47	3.3	3	1	1	206	
Turkee	1 Slice	64	4.7	4	1	1	193	

Turnip

	Serv.	K-Cal.	Fat	Prot.	Carb.	Fib.	Sod.	FAC
Raw	1 Cup	36	0.2	1	8	3	88	A
Diced, Boiled	1 Cup	28	0.1	1	8	3	78	A

Turnip Greens

	Serv.	K-Cal.	Fat	Prot.	Carb.	Fib.	Sod.	FAC
Raw	1 Cup	16	0.2	1	3	1	22	FAC
Boiled	1 Cup	29	0.3	2	6	5	42	FAC
Frozen, Boiled	1 Cup	49	0.7	5	8	6	25	FAC

Turnover (See Pastry, Turnover)

V

	Serv.	K-Cal.	Fat	Prot.	Carb.	Fib.	Sod.	FAC
Vanilla								
Extract	1 Cup	705	0	0	71	0	0	
Extract	1 Tsp	14	0	0	1	0	0	

Veal
(Trimmed = All Separable Fat Removed After Cooking;
Untrimmed = No Fat Removed After Cooking)

	Serv.	K-Cal.	Fat	Prot.	Carb.	Fib.	Sod.	FAC
Leg								
Trimmed, Roasted	3 Oz	128	2.9	24	0	0	58	
Untrimmed, Roasted	3 Oz	136	4	24	0	0	58	
Loin								
Trimmed, Roasted	3 Oz	149	5.9	22	0	0	82	
Untrimmed, Roasted	3 Oz	184	10.5	21	0	0	79	
Rib								
Trimmed, Roasted	3 Oz	150	6.3	22	0	0	83	
Untrimmed, Roasted	3 Oz	194	11.9	20	0	0	78	
Shoulder, Arm								
Untrimmed, Roasted	3 Oz	156	7	22	0	0	77	
Trimmed, Roasted	3 Oz	139	4.9	22	0	0	77	
Shoulder, Blade								
Trimmed, Roasted	3 Oz	145	5.9	22	0	0	87	
Untrimmed, Roasted	3 Oz	158	7.4	21	0	0	85	
Shoulder, Whole								
Trimmed, Roasted	3 Oz	144	5.6	22	0	0	83	
Untrimmed, Roasted	3 Oz	156	7.2	22	0	0	82	
Sirloin								
Trimmed, Roasted	3 Oz	143	5.3	22	0	0	72	
Untrimmed, Roasted	3 Oz	172	8.9	21	0	0	71	
Sweetbreads								
Braised	3 Oz	153	3.8	28	0	0	58	

	Serv.	K-Cal.	Fat	Prot.	Carb.	Fib.	Sod.	FAC
Veal Entree, Alternative								
Veelets (Worthington)	2.5 Oz	171	9	14	10	5	388	

	Serv.	K-Cal.	Fat	Prot.	Carb.	Fib.	Sod.	FAC
Veal Entree, Frozen								
(Classic Lite) Steak	11 Oz	280	8	25	27	6	1,738	FA
(LeMenu) *Lightstyle,*								
Marsala......................	10 Oz	230	3	22	28	NV	700	A
Parmigiana								
(Banquet)	9 Oz	320	14	13	35	7	960	
(Le Menu)	11.5 Oz	390	17	24	36	NV	850	C
(Swanson):								
....	10 Oz	310	12	18	33	4	970	
Hungry Man.................	18.5 Oz	640	23	35	74	7	2,070	AC

Vegemite (See Yeast Extract)

Vegetable (See individual listings)

Vegetable Juice

	Serv.	K-Cal.	Fat	Prot.	Carb.	Fib.	Sod.	FAC
(Campbell's):								
V8...............................	1 Cup	50	0	1	10	1	620	A
V8, LS	1 Cup	60	0	2	11	2	140	A
V8, LT, Tangy	1 Cup	60	0	2	11	1	340	A
V8, Picante..................	1 Cup	50	0	2	10	1	680	A
V8, Spicy Hot	1 Cup	50	0	2	10	1	780	A
(Odwalla) Cocktail	1 Cup	70	0	4	18	2	288	A
(R.W. Knudsen):								
Very Veggie..................	1 Cup	50	1	3	10	NV	610	A
Very Veggie, LS	1 Cup	50	1	3	10	NV	32	A
(Snap-E-Tom)..................	1 Cup	50	0	3	10	2	670	F

Vegetable, Mixed, Canned

	Serv.	K-Cal.	Fat	Prot.	Carb.	Fib.	Sod.	FAC
(Del Monte)	1 Cup	80	0	4	16	4	720	A
(Green Giant) Peas &								
Carrots...........................	1 Cup	100	0	4	22	6	34	A
Peas & Pearl Onions....	1 Cup	120	0	8	8	8	1,040	A
(Luck's) Peas & Corn,								
Blackeye.......................	1 Cup	210	5	9	31	6	500	A
(S & W):								
....	1 Cup	70	0	2	14	4	740	A
Peas & Carrots.............	1 Cup	100	0	6	20	6	660	A
Peas & Onions.............	1 Cup	80	0	6	22	6	1,060	A
(Veg-All)	1 Cup	80	0	2	16	4	580	A

Vegetable, Mixed, Frozen

	Serv.	K-Cal.	Fat	Prot.	Carb.	Fib.	Sod.	FAC
(Flav R Pac):								
Country, Butter Sauce .	1 Cup	180	6.0	4	32	6	1,040	A
Deluxe Stir Fry	1 Cup	40	0	1	7	3	27	A
Fiesta...........................	1 Cup	90	0	6	15	9	195	A
5 Way...........................	1 Cup	90	0.8	5	18	3	75	A
Italian W/Butter Sauce .	1 Cup	100	4	4	16	6	820	A

	Serv.	K-Cal.	Fat	Prot.	Carb.	Fib.	Sod.	FAC
(Vegetable, Mixed, Frozen cont.)								
Omelette Blend............	1 Cup	33	0	1	7	3	20	A
Oriental........................	1 Cup	33	0	1	5	3	20	A
Scandinavian	1 Cup	53	0	3	9	3	60	A
Stew	1 Cup	60	0	2	14	2	68	A
Stew/Soup Blend.........	1 Cup	60	0	2	14	2	68	A
Stir Fry, Asparagus......	1 Cup	25	0	1	4	2	25	A
Stir Fry Blend	1 Cup	33	0	1	7	3	27	A
Stir Fry, Rice	1 Cup	80	0	3	18	2	15	A
Stir Fry W/Noodles	1 Cup	50	0	2	9	2	25	A
Vegetarian	1 Cup	33	0	1	5	3	27	A
(Green Giant):								
Broccoli Fanfare...........	1 Cup	160	4	6	28	6	680	A
California Style.............	1 Cup	33	0	1	7	3	20	A
Heartland Style	1 Cup	30	0	2	6	3	35	A
Manhattan Style...........	1 Cup	25	0	2	4	2	10	A
New England Style	1 Cup	105	2.3	3	20	5	105	A
San Francisco Style	1 Cup	40	0	1	8	3	27	A
Santa Fe Style	1 Cup	80	0	3	17	3	13	A
Seattle Style	1 Cup	33	0	1	7	3	20	A
Western Style	1 Cup	67	2	1	12	3	13	A
W/Butter......................	1 Cup	93	2.7	3	15	4	320	A
W/Cheese.....................	1 Cup	120	4	6	18	4	980	A
(Health Valley) Boiled......	1 Cup	140	2	6	24	4	64	A
(Libby's):								
Italian Style..................	1 Cup	30	0	1	6	2	10	A
Peas and Pearl								
Onions.........................	1 Cup	105	0.8	6	18	6	142	A
(Seneca):								
Broccoli Normandy	1 Cup	30	0	1	5	3	20	A
Capri............................	1 Cup	33	0	1	5	1	33	A
Peas and Carrots	1 Cup	75	0	5	14	5	112	A
Winter Mix	1 Cup	25	0	2	4	2	25	A
Vegetable Oil								
(Also See individual listings)								
(Crisco).......................	1 Tbsp	120	14	0	0	0	0	A
(Wesson)......................	1 Tbsp	122	13.6	0	0	0	0	A
Venison—Deer								
Raw..............................	3 Oz	106	2.4	20	0	0	46	
Chops, Broiled..............	3 Oz	143	3	20	0	0	240	
Dried, Salted	3 Oz	129	0.8	29	0	0	NV	
Ribs, Broiled................	3 Oz	144	3	27	0	0	327	
Stewed, Boneless...........	3 Oz	144	3	27	0	0	309	
Vinegar								
Balsamic								
(Fleischmann's)	3.3 Oz	140	0	0	30	0	20	
(Spectrum) Organic	1 Tbsp	10	0	0	2	0	0	

	Serv.	K-Cal.	Fat	Prot.	Carb.	Fib.	Sod.	FAC
Cider								
(Eden) Organic	1 Tbsp	0	0	0	0	0	0	
(Heinz)	1 Oz	4	0	0	0	0	2	
(Spectrum) Organic	1 Tbsp	7	0	0	2	0	0	
Rice								
(Eden) Brown Rice	1 Tbsp	0	0	0	0	0	0	
(Marukan) Seasoned	1 Tbsp	25	0	0	6	0	530	
(Spectrum) Brown Rice, Organic	1 Tbsp	10	0	0	0	0	0	
White								
White	1 Tbsp	1	0	0	0	0	0	
White, Distilled	1 Cup	29	0	0	12	0	2	
Wine								
(Musselman's) Red	1 Oz	0	0	0	0	0	0	
(Spectrum) Garlic, Organic	1 Tbsp	0	0	0	0	0	0	
Red or White	1 Tbsp	0	0	0	0	0	0	

W

	Serv.	K-Cal.	Fat	Prot.	Carb.	Fib.	Sod.	FAC
Waffles, Frozen								
(Aunt Jemima):								
Blueberry	1 Item	95	3.5	2	14	1	265	
Buttermilk	1 Item	85	3	2	14	1	205	
Cinnamon	1 Item	90	3	2	14	1	235	
LF	1 Item	80	5.5	0	0	0	0	
Oatmeal	1 Item	85	3.5	2	14	2	330	
Whole Grain	1 Item	85	3.5	3	12	1	225	
(Ener-G) Belgium,								
Gluten-Free	1 Item	237	7	0	46	0	14	C
(Krusteaz):								
Belgium	1 Item	170	5	4	26	1	440	
Blueberry	1 Item	115	4	2	17	1	210	
(Kellogg's) *Eggo*:								
Blueberry	1 Item	110	4	3	17	0	225	F
Buttermilk	1 Item	110	4	3	15	0	240	F
Cinnamon	1 Item	23	0.8	0	4	0	39	
Homestyle	1 Item	110	4	3	15	0	235	F
Nut & Honey	1 Item	120	5	3	16	0	240	F
Oat Bran, Common								
Sense	1 Item	100	3.5	3	14	2	175	F
Oat Bran, Fruit/Nut	1 Item	110	4	3	16	2	170	F
Special K	1 Item	70	0	3	15	0	125	F
(Kellogg's) *Nutri-Grain*:								
Multibran	1 Item	90	3	3	16	3	200	F
Plain	1 Item	95	3	3	15	2	215	F
Raisin Bran	1 Item	105	3	3	18	3	195	F
Walnut								
(1 cup weighs approximately 4 Oz)								
Black								
Raw	1 Oz	180	17	7	3	NV	0	
Chopped	1 Cup	759	70.7	30	15	6	1	FA
Persian or English								
Raw	1 Oz	180	18	4	5	1	2	
Chopped	1 Cup	770	74.2	17	22	6	12	FA

	Serv.	K-Cal.	Fat	Prot.	Carb.	Fib.	Sod.	FAC
Whole	1 Oz	178	15.2	4	6	1	2	

Walnut Oil
(Spectrum)	1 Tbsp	120	13.6	0	0	0	0	A

Wasabi—Japanese Horseradish
Raw	1 Oz	21	0	1	5	NV	0	A
Dry	1 Tbsp	24	0.1	1	5	NV	2	

Water
(Calistoga) All Flavors, Sparkling	1 Cup	0	0	0	0	0	40	
(Crystal Geyser):								
All Flavors, Sparkling	1 Cup	0	0	0	0	0	45	
Spring	1 Cup	0	0	0	0	0	0	
Municipal Tap	1 Cup	0	0	0	0	0	7	
(Perrier) Mineral, Sparkling	1 Cup	0	0	0	0	0	2	

Water Chestnut, Chinese
Fresh
Raw	1 Cup	131	0.1	2	30	4	17	
Canned								
Chinese	1 Cup	70	0.1	1	17	4	11	
Sliced (La Choy)	1 Tbsp	6	0	0	1	1	1	
Whole (La Choy)	1 Item	5	0	0	1	0	1	

Watercress
Raw	1 Oz	6	0	1	1	0	7	A
Raw	1 Cup	4	0	1	0	1	14	A

Watermelon
Raw	1 Oz	8	0	0	2	0	1	
Raw	1 Cup	51	0.7	1	12	1	3	A

Watermelon Seed, Kernels
Dried	1 Oz	150	12.2	6	4	4	38	
Dried	1 Cup	600	51	31	17	NV	100	F

Wax Bean—Yellow Wax
Boiled	1 Cup	43	0.4	2	10	4	4	FA
Canned (S & W)	1 Cup	40	0	2	8	2	800	FA
Canned (Del Monte)	1 Cup	40	0	2	8	4	720	FA
Frozen, Boiled	1 Cup	39	0.2	23	9	4	12	FA

Wheat
Cracked	1 Cup	700	4	26	140	6	6	FA
Durum	1 Cup	651	4.7	26	137	23	4	FA

	Serv.	K-Cal.	Fat	Prot.	Carb.	Fib.	Sod.	FAC
(Wheat cont.)								
Hard Red, Spring	1 Cup	632	3.7	30	131	23	4	**FA**
Hard Red, Winter	1 Cup	628	3	24	137	23	4	**FA**
Hard White	1 Cup	657	3.3	22	146	23	4	**FA**
Soft Red, Winter	1 Cup	556	2.6	17	125	21	3	**FA**
Soft White	1 Cup	571	3.3	18	127	21	3	**FA**
Sprouted	1 Cup	214	1.4	8	46	1	17	**FA**
Whole Course	1 Cup	476	2.7	19	95	4	4	**FA**
Whole Grain	1 Oz	99	0.6	4	20	1	3	
Whole Regular	1 Cup	511	2.9	20	102	4	4	**FA**

Wheat Bran

Crude	1 Cup	130	2.6	9	39	26	1	**F**
Toasted (Kretschmer)	1 Cup	120	4	12	40	28	0	**F**
Unprocessed (Quaker)	1 Cup	90	0	9	33	24	0	

Wheat Flour
(1 cup weighs approximately 5 Oz)
All-Purpose White
(Arrowhead Mills)

Unbleached	1 Cup	480	1.5	15	99	0	0	
(General Mills) *Gold*								
Medal	1 Oz	100	0	3	22	1	0	
(Pillsbury) Unbleached	1 Cup	400	1	12	86	0	0	
Bread, White								
Enriched	1 Cup	495	2.3	16	99	4	3	**F**
(Ener-G) Unbleached	1 Cup	479	1.4	16	101	0	3	
(General Mills) *Gold*								
Medal	1 Oz	100	0	4	22	1	0	
(Pillsbury)	1 Cup	400	2	14	83	0	0	
Cake, White								
Enriched	1 Cup	395	0.9	9	85	2	2	
(Arrowhead Mills)								
Unbleached	1 Cup	400	2	12	92	16	0	
Self-Rising, White								
(Aunt Jemima) Enriched	1 Cup	480	0	16	107	5	1,648	**FC**
(General Mills) *Gold*								
Medal	1 Oz	100	0	3	22	1	400	
(Pillsbury) Unbleached	1 Cup	380	1	9	84	2	1,290	
Tortilla Mix, White								
Enriched	1 Cup	450	11.8	11	75	3	751	**C**
Whole Grain								
(Arrowhead Mills):								
....	1 Cup	440	2	16	96	16	0	**F**
Stoneground	1 Cup	390	2	20	100	20	0	**F**
(Bob's Red Mill):								
....	1 Cup	400	2	20	80	8	0	**F**
Pastry	1 Cup	440	2	20	92	20	0	**F**

	Serv.	K-Cal.	Fat	Prot.	Carb.	Fib.	Sod.	FAC
(General Mills):								
Gold Medal	1 Cup	350	2	16	78	10	0	F
Gold Medal, Blend	1 Cup	400	2	12	80	8	0	F
(Pillsbury)	1 Oz	120	1	5	7	16	0	
(Robin Hood)	1 Oz	90	0.5	4	18	3	0	

Wheat Germ

	Serv.	K-Cal.	Fat	Prot.	Carb.	Fib.	Sod.	FAC
Crude	1 Cup	414	11.2	27	60	15	14	F
Toasted	1 Cup	431	12	33	56	15	4	F
(Arrowhead Mills) Raw	1 Cup	120	2	12	28	24	0	F
(Kretschmer):								
	1 Tbsp	25	0.5	2	3	1	0	
Honey Crunch	1 Tbsp	30	0.6	2	6	1	0	

Wheat Germ Oil

	Serv.	K-Cal.	Fat	Prot.	Carb.	Fib.	Sod.	FAC
(Spectrum)	1 Tbsp	120	13.6	0	0	0	0	A

Wheat, Gluten

	Serv.	K-Cal.	Fat	Prot.	Carb.	Fib.	Sod.	FAC
(Arrowhead Mills)	3 Tbsp	35	0	5	3	0	0	
(Bob's Red Mill)	1 Oz	120	0.5	23	6	0	9	

Whey

	Serv.	K-Cal.	Fat	Prot.	Carb.	Fib.	Sod.	FAC
Acid, Dry	1 Tbsp	10	0	0	2	0	28	C
Acid, Fluid	1 Cup	59	0.2	2	13	0	118	
Sweet, Dry	1 Tbsp	27	0.1	1	6	0	81	C
Sweet, Fluid	1 Cup	66	0	2	13	0	132	

Whiskey (See Alcoholic Beverage, Liqueur)

White Bean (See Bean, White)

Whitefish

	Serv.	K-Cal.	Fat	Prot.	Carb.	Fib.	Sod.	FAC
Raw	3 Oz	114	4.8	16	0	0	43	
Broiled	3 Oz	149	6.4	21	0	0	58	
Dry Flesh (Alaska)	3 Oz	320	10	56	1	0	NV	
Smoked	1 Oz	30	0.3	7	0	0	285	

Whiting

	Serv.	K-Cal.	Fat	Prot.	Carb.	Fib.	Sod.	FAC
Raw	3 Oz	75	1.1	15	0	0	66	
Broiled	3 Oz	910	1.5	20	0	0	114	

Winged Bean—Goa Bean (See Bean, Winged)

Wine (See Alcoholic Beverage, Wine)

Winter Melon

	Serv.	K-Cal.	Fat	Prot.	Carb.	Fib.	Sod.	FAC
Cooked	1 Cup	23	0.4	1	5	2	591	A

	Serv.	K-Cal.	Fat	Prot.	Carb.	Flb.	Sod.	FAC
Won Ton Wrapper								
(Nasoya)	1 Item	20	0	1	4	0	32	
Worcestershire Sauce								
(Crosse & Blackwell)......	1 Tsp	5	0	0	0	0	65	
(French's)	1 Tsp	3	0	0	1	0	53	
(Heinz)	1 Tsp	0	0	0	0	0	55	
(Lea & Perrins)...............	1 Tsp	5	0.9	<1	1	0	55	

Y

	Serv.	K-Cal.	Fat	Prot.	Carb.	Fib.	Sod.	FAC
Yam								
Fresh								
Raw	1 Cup	180	0.2	2	42	6	14	
Baked	1 Cup	158	0.2	2	38	5	11	
Boiled	8 Oz	264	0.4	3	62	NV	18	
Canned								
(Princella)	1 Cup	256	0.8	0	60	5	53	**A**
(S & W) Candied	1 Cup	340	0	4	92	8	720	**A**
Frozen								
Patties	1 Piece	75	0.5	1	17	2	100	

Yard-Long Bean—Asparagus Bean (See Green Bean)

Yeast, Baker's

	Serv.	K-Cal.	Fat	Prot.	Carb.	Fib.	Sod.	FAC
Compressed	1 Oz	24	0.1	3	3	2	5	
Compressed, Cake	0.6 Oz	18	0.3	1	3	1	5	
Dry, Active	1 Tbsp	35	0.6	5	5	3	6	
Dry, Active, Package	0.25 Oz	21	0.3	3	3	1	4	

Yeast, Brewer's

	Serv.	K-Cal.	Fat	Prot.	Carb.	Fib.	Sod.	FAC
Debittered	1 Tbsp	23	0.1	3	3	NV	10	**F**
Dry	1 Tbsp	25	0	3	3	3	10	**F**

Yeast Extract

	Serv.	K-Cal.	Fat	Prot.	Carb.	Fib.	Sod.	FAC
(Vegemite)	1 Tsp	10	0	2	1	0	160	
(Marmite)	1 Tsp	20	0	4	0	0	400	

Yellowtail

	Serv.	K-Cal.	Fat	Prot.	Carb.	Fib.	Sod.	FAC
Raw	3 Oz	124	4.3	20	0	0	33	
Broiled	3 Oz	156	6	25	0	0	43	

Yellow Wax Bean (See Wax Bean)

	Serv.	K-Cal.	Fat	Prot.	Carb.	Fib.	Sod.	FAC
Yogurt								
Almond								
(Yoplait)	8 Oz	280	2.7	12	55	NV	133	C
Apple								
(Dannon) W/Cinnamon, LF	8 Oz	240	3	9	46	1	140	C
Berry, Mixed								
(Dannon) LF	8 Oz	240	3	9	45	1	150	C
(Yoplait) LF	8 Oz	267	2.7	11	53	3	167	C
Blueberry								
(Dannon) LF	8 Oz	240	3	9	46	1	140	C
(R.W. Knudsen), FF	6 Oz	70	0	7	12	0	80	C
(Wt Watchers) W/ Creme, FF	8 Oz	90	0	8	14	3	140	C
Coffee								
(Dannon) LF	8 Oz	210	3	10	36	0	160	C
(Wt Watchers) Ult 90, FF	8 Oz	90	0	8	14	0	140	C
Cranberry								
(Dannon) W/Raspberry, LF	8 Oz	210	3	10	36	0	160	C
(Wt Watchers) W/Raspberry, FF	8 Oz	90	0	8	14	0	140	C
Lemon								
(Dannon) LF	8 Oz	210	3	10	36	0	160	C
(Wt Watchers) Ult 90, FF	8 Oz	90	0	8	14	1	140	C
Orange								
(Dannon) LF	8 Oz	240	3	9	45	0	135	C
Peach								
(Dannon) LF	8 Oz	240	3	9	45	1	140	C
(Wt Watchers) Ult 90	8 Oz	90	0	8	14	0	140	C
Plain								
(Brown Cow) Whole	8 Oz	160	10	8	11	0	105	C
(Continental) FF	8 Oz	120	0	12	19	0	150	C
(Nancy's) LF	8 Oz	150	3	11	16	0	170	C
(Pavel's):								
	8 Oz	140	8	8	10	0	150	C
FF	8 Oz	110	0	11	15	0	220	C
(Wt Watchers) Ult 90, FF	8 Oz	90	0	8	14	0	150	C
(Yoplait):								
	6 Oz	180	1.5	7	33	0	125	C
Creamy, FF	8 Oz	130	0	13	19	0	170	C
Custard	6 Oz	190	3	8	32	0	100	C
FF	6 Oz	160	0	7	34	0	95	C
Raspberry								
(Dannon) LF	8 Oz	240	3	9	45	1	150	C
(Wt Watchers) Creme, FF	8 Oz	90	0	8	14	0	140	C

	Serv.	K-Cal.	Fat	Prot.	Carb.	Flb.	Sod.	FAC
Strawberry								
(Dannon):								
LF	8 Oz	240	3	9	46	1	135	C
W/Banana, LF	8 Oz	240	3	9	43	1	140	C
(Wt Watchers) Ult 90, FF	8 Oz	90	0	8	14	2	140	C
(Yoplait) W/Almonds	8 Oz	267	2.7	12	51	NV	140	C
Vanilla								
(Dannon) LF	8 Oz	210	3	10	36	0	160	C
(Wt Watchers) ULT 90,								
FF	8 Oz	90	0	8	14	0	140	C
(Yoplait):								
	6 Oz	180	1.5	7	33	0	125	C
Custard Style	6 Oz	190	3	8	32	0	95	C
FF	8 Oz	210	0	11	41	0	140	C
Yogurt, Alternative								
Goat Milk								
(Red Hill Farm)								
Blueberry	1 Cup	180	5	6	28	0	110	C
Vanilla	1 Cup	190	6	7	28	0	110	C
(SkyHill) Plain	6 Oz	120	7	6	8	0	75	C
Soy								
(Nancy's) Blackberry	1 Cup	210	4	7	37	4	25	A
Plain	1 Cup	190	4	6	35	2	25	A
(White Wave):								
Lemon	6 Oz	180	2.5	6	33	1	40	
Plain	6 Oz	140	5	9	13	4	55	
Raspberry	6 Oz	150	1	5	30	3	50	
Vanilla	6 Oz	140	2.5	6	23	1	45	
Yogurt, Frozen								
Apple								
(Ben & Jerry's) Pie	1 Cup	340	6	8	64	0	180	C
Banana W/Strawberry								
(Ben & Jerry's)	1 Cup	320	4	8	64	2	120	AC
(Dreyers) FF	1 Cup	160	0	6	36	NV	100	
Blueberry								
(Baskin Robbins) LF	1 Cup	240	3	8	48	0	140	C
(Ben & Jerry's)	1 Cup	320	4	8	64	2	120	AC
Cheesecake								
(Baskin Robbins) LF	1 Cup	240	3	8	42	0	150	C
Cherry								
(Baskin Robbins) Black,								
FF	1 Cup	220	0	6	48	0	100	C
(Ben & Jerry's) Cherry								
Garcia	1 Cup	340	7	6	60	0	140	
(Edy's) Vanilla Swirl, FF	1 Cup	180	0	8	38	NV	130	

	Serv.	K-Cal.	Fat	Prot.	Carb.	Fib.	Sod.	FAC
(*Yogurt, Frozen cont.*)								
Chocolate								
(Baskin Robbins):								
Choco Laka	1 Cup	320	10	8	48	2	150	
Dutch, FF....................	1 Cup	200	0	8	46	2	120	C
LF................................	1 Cup	240	3	10	46	0	150	C
W/Mint, FF..................	1 Cup	200	0	8	46	2	120	C
(Ben & Jerry's):								
Fudge Brownie	1 Cup	360	4	12	68	4	230	C
FF................................	1 Cup	260	0	6	58	2	100	C
W/Raspberry	1 Cup	400	5	10	80	2	150	C
(Dreyers):								
....	1 Cup	200	6	6	34	NV	60	
Brownie Chunk	1 Cup	220	8	6	36	NV	60	
FF................................	1 Cup	180	0	8	36	NV	130	
Fudge, FF....................	1 Cup	200	0	6	42	NV	150	
(Edy's) Marble Fudge	1 Cup	220	6	6	38	NV	70	
(Häagen-Dazs)	1 Cup	314	5.1	16	52	2	116	C
Coffee								
(Baskin Robbins) Kah-								
lua, FF	1 Cup	200	0	6	42	0	110	C
(Ben & Jerry's) Cappuc-								
cino, FF......................	1 Cup	280	0	6	64	0	170	C
W/Almond Fudge........	1 Cup	400	10	10	60	2	150	C
(Dreyers) Espresso Chip	1 Cup	220	8	6	38	NV	60	
(Häagen-Dazs)	1 Cup	316	5.1	16	51	0	110	C
Cookies 'N Cream								
(Dreyers)........................	1 Cup	240	8	6	40	NV	140	
Orange								
(Dreyers) Van Swirl........	1 Cup	200	5	6	34	NV	60	
(Häagen-Dazs) Tango....	1 Cup	261	2.4	8	53	1	52	C
Peach								
(Baskin Robbins) FF......	1 Cup	200	0	6	44	0	100	C
(Dreyers) Perfectly	1 Cup	200	5	4	34	NV	50	
Piña Colada								
(Baskin Robbins) FF......	1 Cup	220	0	6	44	0	100	AC
(Häagen-Dazs)	1 Cup	270	3.5	7	52	1	52	AC
Raspberry								
(Baskin Robbins):								
Cheese Louise............	1 Cup	260	6	8	48	0	190	C
FF................................	1 Cup	200	0	6	46	0	110	C
LF................................	1 Cup	240	2	8	48	NV	80	C
(Ben & Jerry's) FF	1 Cup	240	0	6	54	0	120	C
(Dreyers)........................	1 Cup	200	5	4	34	NV	50	
Duet (Häagen-Dazs)	1 Cup	262	3.5	5	53	2	47	C
(Edy's):								
FF................................	1 Cup	180	0	6	36	NV	110	
Vanilla Swirl	1 Cup	200	5	6	34	NV	60	
W/Choc Chip	1 Cup	240	8	6	38	NV	50	

	Serv.	K-Cal.	Fat	Prot.	Carb.	Fib.	Sod.	FAC
(Häagen-Dazs)	1 Cup	261	2.6	8	52	3	54	C
Strawberry								
(Baskin Robbins) FF	1 Cup	200	0	6	46	0	110	C
LF	1 Cup	240	2	8	48	0	80	C
(Ben & Jerry's)	1 Cup	240	0	6	54	0	120	AC
(Edy's) FF	1 Cup	180	0	6	36	0	110	
Vanilla								
(Baskin Robbins) FF	1 Cup	220	0	8	46	0	130	C
LF	1 Cup	240	4	8	44	0	150	C
(Ben & Jerry's) Fudge,								
FF	1 Cup	300	0	6	64	0	160	C
(Dreyers) FF	1 Cup	180	0	8	38	NV	130	
(Edy's)	1 Cup	200	5	6	34	NV	60	
Chocolate Swirl, FF	1 Cup	180	0	8	36	NV	130	
(Häagen-Dazs)	1 Cup	318	5.1	17	51	0	114	C

Yogurt, Frozen Bar

(Ben & Jerry's) Cherry								
Garcia	1 Item	270	15	5	33	2	60	
(Häagen-Dazs):								
Peach	1 Item	97	1.2	2	19	0	19	
Piña Colada	1 Item	98	1.2	3	19	0	43	
Raspberry Vanilla	1 Item	95	1.1	3	19	0	23	
Strawberry Daiquiri	1 Item	90	1	2	18	0	22	
Tropical Orange	1 Item	99	1.3	2	20	0	20	

Yuca
(See Cassava)

Z

	Serv.	K-Cal.	Fat	Prot.	Carb.	Fib.	Sod.	FAC

Zucchini (See Squash, Summer, Zucchini)

Zwieback (See Baby Food, Dessert, Cookie)